Surgical Approaches to Esophageal Disease

Editor

DMITRY OLEYNIKOV

SURGICAL CLINICS
OF NORTH AMERICA

www.surgical.theclinics.com

Consulting Editor
RONALD F. MARTIN

June 2015 • Volume 95 • Number 3

ELSEVIER

1600 John F. Kennedy Boulevard • Suite 1800 • Philadelphia, Pennsylvania, 19103-2899

http://www.surgical.theclinics.com

SURGICAL CLINICS OF NORTH AMERICA Volume 95, Number 3
June 2015 ISSN 0039–6109, ISBN-13: 978-0-323-38908-2

Editor: John Vassallo, j.vassallo@elsevier.com

Developmental Editor: Colleen Viola

Surgical Clinics of North America (ISSN 0039–6109) is published bimonthly by Elsevier Inc., 360 Park Avenue South, New York, NY 10010-1710. Months of publication are February, April, June, August, October, and December. Business and Editorial Offices: 1600 John F. Kennedy Blvd., Suite 1800, Philadelphia, PA 19103-2899. Periodicals postage paid at New York, NY and additional mailing offices. Subscription prices are $370.00 per year for US individuals, $627.00 per year for US institutions, $180.00 per year for US students and residents, $455.00 per year for Canadian individuals, $793.00 per year for Canadian institutions, $510.00 for international individuals, $793.00 per year for international institutions and $250.00 per year for Canadian and foreign students/residents. To receive student/resident rate, orders must be accompanied by name of affiliated institution, date of term, and the *signature* of program/residency coordinator on institution letterhead. Orders will be billed at individual rate until proof of status is received. Foreign air speed delivery is included in all *Clinics* subscription prices. All prices are subject to change without notice. POSTMASTER: Send address changes to *Surgical Clinics*, Elsevier Health Sciences Division, Subscription Customer Service, 3251 Riverport Lane, Maryland Heights, MO 63043. **Customer Service (orders, claims, online, change of address): Telephone: 1-800-654-2452 (U.S. and Canada); 314-447-8871 (outside U.S. and Canada). Fax: 314-447-8029. E-mail: journalscustomerservice-usa@elsevier.com (for print support); journalsonlinesupport-usa@elsevier.com (for online support).**

Reprints. For copies of 100 or more, of articles in this publication, please contact the Commercial Reprints Department, Elsevier Inc., 360 Park Avenue South, New York, New York 10010-1710. Tel. 212-633-3874, Fax: 212-633-3820, E-mail: reprints@elsevier.com.

The Surgical Clinics of North America is also published in Spanish by McGraw-Hill Interamericana Editores S.A., P.O. Box 5-237 06500 Mexico D.F. Mexico; and in Portuguese by Interlivros Edicoes Ltda., Rua Comandante Coelho 1085, CEP 21250, Rio de Janeiro, Brazil; and in Greek by Paschalidis Medical Publications, Athens Greece.

The Surgical Clinics of North America is covered in *MEDLINE/PubMed (Index Medicus), EMBASE/Excerpta Medica, Current Contents/Clinical Medicine, Current Contents/Life Sciences, Science Citation Index,* and *ISI/BIOMED.*

Contributors

CONSULTING EDITOR

RONALD F. MARTIN, MD
Staff Surgeon, Department of Surgery, Marshfield Clinic, Marshfield, Wisconsin; Clinical Associate Professor, University of Wisconsin School of Medicine and Public Health, Madison, Wisconsin; Colonel, Medical Corps, United States Army Reserve

EDITOR

DMITRY OLEYNIKOV, MD, FACS
Professor of Surgery; Chief, Minimally Invasive and Bariatric Surgery, Director, Minimally Invasive and Robotic Surgery, Director, Center for Advanced Surgical Technology, Nebraska Medical Center, Omaha, Nebraska

AUTHORS

AMAN ALI, MD
Assistant Professor of Gastroenterology, Southern Illinois University School of Medicine, Springfield, Illinois

MARCO E. ALLAIX, MD, PhD
Department of Surgical Sciences, University of Torino, Torino, Italy

MARIA S. ALTIERI, MD, MS
Division of Bariatric, Foregut and Advanced Gastrointestinal Surgery, Department of Surgery, Stony Brook University Medical Center, Stony Brook, New York

STEVEN P. BOWERS, MD, FACS
Associate Professor of Surgery, Mayo Clinic Florida, Jacksonville, Florida

IBRAHIM BULENT CETINDAG, MD
Assistant Professor of Surgery, Southern Illinois University School of Medicine, Springfield, Illinois

JAMES P. DOLAN, MD, FACS
Associate Professor of Surgery, Division of Gastrointestinal and General Surgery, Digestive Health Center, Oregon Health and Science University, Portland, Oregon

STEVE EUBANKS, MD
Director of Academic Surgery; Medical Director of the Institute for Surgical Advancement, Center for Interventional Endoscopy, Florida Hospital Institute for Minimally Invasive Therapy; Professor of Surgery, University of Central Florida, Orlando, Florida

BRANDON T. GROVER, DO, FACS
Department of General and Vascular Surgery, Gundersen Health System, La Crosse, Wisconsin

CINDY HA, MD
Resident in General Surgery, Southern Illinois University School of Medicine, Springfield, Illinois

KRISTIN HUMMEL, DO
PGY5 General Surgery Resident, Department of Surgery, University of South Alabama College of Medicine, Mobile, Alabama

JOHN G. HUNTER, MD, FACS
Mackenzie Professor and Chair, Division of Gastrointestinal and General Surgery, Digestive Health Center, Oregon Health and Science University, Portland, Oregon

BLAIR A. JOBE, MD, FACS
Director, Esophageal and Lung Institute, Allegheny Health Network, Pittsburgh, Pennsylvania

JENNIFER M. JOLLEY, MD
MIS Fellow, Department of Surgery, Nebraska Medical Center, University of Nebraska Medical Center, Omaha, Nebraska

LEENA KHAITAN, MD, MPA, FACS
Associate Professor, Department of Surgery, University Hospitals Case Medical Center, Cleveland, Ohio

SHANU N. KOTHARI, MD, FACS
Department of General and Vascular Surgery, Gundersen Health System, La Crosse, Wisconsin

NICHOLAS R. KUNIO, MD
Division of General and Vascular Surgery, Advocate Medical Group, Elgin, Illinois

JOHN D. MELLINGER, MD, FACS
Professor of Surgery, J. Roland Folse Endowed Chair in Surgery, Chair of General Surgery, Residency Program Director, Southern Illinois University School of Medicine, Springfield, Illinois

DEAN J. MIKAMI, MD, FACS
Associate Professor of Surgery; Associate Director of Education, Center for Minimally Invasive Surgery; Director International Scholar Program; Division of Gastrointestinal Surgery, The Ohio State University Wexner Medical Center, Columbus, Ohio

KENRIC M. MURAYAMA, MD, FACS
Chairman and Program Director; Department of Surgery, Abington Memorial Hospital, Abington, Pennsylvania; Professor of Surgery, Drexel University College of Medicine, Philadelphia, Pennsylvania

UDAYAKUMAR NAVANEETHAN, MD
Assistant Professor of Internal Medicine, University of Central Florida; Center for Interventional Endoscopy, Florida Hospital Institute for Minimally Invasive Therapy, Orlando, Florida

BRANT K. OELSCHLAGER, MD
Byers Endowed Professor in Esophageal Research; Chief, Division of General Surgery, Department of Surgery; Director, Center for Esophageal and Gastric Surgery, University of Washington, Seattle, Washington

DMITRY OLEYNIKOV, MD, FACS
Professor of Surgery; Chief, Minimally Invasive and Bariatric Surgery, Director, Minimally Invasive and Robotic Surgery, Director, Center for Advanced Surgical Technology, Nebraska Medical Center, Omaha, Nebraska

MARCO G. PATTI, MD
Center for Esophageal Diseases, Department of Surgery, University of Chicago Pritzker School of Medicine, Chicago, Illinois

AURORA D. PRYOR, MD
Division of Bariatric, Foregut and Advanced Gastrointestinal Surgery, Department of Surgery, Stony Brook University Medical Center, Stony Brook, New York

JAMES REGAN, MD
Resident in General Surgery, Southern Illinois University School of Medicine, Springfield, Illinois

WILLIAM RICHARDS, MD, FACS
Professor and Chair of Surgery, Department of Surgery, University of South Alabama College of Medicine, Mobile, Alabama

VIKAS SINGHAL, MBBS
Executive Consultant, Department of GI and Bariatric Surgery, Jaypee Hospital, Noida, Uttar Pradesh

C. DANIEL SMITH, MD
Professor of Surgery, Mayo Clinic, Atlanta, Georgia

MARK SPLITTGERBER, MD
Division of General Surgery, University of South Florida, Tampa, Florida

VIC VELANOVICH, MD
Division of General Surgery, University of South Florida, Tampa, Florida

ROBERT B. YATES, MD
Acting Instructor and Senior Fellow, Department of Surgery, Center for Videoendoscopic Surgery, University of Washington, Seattle, Washington

Contents

> The diagnosis of esophageal motility disorders has been greatly enhanced with the development of high-resolution esophageal manometry studies and the Chicago Classification. Both hypomotility disorders and hypercontractility disorders of the esophagus have new diagnostic criteria. For the foregut surgeon, new diagnostic criteria for esophageal motility disorders have implications for decision-making during fundoplication and may expand the role of surgical therapy for esophageal achalasia by clarifying diagnostic criteria.

> Patients frequently present to a physician with complaints of difficulty swallowing. The approach to systematically evaluating these problems can be challenging for those who do not manage this type of patient regularly. The potential for life-threatening malignancies is present and makes this evaluation a priority. Numerous excellent tools are available to aid with the determination of the cause of dysphagia and assist with the formulation of a logical treatment algorithm.

> Benign esophageal and paraesophageal masses and cysts are a rare but important group of pathologies. Although often asymptomatic, these lesions can cause a variety of symptoms and, in some cases, demonstrate variable biological behavior. Contemporary categorization relies heavily on endoscopic ultrasound and other imaging modalities and immunohistochemical analysis when appropriate. Minimally invasive options including endoscopic, laparoscopic, and thoracoscopic methods are increasingly used for symptomatic or indeterminate lesions.

> Gastroesophageal reflux disease (GERD) is one of the most common problems treated by primary care physicians. Almost 20% of the population in

the United States experiences occasional regurgitation, heartburn, or retrosternal pain because of GERD. Reflux disease is complex, and the physiology and pathogenesis are still incompletely understood. However, abnormalities of any one or a combination of the three physiologic processes, namely, esophageal motility, lower esophageal sphincter function, and gastric motility or emptying, can lead to GERD. There are many diagnostic and therapeutic approaches to GERD today, but more studies are needed to better understand this complex disease process.

Gastroesophageal reflux disease (GERD) is the most common benign medical condition of the stomach and esophagus. For patients that experience life-limiting symptoms of GERD despite medical therapy, antireflux surgery should be considered. The application of laparoscopy to antireflux surgery has decreased perioperative morbidity, hospital length of stay, and cost compared with open operations. Laparoscopic antireflux surgery (LARS) is a safe operation that provides durable improvement in typical symptoms of GERD. Careful patient selection based on symptoms, response to medical therapy, and preoperative testing will optimize chances for effective and durable postoperative control of symptoms. Complications of LARS are rare.

Minimally invasive surgery is the mainstay of treatment for symptomatic hiatal hernia. Laparoscopic paraesophageal hernia (PEH) repair includes certain key steps such as complete reduction of the hernia sac, identification of both crura and the gastroesophageal junction, obtaining at least 3 cm of intra-abdominal esophageal length, tension-free re-approximation of the crura utilizing an absorbable mesh onlay, creation of an anti-reflux procedure, and diagnostic endoscopy at the end of the procedure. This article reviews various aspects of managing a patient who presents with a paraesophageal hernia and examines the current controversies in surgical technique with regards to laparoscopic PEH repair.

Esophageal achalasia is a primary esophageal motility disorder characterized by the absence of esophageal peristalsis and failure of the lower esophageal sphincter to relax in response to swallowing. This article reviews the most clinically relevant aspects of diagnosis and management of patients with achalasia, focusing on the several treatment modalities available. At present, laparoscopic Heller myotomy with partial fundoplication is considered the gold standard for the treatment. Endoscopic procedures such as endoscopic botulinum toxin injection and pneumatic dilatation should be considered as primary treatment modalities only in frail patients. Peroral endoscopic myotomy is a new approach with promising short-term results.

reoperation. The major anatomic causes of failed fundoplication are slipped fundoplication, failure to identify a short esophagus, and problems with the wrap. Minimally invasive surgery has become more common for these procedures. Options for surgery include redo fundoplication with hiatal hernia repair if needed, conversion to Roux-en-Y anatomy, or, as a last resort, esophagectomy. Conversion to Roux-en-Y anatomy has a high rate of success, making this approach an important option in the properly selected patient.

In the presence of long-standing and severe gastroesophageal reflux disease, patients can develop various complications, including a shortened esophagus. Standard preoperative testing in these patients should include endoscopy, esophagography, and manometry, whereas the objective diagnosis of a short esophagus must be made intraoperatively following adequate mediastinal mobilization. If left untreated, it is a contributing factor to the high recurrence rate following fundoplications or repair of large hiatal hernias. A laparoscopic Collis gastroplasty combined with an antireflux procedure offers safe and effective therapy.

Multiple new endoluminal devices and therapies have been devised to create a more effective antireflux barrier in patients with gastroesophageal reflux disease (GERD). Most of these therapies have been abandoned, because they were ineffective and/or had significant adverse effects. However, there are currently two therapies (Stretta, EsophyX) that have US Food and Drug Administration approval and continue to be used in select patients with GERD. The clinical management of GERD, disease complications, endoluminal techniques, evidence for efficacy, and controversies concerning endoluminal therapy for GERD are reviewed and discussed.

Esophageal disease and dysfunction of the lower esophageal sphincter (LES) manifesting as gastroesophageal reflux disease (GERD) particularly, is the most common of all gastrointestinal conditions impacting patients on a day-to-day basis. LES dysfunction can lead to anatomic changes to the distal esophagus, with GERD-mediated changes being benign stricture or progression of GERD to Barrett's esophagus and even esophageal cancer, and LES hypertension impairing esophageal emptying with subsequent development of pulsion esophageal diverticulum. This article details the causes, clinical presentation, workup, and treatment of esophageal stricture and epiphrenic esophageal diverticulum. Other types of esophageal diverticula (Zenker's and midesophageal) are also covered.

SURGICAL CLINICS
OF NORTH AMERICA

VISIT THE CLINICS ONLINE!
Access your subscription at:
www.theclinics.com

Foreword
Esophageal Disease

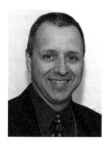

Ronald F. Martin, MD
Consulting Editor

Surgeons love to fix things. It's in our nature. It must be true because I read it in almost every personal statement written by an applicant to our training program each year. Even if it were not true, it is clear that most, if not all, of the young people who are attracted to the discipline of surgery either think it is true or want me to believe that they do. And they must have gotten that impression from somewhere—probably from working with us.

Yet, sometimes I am not sure if we know what it means to "fix things." I will grant you, dear reader, that I may have a skewed view, as a sizable fraction of what I do for a living is to modify, redo, or undo some "fix" that was already implemented. The problems I tackle were sometimes created decades ago and were sometimes created hours (or less) ago; fortunately, the former is far more common. Most of the "reinterventions" need to be undertaken for good reasons: our basic understanding has changed; the patient has aged and changed; the underlying disease has progressed; some device has failed; some unintended and unforeseeable consequence has occurred. And most of the immediate reoperations stem from rapidly changing clinical scenarios or time-sensitive limitations in resources—frequently personnel. Occasionally, however, both in the remote past and in the immediate past group, we need to intervene because someone did something that just plain did not make sense, even in light of the understanding of the day.

One could argue that the greatest example of long-term scientific improvement in surgical thinking was the development of our understanding of the anatomy, physiology, and pathophysiology of the stomach. It would probably be fair to extend that line of inquiry to include the esophagus, as the two are profoundly interconnected. From the last part of the nineteenth century to the present, there was a sustained acquisition and refinement of our understanding of not just the structure and function of these organs, but also how our operative changes could and would modify how these organs would work—or fail. Most of the knowledge has been around longer than many of us have been in practice, though there are plenty of newer bits of

Surg Clin N Am 95 (2015) xiii–xiv
http://dx.doi.org/10.1016/j.suc.2015.03.007
0039-6109/15/$ – see front matter © 2015 Published by Elsevier Inc.

surgical.theclinics.com

knowledge as well. Yet, somehow we still see many examples of people performing operations that seem to ignore what we know already.

I suspect there are lots of reasons for this. Anatomy and physiology are not taught the same way in medical school as they once were. Process knowledge has become more emphasized and fact-based knowledge has been de-emphasized a bit. Team-based care has replaced individual-driven care. People seem more likely to read reports than to review the primary data and decide whether they agree with the initial interpretation of the report. Even among surgeons, gastric and esophageal surgery is considered perhaps more specialty surgery than general surgery. All of these may contribute to a more superficial knowledge than is required to be maximally effective. I shall leave each of you to contemplate which, if any, of the above assertions is true.

One incontrovertible fact regarding surgery of the foregut remains: if you want a good operative result, you need to understand the problem you are trying to resolve, and you must choose and properly conduct the right operative solution. It sounds simple enough, but apparently it is not.

Dr Oleynikov and his colleagues have assembled an impressive collection of articles that should help the reader to understand not only which procedures we can perform but also how we assess the structure and function of the esophagus and associated organs so that we understand which operation (or procedure or neither) should be done. There is an adage I learned while working construction earlier in my life: measure twice, cut once. Perhaps in surgery we should think twice and operate once. One's best chance to solve a problem with an operative solution is most likely to be at the first operation. One will be far better positioned to think clearly and effectively about how to view problems that patients have with their esophagus if one takes these articles to heart. We are indebted to Dr Oleynikov and his colleagues for their efforts in reviewing these topics.

Ronald F. Martin, MD
Department of Surgery
Marshfield Clinic
1000 North Oak Avenue
Marshfield, WI 54449, USA

E-mail address:
martin.ronald@marshfieldclinic.org

Preface

Esophageal Disease

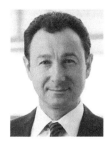

Dmitry Oleynikov, MD, FACS
Editor

Esophageal surgery, in many ways, remains very similar to principles and techniques written about in the 1997 "Surgery of the Esophagus" issue of *Surgical Clinics of North America*. But when you compare that publication and this current update, you realize just how much technology has changed the approach to diseases of the esophagus. From diagnosis of esophageal problems using new high-resolution manometry to the use of new wireless pH probes, and new methods of approaching esophageal disease endoluminally, we have rethought many concepts about esophageal surgery and the diseases that we treat. For instance, increasing use of higher-resolution manometry has revolutionized a more exact diagnosis of multiple disease states. The use of this higher-resolution manometry in conjunction with the newly revised Chicago Classification has resulted in newer diagnostic criteria for both hypomotility disorders and hypercontractility disorders and has potentially expanded surgical therapy for achalasia. Initial results from POEM (per oral endoscopic mytotomy) are promising and represent a monumental shift in how endoluminal surgery has changed our approach to this clinical entity.

Newer diagnostic approaches to benign esophageal tumors include endoscopic ultrasound and a combination of endoluminal, laparoscopic, and thoracoscopic approaches used much more frequently than in the past for these tumors. Gastro-esophageal reflux disease (GERD) continues to be the most commonly encountered gastrointestinal disease, and significant resources are still being expended to effectively treat this burden on our health care system. In patients with potential GERD, diagnostic testing now includes wireless pH monitoring.

While the incidence of Barrett esophagus continues to rise concomitantly with the increase in GERD, newer treatment modalities have also come on the market. These include endoluminal ablation and endoscopic mucosal resection as a major change in how we approach dysplasia. Multiple endoluminal devices and therapies have been introduced for GERD management and maybe one day will be positioned well to replace the venerable laparoscopic Nissen.

Surg Clin N Am 95 (2015) xv–xvi
http://dx.doi.org/10.1016/j.suc.2015.03.006
0039-6109/15/$ – see front matter © 2015 Published by Elsevier Inc.

surgical.theclinics.com

The increasing use of sleeve gastrectomy as a bariatric surgery of choice is probably leading to an increase in de novo postsurgical GERD, resulting in the need for Roux-en-Y gastric bypass procedures or other as yet to be developed therapies for symptomatic GERD.

In conclusion, it is indeed my distinct pleasure to have a very distinguished group of scientists contribute to this issue, which includes two authors and one editor of the 1997 issue mentioned above. Each of them discusses an important topic that speaks to us all about the continuing changes and improvements that are happening in the management of esophageal disease.

Dmitry Oleynikov, MD, FACS
Department of Surgery
986245 Nebraska Medical Center
Omaha, NE 68198-6245, USA

E-mail address:
doleynik@unmc.edu

Esophageal Motility Disorders

Steven P. Bowers, MD

KEYWORDS

- High-resolution manometry • Esophageal motility • Achalasia
- Spastic motility disorder • Peristalsis • Fundoplication

KEY POINTS

- The esophageal motility study is an important component of the evaluation of patients presenting with thoracic dysphagia.
- The Chicago classification includes an algorithm for diagnosis of primary esophageal motility disorders, designed primarily to be more clinically relevant and identify motility disorders that are pathologic or not found in normal patients.
- High-resolution esophageal motility studies and the Chicago classification have clarified the definitions of spastic esophageal motility disorders; however, it is not clear if revised definitions of hypomotility disorders will or have affected surgical decision making.
- The esophageal motility disorder is still thought to be an essential part of the evaluation of any patient considered for antireflux surgery.
- Achalasia has a revised classification scheme that has a correlation with surgical and medical therapies.

INTRODUCTION: NATURE OF THE PROBLEM

The diagnosis of esophageal motility disorders has historically been closely linked to the development of technology, with diagnostic criteria changing at each technological breakthrough. For most of the modern era of laparoscopic foregut surgery, esophageal motility disorders were defined in terms of water-perfused catheters using a hydraulic capillary infusion system developed in 1977.[1] Careful manometric evaluation of the esophagus and the lower esophageal sphincter (LES) became an essential part of the preoperative evaluation before antireflux surgery and surgeons used the study of esophageal motility to guide which antireflux operation best suited their respective patients. Because more than 50% of patients presenting with dysphagia without signs of mechanical esophageal obstruction have been found to have abnormal esophageal motility, the esophageal manometry study (EMS) became an essential diagnostic test in the study of patients with esophageal origin chest pain and/or dysphagia.[2]

Mayo Clinic Florida, Department of Surgery, 4500 San Pablo Road, Jacksonville, FL 32224, USA
E-mail address: bowers.steven@mayo.edu

Surg Clin N Am 95 (2015) 467–482
http://dx.doi.org/10.1016/j.suc.2015.02.003   surgical.theclinics.com

Abbreviations	
CDP	Contractile deceleration point
CFV	Contractile front velocity
DCI	Distal contractile integral
DES	Distal esophageal spasm
DL	Distal latency
EMS	Esophageal manometry study
EPT	Esophageal pressure topography
GEJ	Gastroesophageal junction
GERD	Gastroesophageal reflux disease
IEMD	Ineffective esophageal motility disorder
IRP	Integrated relaxation pressure
LES	Lower esophageal sphincter
POEM	Peroral endoscopic myotomy

With the exception of esophageal achalasia and scleroderma esophagus, disorders that are associated with distinct pathologic findings designating them as disease processes, all esophageal motility disorders are defined by the use of the EMS. Thus, the development of the high-resolution manometry study obligated the redefinition of all esophageal motility disorders. This article discusses esophageal motility disorders in the light of 2 important breakthroughs: high-resolution manometry studies and the diagnostic algorithm of the Chicago classification.[3]

Esophageal motility disorders have been classified as primary or secondary, or as hypocontractility, disordered contractility, or hypercontractility disorders. For the surgeon it is far more rational to group these in terms of the impact they have on surgical decision making, either as part of the evaluation for antireflux surgery or for planning operations for the relief of dysphagia. The author has grouped the esophageal motility disorders according to diagnostic criteria included in the Chicago classification.

HIGH-RESOLUTION MANOMETRY

The high-resolution manometry catheter is a solid state pressure detection system, with sensors closely spaced (1 cm or less) along the length of the catheter and radially, allowing simultaneous pressure readings of the lower and upper esophageal sphincters and the esophageal body. The high-resolution manometry systems allow pressures interpolated between measurement points to create a continuous 3-dimensional (time, distance down the axis of the esophagus, and pressure) graphic display called esophageal pressure topography (EPT).[4] Whereas water-perfused catheter systems reported esophageal pressures in terms of mm Hg of amplitude, analysis of high-resolution manometry is done by integrating the volume under the isobaric map for a given esophageal segment. Isobaric curves are created and, for ease of use, the color green is designated as 30 mm Hg pressure, based on the simultaneous video-radiographic and manometric data showing that ineffective bolus movement is associated with distal esophageal contraction amplitudes of less than 30 mm Hg.[5]

Aside from the diagnostic calculations, which must be done using a computer interface, the process of performing the study has been simplified by eliminating the need for multiple catheter manipulations (pull-throughs). Once the catheter has been placed through the gastroesophageal junction (GEJ) and into the intraabdominal stomach, the patient is placed supine and given 10 5 mL aliquots of fluid to swallow. The analysis of the study consists of evaluation (similar to water-perfused EMS) of the GEJ with measurement of LES pressure and length, assessment of the adequacy of LES deglutitive relaxation, and assessment of esophageal body function and adequacy of propagation of peristalsis.[6]

To better understand the assessment of esophageal body function, it is important to understand the metrics that have been developed to quantify esophageal function in the setting of EPT.[7] Propagation of esophageal peristalsis is faster in the more proximal esophagus and midesophagus, and slows in the distal esophagus (the ampulla of the esophagus). The contractile deceleration point (CDP) is calculated as the point where the slope of the isobaric contour line of the upper esophagus meets that of the lower esophagus. The speed of the propagation of the peristaltic wave is called the contractile front velocity (CFV), which is the slope of the 30 mm Hg isobaric curve proximal to the CDP. Distal latency (DL) is calculated as the time between upper esophageal sphincter relaxation and the CDP, and is a measure of deglutitive inhibition. DL has been found to be a more consistent measure of the simultaneous or premature nature of a peristaltic wave.

The amplitude of esophageal peristalsis is measured as the distal contractile integral (DCI), which is the integrated volume under the EPT map of that respective esophageal segment (measured as mm Hg × centimeter × second). For assessment of LES relaxation, esophageal manometry cannot distinguish pressures caused by the diaphragmatic crura (or other external compressive force such as fundoplication wrap) as being separate from the LES, thus the metric used is called the integrated relaxation pressure (IRP). The IRP is the average from 10 swallows of the lowest mean pressure at the GEJ during a 4-second period after deglutition.

Assessment of adequacy of esophageal body peristalsis includes visualization of continuity of the 20 mm Hg isobaric curve and assessment of each swallow as intact peristalsis, weak peristalsis (with discontinuity of the 20 mm Hg IBC in either small [2–5 cm] or large [>5 cm] breaks), or failed peristalsis. Intact peristaltic waves are further characterized by the above metrics and each peristaltic wave is assessed for esophageal pressurization to greater than 30 mm Hg. Esophageal pressurization is further assessed as being panesophageal or compartmentalized. Esophageal impedance can also be also measured during the high-resolution manometry study and each peristaltic wave is assessed by whether there is associated complete bolus clearance.

Chicago Classification Scheme

Based on the categorical assessment of 10 swallows, the manometry studies are applied to the Chicago classification scheme. Most patients can be classified as having normal esophageal motility, having an abnormal GEJ relaxation state, a major motility disorder with normal GEJ relaxation, or borderline peristaltic function (**Fig. 1**).

The Chicago classification prioritizes the identification of abnormal EPT metrics into a hierarchy. The highest priority is given to identification of abnormal IRP-designating disorders of GEJ relaxation. This would serve to reduce the frequency of misdiagnosed esophageal achalasia variants. If IRP and, therefore, GEJ relaxation are normal, then priority is given to identification of the 3 major esophageal body motility disorders not seen in normal individuals. These include absent peristalsis, distal esophageal spasm (DES), and hypercontractile or jackhammer esophagus. Finally, the Chicago classification designates as borderline esophageal motility those abnormalities that can be seen in fewer than 5% of normal asymptomatic individuals.[7] Borderline esophageal motility includes weak peristalsis and frequent failed peristalsis (previously known as ineffective esophageal motility disorder [IEMD]), hypertensive peristalsis or nutcracker esophagus, and rapid contraction (previously known as nonspecific spastic motility disorder).

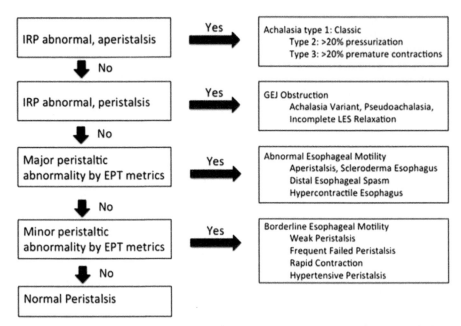

Fig. 1. Chicago classification diagnostic algorithm. The Chicago classification includes a diagnostic algorithm based on hierarchical analysis of EPT metrics. (*Adapted from* Bredenoord AJ, Fox M, Kahrilas PJ, et al. Chicago classification criteria of esophageal motility disorders defined in high resolution esophageal pressure topography. Neurogastroenterol Motil 2012;24(Suppl 1):57; with permission.)

Implications for the Surgeon

In patients considered for antireflux surgery, an assessment of esophageal motility is considered the standard of practice. This is primarily done to identify patients for whom antireflux surgery is contraindicated. The motility study is also very useful in identifying the cause of nonreflux esophageal symptoms and setting patient expectations for recovery after antireflux surgery. Using high-resolution motility study as a preoperative test before proposed antireflux surgery, up to 7% of patients were identified as having an esophageal motility disorder that contraindicated Nissen fundoplication.[8] There is a significant correlation between preoperative dysphagia and the presence of a hypocontractile esophageal motility disorder.[9] Also, it has been demonstrated that patients with nonspecific spastic esophageal motility disorders are more likely to have postoperative typical reflux symptoms after antireflux surgery.[10] When also considering the disastrous consequences of performing fundoplication in a patient with achalasia, there can be little doubt of the benefit of routine esophageal motility assessment before antireflux surgery.

Compared with the water-perfused esophageal motility systems of the past, high-resolution esophageal manometry studies have some distinct advantages but also some disadvantages. The EPT graphics do not reproduce by copy or transmit by facsimile well. A computer interface is required to interpret the EPT data. Thus, the surgeon depends more on interpretation by the provider reading the study. The summary EPT, an average of the 10 swallows, is generally not helpful for surgical planning. Thus, from the high-resolution motility study report, the surgeon still is required to make decisions mainly based on the reported LES pressure, LES relaxation pressure (IRP), the classification of peristaltic waves, and the final diagnosis according to the Chicago classification. Disorder-specific surgical implications are separately discussed.

ESOPHAGEAL ACHALASIA

Esophageal achalasia is a disease characterized by esophageal outflow obstruction caused by inadequate relaxation of the LES and a pressurized and dilated hypomotile esophagus with nonprogressive swallow responses. Pathophysiologically, there is degeneration of ganglion cells in the myenteric plexus of the esophageal wall, related to absence in the LES of the neurotransmitters nitric oxide and vasoactive intestinal polypeptide.[11] Experimental models have long suggested that the peristaltic abnormalities seen in esophageal achalasia are secondary to the outflow obstruction.[12] However, by the water-perfused manometry study and standard motility classification, aperistalsis was used as the most important motility abnormality identified in achalasia. Use of high-resolution manometry studies and the Chicago classification have redirected the diagnosis to reflect the pathophysiologic findings of achalasia.[7]

Esophageal achalasia had previously been classified into subtypes, classic and vigorous achalasia, based on the finding in the esophageal body of vigorous repetitive and high-amplitude swallow responses. This classification had no clinical significance, however. The Chicago classification has refined the subclassification of achalasia into subtypes based on the finding of esophageal pressurization and premature contractions.[13–15] Whereas type 1 represents classic achalasia, type 2 identifies patients with panesophageal pressurization (to >30 mm Hg) in 20% or greater swallows. Type 3, or spastic achalasia identifies patients who have no intact peristalsis but have the finding, in 20% or greater swallows, of premature or simultaneous contractions (with DL <4.5 seconds). Further, type 3 achalasia represents patients who may have been previously diagnosed as having diffuse esophageal spasm with incomplete LES relaxation. These patients are more likely to present with chest pain as a prominent symptom. Of these subtypes, type 2 seems to be slightly more common than type 1, and type 3 is infrequent in most reported series (**Fig. 2**).

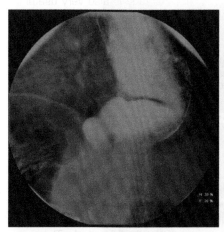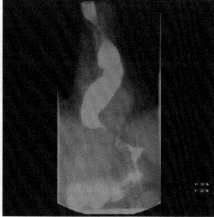

Fig. 2. Esophageal achalasia subtype I and II. Contrast esophagrams of patients with classic achalasia, subtype I (*left*) and achalasia with pressurization, subtype II (*right*). The greater esophageal body tone seen in subtype II may be preventative of esophageal dilation, and thus responsible for the observed better outcomes of therapy.

Additionally, the Chicago classification has allowed for the identification of patients with an achalasia variant, so designated because of the finding of nonrelaxing LES and some preservation of peristalsis.[16] The classification EGJ (esophagogastric junction) relaxation abnormality includes patients who are found on later study to have achalasia with aperistalsis, as well as those with pseudoachalasia and postoperative (postfundoplication) states, and those with incomplete LES relaxation as the sole identified abnormality (**Fig. 3**).

Implications for the Surgeon

The development of high-resolution manometry and the Chicago classification has both broadened and simplified the definitions of achalasia and its subtypes. Additionally, the Chicago classification subtypes have some added prognostic value that may aid in the formulation of surgical planning. Type 1 achalasia seems to have better outcomes with myotomy as the initial treatment when compared with endoscopic therapies (botulinum toxin injection or pneumatic balloon dilation).[13] Type 2 achalasia seems to have the best outcomes regardless of the initial treatment strategy and type 3 has the worst outcomes irrespective of treatment strategy (botulinum toxin, pneumatic dilation, and myotomy). There are no available data on the association of type 1 achalasia with greater esophageal dilation than that seen in type 2 but it is intuitive that a greater degree of esophageal dilation would be associated with a decreased symptomatic response to treatment.

High-quality studies demonstrating greater effectiveness of surgical myotomy compared with botulinum toxin injection and pneumatic dilation were reported without the benefit of the Chicago classification. Based on the improved response of type 2 patients to any initial treatment, there is greater support among gastroenterologists for initial endoscopic therapy in type 2 achalasia patients, with myotomy relegated to treatment failures in type 2 patients. However, because there is a continuum between type 1 cases with pressurization to just below 30 mm Hg and type 2 cases,

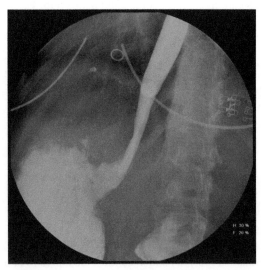

Fig. 3. EGJ outflow obstruction, achalasia variant. Contrast esophagram of a patient presenting with dysphagia-note presence of 12.5 mm barium pill above LES. HRM revealed preserved peristalsis but elevated IRP, consistent with achalasia variant.

and marginal differences between type 3 cases and some achalasia variants, it is unrealistic to make a firm algorithm regarding treatment based on achalasia types.

Although laparoscopic Heller myotomy with partial fundoplication is accessible to most patients with achalasia in North America, the diffusion of centers offering peroral endoscopic myotomy (POEM) as a definitive treatment of achalasia has made this an option for most regions. Because POEM is reflexogenic in one-third of patients without hiatal hernia, the presence of a hiatal hernia should be seen as a relative contraindication for the POEM procedure.[17] Otherwise, analysis of the outcomes for POEM based on reports from high-volume centers and the growing international experience essentially equates POEM outcomes with surgical myotomy without fundoplication by other approach.[17–20]

In the setting of prefundoplication evaluation, the finding on high-resolution manometry of GEJ obstruction and intact peristalsis in a patient without dysphagia may be a false-positive, and the surgeon may consider a contrast esophagram with barium tablet to confirm that there is a functional delay in esophageal emptying before changing the surgical plan.

HYPERCONTRACTILITY STATES

Gastroesophageal reflux disease (GERD) is the most common cause of noncardiac chest pain and hypercontractile motility disorders are rare; however, the symptoms of dysphagia and chest pain are clinical scenarios that are suspicious for hypercontractile esophageal motility disorders. Patients with chest pain usually have undergone a cardiac evaluation that is not consistent with coronary origin chest pain. All patients with dysphagia should have esophageal obstruction ruled out by upper endoscopy or contrast esophagram.

Although contrast esophagram may confirm a hypercontractile esophageal motility disorder, it is not sensitive enough to be used as a screening test. An esophageal motility study is required to establish a diagnosis and initiate treatment. The natural history of these disorders has seen some overlap and, classically, there were a substantial number of hypercontractile motility disorders identified in asymptomatic patients.[21] By classic water-perfused manometry, the clinical relevance of hypercontractile esophageal motility disorders could only be established when therapy based on motility study finding and directed at patient symptoms was successful in symptom resolution. Based on the Chicago classification and analysis of high-resolution manometry EPT metrics, there are 2 identified major hypercontractile abnormalities that are always associated with patient symptoms and never identified in normal individuals.[22] Using the new classification scheme, the number of patients diagnosed with hypercontracting motility disorders is markedly reduced and, because the most extreme cases have been selected, response to medications and natural history of the disorders as currently diagnosed are unknown.

Distal Esophageal Spasm

The name diffuse esophageal spasm has been something of a misnomer because it is the distal esophagus that is spastic.[23] DES is now the preferred terminology but both are used interchangeably. Patients with DES commonly present with dysphagia. Because of the observed response in DES patients to nitroglycerin, it is thought that DES may be pathophysiologically linked to a defect in esophageal nitric oxide production.[24,25] Contrast esophagram may demonstrate the classic corkscrew esophagus or rosary bead esophagus; however, a normal contrast esophagram does not exclude DES (**Fig. 4**). The hallmark of DES by classic esophageal motility study has been the

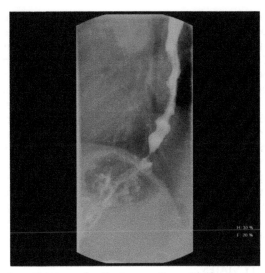

Fig. 4. DES. Contrast esophagram of patient presenting with chest pain and dysphagia. HRM revealed normal IRP, but 30% of peristaltic waves had DL less than 4.5 seconds and 50% of waves with CFV greater than 9 cm/s, consistent with DES. Corkscrew pattern of esophageal contraction can also be seen with any hypercontracting esophageal motility disorder.

finding of frequent simultaneous peristalsis. Classically, in one-third of patients there has been some abnormality of the LES (either hypertensive LES or incompletely relaxing LES).[26,27] However, with high-resolution manometry and interpreted by the Chicago classification, some of these latter patients are now considered to have type 3 achalasia or an achalasia variant.

High-resolution manometry diagnostic criteria rely on measurement of DL to determine whether a peristaltic contraction is considered premature or simultaneous (DL <4.5 seconds). The Chicago classification designates DES as having 20% or greater of swallows with DL less than 4.5 seconds. This is in contrast to the characteristic manometry finding of high-velocity peristalsis (CFV > 8–9 cm/s) to identify simultaneous contractions, or the findings of repetitive contractions or contractions of long duration (>6 seconds) in greater than 20% of peristaltic waves that previously constituted DES. The Chicago classification requires that there also be normal LES relaxation to distinguish DES from achalasia variants. Greater than two-thirds of patients previously diagnosed as having DES will now receive a different diagnosis using the Chicago classification.[28] Rapid contraction, defined as 20% or greater swallows with CFV greater than 9 cm/s is considered borderline motility by the Chicago classification.[7]

Although patients with classically defined DES followed longitudinally show that the majority improve somewhat with time without directed medical therapy,[29] there are several classes of medication that have proven to be somewhat helpful in managing the disorder. The antidepressants trazodone and imipramine were found to decrease chest pain with DES, likely by modifying esophageal sensitivity.[30,31] The phosphodiesterase inhibitor sildenafil has been associated with symptoms relief.[32] Botulinum toxin delivered by endoscopic injection was found to decrease dysphagia.[33]

Implications for the surgeon
The diagnostic criteria for DES are now more restrictive and DES now refers to a more distinct clinical phenotype. With the more restrictive definition, it should be

infrequent that the surgeon encounters a patient with documented GERD and DES. In a patient with documented GERD who has diagnostic criteria for DES on preoperative high-resolution manometry, the surgeon should reassess which symptoms may be due to DES and, therefore, unlikely to respond to antireflux therapy. For patients with GERD who have prominent dysphagia symptoms and DES, Nissen fundoplication is not recommended. In patients with noncardiac chest pain found to have DES and GERD that are failing medical therapy, the surgeon should consider starting an antidepressant before or after antireflux surgery.

More commonly, the surgeon encounters patients who previously would have been diagnosed with DES but are now classified as having a nonspecific spastic motility disorder or rapid contraction (CFV > 9 cm/s) because of rapid or simultaneous contractions not fulfilling criteria for DES (90% of swallows with DL > 4.5 seconds). Expectations should be revisited as to which symptoms are likely to improve after operation.

In patients presenting with DES and refractory symptoms of dysphagia and chest pain, it is reasonable to perform endoscopic botulinum toxin injection. Although there are reported small series of POEM surgery for DES,[19,34] this should be viewed as experimental and caution should be exercised because of the propensity for DES symptoms to lessen over time without intervention.

Jackhammer Esophagus

The hypercontractile esophagus is characterized by high-amplitude esophageal body peristaltic contractions associated with chest pain and/or dysphagia (**Fig. 5**). Using the water-perfused manometry system, the criteria for defining the disorder as nutcracker esophagus had undergone some evolution to a higher mean amplitude (from 180 mm Hg to 220 mm Hg) to decrease the number of patients diagnosed with the disorder who had reflux symptoms rather than chest pain.[35] Using the high-resolution manometry system, the Chicago classification used an entirely new metric, the DCI, and identified the threshold for which a single swallow with elevated DCI was always associated with dysphagia (DCI >8000 mm Hg/cm/s) and termed this disorder jackhammer

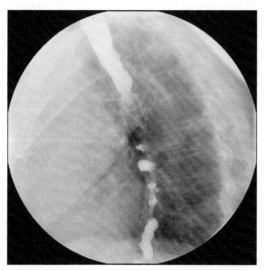

Fig. 5. Hypercontractile or jackhammer esophagus. Contrast esophagram showing rosary bead esophagus in a patient presenting with chest pain and dysphagia. HRM revealed 20% of swallows with DCI greater than 9000, consistent with hypercontractile esophagus.

esophagus. This is reflective of the finding of repetitive contractions in most spastic hypercontractile waves. Mean DCI greater than 5000 mm Hg/cm/s based on 10 swallows is termed hypertensive peristalsis and still nicknamed nutcracker esophagus; however, with the assumption that it is possible in asymptomatic patients.

The pathophysiology of the hypercontractile esophageal disorders is thought to be due to asynchrony in the circular and longitudinal smooth muscle of the esophagus during contraction. Because this is reversible with atropine, it thought to be due in part to a hypercholinergic state.[36] When using a mean amplitude of greater than 180 mm Hg as a threshold for defining nutcracker esophagus, there was an association with GERD.[35]

Classically, the nutcracker esophagus has been associated with hypertensive LES. Almost 50% of patients with hypertensive LES were found to have nutcracker esophagus and hypertensive LES was formerly classified as a hypercontracting motility disorder.[37]

Treatment of hypercontractile esophagus is similar to treatment of DES. Diltiazem was found to relieve chest pain in patients with nutcracker esophagus.[38] Sildenafil, trazodone, and imipramine have also been found to be helpful.[30–32] Based on the pathophysiology of the disorder, anticholinergics would be expected to have treatment benefit. Endoscopic botulinum toxin injection has a response rate greater than 70% and half of treated patients have, at least temporarily, complete relief of chest pain.[39] Failing medical therapy, patients with nutcracker esophagus with severe dysphagia may undergo Heller myotomy with good relief of dysphagia; however, relief of chest pain is less certain with laparoscopic Heller myotomy.[40] Small series of POEM for hypercontractile esophagus show promise, with high rates of relief of chest pain.[19]

Implications for the surgeon
The classically described nutcracker esophagus has been associated with GERD. The finding of hypertensive peristalsis in a patient with GERD should not alter the treatment plan for antireflux surgery. Because jackhammer esophagus is a finding always associated with chest pain or dysphagia, the treatment plan should reflect the expectation that this disorder will not resolve with treatment of GERD and should be specifically addressed. However, definitive treatment studies have not been performed using these specific criteria for hypercontractile esophagus.

HYPOCONTRACTILE STATES
Aperistalsis or Scleroderma Esophagus

Esophageal manifestations of systemic sclerosis or scleroderma and collagen vascular disease should be considered separately from ineffective esophageal motility associated with GERD. Scleroderma esophagus is defined as aperistalsis with low or absent LES pressure (resting pressure <10 mm Hg). Esophageal findings are present in more than 70% of patients with typical skin manifestations of scleroderma.[41,42] Scleroderma esophagus is caused by atrophy and sclerosis of the smooth muscle of the esophagus; the striated proximal esophageal muscle is spared. Esophageal manometry findings similar to scleroderma esophagus may be found in other connective tissue diseases, such as polymyositis, dermatomyositis, and mixed connective tissue disorder.

Implications for the surgeon
The primary consideration in managing scleroderma esophagus is preventing development of peptic esophageal stricture and recurrent aspiration pneumonia and malnutrition. Although a loose Nissen fundoplication may be used,[43] more recent reports

recommend partial fundoplication,[44] and some consideration should be given to placement of feeding access via gastrostomy tube during antireflux surgery.[45]

Weak Peristalsis and Frequent Failed Peristalsis

Gastroesophageal reflux disease is associated with hypocontractile states and GERD is likely causative of impaired peristalsis and decreased peristaltic amplitude. Hypotensive LES and inappropriate LES relaxation are similarly causative of GERD.

The most common hypocontractile conditions of the esophagus were grouped as IEMDs, the definition of which has changed several times during the era of laparoscopic antireflux surgery. Initially, the percentage of propagation of peristalsis and the mean distal esophageal pressures were reported. Abnormal esophageal peristalsis corresponded to propagation of peristalsis in fewer than 80% of swallows, or mean distal amplitude of less than 30 mm Hg.[46] Eventually these 2 metrics were combined with the concept of effective esophageal peristalsis, which is a continuous peristaltic wave with distal amplitude of greater than 30 mm Hg, and IEMD was defined as ineffective esophageal peristaltic waves in 30% or greater of swallows.[47]

Approximately 30% of patients with IEMD report dysphagia, whereas most patients with IEMD are asymptomatic of the motility disorder. When patients with IEMD were studied with simultaneous esophageal impedance, more than 30% had normal esophageal bolus clearance.[47] Manometric diagnosis of ineffective esophageal motility may not always correlate with the effectiveness of esophageal function and may be present in normal individuals.

By high-resolution manometry testing and interpretation using the EPT metrics, there are 2 categories of ineffective peristalsis: weak peristalsis and frequent failed peristalsis.[7] A weak peristaltic wave has been defined as a greater than 2 cm break in the 20 mm Hg isobaric contour line. This is based on the finding of incomplete bolus transport on simultaneous intraluminal impedance.[48] A diagnosis of weak peristalsis is given with 30% or greater swallows having small breaks (2–5 cm) or 20% or greater large breaks (>5 cm) in the 20 mm Hg isobaric contour line. Frequent failed peristalsis is defined as failed peristalsis in 30% to 90% of swallows. Interestingly, patients with weak peristalsis were more likely to be symptomatic than patients with a similar degree of failed peristaltic waves.[48] Whereas IEMD was graded as mild or severe based on the frequency of ineffective peristalsis (30% or greater vs 70% or greater, respectively), no such gradations of weak or failed peristalsis are considered in the Chicago classification.

Implications for the surgeon

Tailoring of the fundoplication in patients with GERD and ineffective esophageal motility has been long debated. This concept involved using Nissen fundoplication for patients with normal esophageal motility (defined as normal propagation of peristalsis in >80% of swallows and normal distal mean amplitude > 30 mm Hg) but using partial fundoplication for patients with demonstrated abnormal esophageal motility.[49] Because there is an association between severe GERD and esophageal hypomotility, tailoring the fundoplication in this way selected patients with the most severe GERD for partial fundoplication. Many large North American centers reported higher rates of failure of partial fundoplication when assessed at longer follow-up intervals.[50–53]

A large randomized trial comparing Nissen and Toupet fundoplication was conducted in Hamburg, Germany.[9,54] The investigators stratified subjects based on the presence of abnormal esophageal motility (defined somewhat liberally as mean distal amplitude <40 mm Hg). The investigators concluded that esophageal motility testing was not helpful in predicting dysphagia-related outcomes and that outcomes with Toupet fundoplication were superior. This study also established that preoperative dysphagia was more likely to improve with partial fundoplication and that the frequency of abnormal esophageal peristalsis is not likely to improve with Nissen but may improve with partial fundoplication.

From a randomized trial of achalasia patients treated with Heller myotomy, Nissen fundoplication was associated with greater severe, long-term dysphagia compared with partial fundoplication.[55] Therefore, for patients with aperistalsis due to scleroderma esophagus and severe GERD, partial fundoplication is also indicated. Patients with aperistalsis thought due to severe GERD, without any findings consistent with connective tissue disorder, may be treated intensively with proton pump inhibitor therapy for 3 to 4 months and a motility study repeated. If there is significant improvement in esophageal peristalsis, then Nissen fundoplication can be considered. Patients who have dysphagia and esophageal hypocontractile disorders, which are out of proportion to the severity of GERD, may have a primary esophageal motility disorder, and the motility disorder may be partially causative of GERD due to abnormal esophageal clearance. In such patients, a partial fundoplication may also be indicated.

The concept of tailoring a Nissen fundoplication, constructing the wrap to be more loose or floppy based on preoperative esophageal motility, has not been systematically studied. The novel technology of impedance planimetry has been used to measure the distensibility of the GEJ via the use of a functional luminal imaging probe.[56,57] It remains to be seen if this technology can add to surgeon experience in creating a fundoplication that is appropriate for patients with varying levels of esophageal peristaltic dysfunction.

HYPERTENSIVE LOWER ESOPHAGEAL SPHINCTER

The upper limit of normal LES pressure by high-resolution manometry is 35 mm Hg (45 mm Hg by water perfused systems). Although no longer considered an esophageal motility disorder by the Chicago classification, it important for the surgeon to recognize the importance of this finding. Hypertensive LES had been grouped with DES

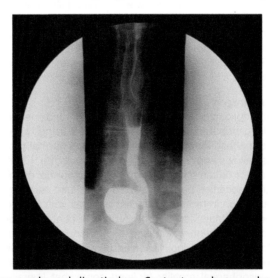

Fig. 6. Pulsion-type esophageal diverticulum. Contrast esophagram showing pulsion-type esophageal diverticulum. Water perfused esophageal motility study revealed resting LES pressure of 48 with normal LES relaxation, and 50% of swallows with CFV greater than 8 cm/s, consistent with hypertensive LES.

and nutcracker esophagus as a hypercontractile primary esophageal motility disorder, and has been found associated with epiphrenic diverticulum in up to 20% of reported cases (**Fig. 6**).[58] Hypertensive LES has been associated with dysphagia, particularly after Nissen fundoplication. In fact, even when measured to be within normal range, there is an association of increasing LES baseline pressure to postoperative dysphagia after Nissen fundoplication.[59]

SUMMARY

Reports of outcomes are needed in patients treated with motility disorders diagnosed using high-resolution manometry and the Chicago classification. The new classification of achalasia has been associated with some prognostic value, and will increase the number of patients diagnosed with early achalasia rather than other spastic esophageal motor disorders, potentially increasing the frequency of surgical esophagogastric myotomy. Clarification of the diagnoses of DES and hypercontractility has decreased the overlap of these disorders with GERD, and it is hoped will eventually clarify the role of a surgical approach to these disorders. Surgeons reporting their results using the diagnostic criteria according to EPT metrics and the Chicago classification will enhance this effort. As for hypomotility of the esophagus, the Chicago classification has, if anything, muddied the water, creating an additional category, weak peristalsis, and eliminating gradations of peristaltic failure. Although weak peristalsis may have had a stronger association with dysphagia than frequent failed peristalsis, the diagnostic criteria seem overly sensitive and the disorder is likely to be underappreciated by surgeons.

REFERENCES

1. Arndorfer RC, Steff JJ, Dodds WJ, et al. Improved infusion system for intraluminal esophageal manometry. Gastroenterology 1977;73:23–7.
2. Katz PO, Dalton CB, Richter JE, et al. Esophageal testing of patients with noncardiac chest pain or dysphagia. Results of three years' experience with 1161 patients. Ann Intern Med 1987;106:593.
3. Kahrilas PJ, Ghosh SK, Pandolfino JE. Esophageal motility disorders in terms of pressure topography: the Chicago Classification. J Clin Gastroenterol 2008; 42:627.
4. Clouse RE, Prakash C. Topographic esophageal manometry: an emerging clinical and investigative approach. Dig Dis 2000;18:64.
5. Kahrilas PJ, Dodds WJ, Hogan WJ. Effect of peristaltic dysfunction on esophageal volume clearance. Gastroenterology 1988;94(1):73–80.
6. ASGE Technology Committee, Wang A, Pleskow DK, et al. Esophageal function testing. Gastrointest Endosc 2012;76:231.
7. Bredenoord AJ, Fox M, Kahrilas PJ, et al. Chicago classification criteria of esophageal motility disorders defined in high resolution esophageal pressure topography. Neurogastroenterol Motil 2012;24(Suppl 1):57.
8. Chan WW, Haroian LR, Gyawali CP. Value of preoperative esophageal function studies before laparoscopic antireflux surgery. Surg Endosc 2011;25:2943–9.
9. Fibbe C, Layer P, Keller J, et al. Esophageal motility in reflux disease before and after fundoplication: a prospective, randomized, clinical, and manometric study. Gastroenterology 2001;121:5.
10. Winslow ER, Clouse RE, Desai KM, et al. Influence of spastic motor disorders of the esophageal body on outcomes from antireflux surgery. Surg Endosc 2003;17: 738–45.

11. Ghoshal UC, Daschakraborty SB, Singh R. Pathogenesis of achalasia cardia. World J Gastroenterol 2012;18(4):3050–7.
12. Khajanchee YS, VanAndel R, Jobe BA, et al. Electrical stimulation of the vagus nerve restores motility in an animal model of achalasia. J Gastrointest Surg 2003;7(7):843–9.
13. Pandolfino JE, Kwiatek MA, Nealis T, et al. Achalasia: a new clinically relevant classification by high-resolution manometry. Gastroenterology 2008;135:1526.
14. Salvador R, Costantini M, Zaninotto G, et al. The preoperative manometric pattern predicts the outcome of surgical treatment for esophageal achalasia. J Gastrointest Surg 2010;14(11):1635–45.
15. Pratap N, Kalapala R, Darisetty S, et al. Achalasia cardia subtyping by high-resolution manometry predicts the therapeutic outcome of pneumatic balloon dilatation. J Neurogastroenterol Motil 2011;17(1):48–53.
16. Scherer JR, Kwiatek MA, Soper NJ, et al. Functional esophagogastric junction obstruction with intact peristalsis: a heterogeneous syndrome sometimes akin to achalasia. J Gastrointest Surg 2009;13:2219.
17. Sharata AM, Dunst CM, Pescarus R, et al. Peroral Endoscopic Myotomy (POEM) for Esophageal Primary Motility Disorders: Analysis of 100 Consecutive Patients. J Gastrointest Surg 2015;19:161–70.
18. Inoue H, Tianle KM, Ikeda H, et al. Peroral endoscopic myotomy for esophageal achalasia: technique, indication and outcomes. Thorac Surg Clin 2011;21(4):519–25.
19. Ling TS, Guo HM, Yang T, et al. Effectiveness of peroral endoscopic myotomy in the treatment of achalasia: a pilot trial in Chinese Han population with a minimum of one-year follow-up. J Dig Dis 2014;15(7):352–8.
20. Von Renteln D, Fuchs KH, Breithaupt W, et al. Peroral endoscopic myotomy for the treatment of esophageal achalasia: an international multicenter study. Gastroenterology 2013;145(2):309–11.
21. Achem SR, Crittenden J, Kolts B, et al. Long-term clinical and manometric follow-up of patients with nonspecific esophageal motor disorders. Am J Gastroenterol 1992;87:825.
22. Roman S, Pandolfino JE, Chen J, et al. Phenotypes and clinical context of hyper-contractility in high-resolution esophageal pressure topography (EPT). Am J Gastroenterol 2012;107(1):37–45.
23. Sperandio M, Tutuian R, Gideon RM, et al. Diffuse esophageal spasm: not diffuse but distal esophageal spasm (DES). Dig Dis Sci 2003;48:1380.
24. Orlando RC, Bozymski EM. Clinical and manometric effects of nitroglycerin in diffuse esophageal spasm. N Engl J Med 1973;289:23.
25. Swamy N. Esophageal spasm: clinical and manometric response to nitroglycerine and long acting nitrites. Gastroenterology 1977;72:23.
26. DiMarino AJ Jr. Characteristics of lower esophageal sphincter function in symptomatic diffuse esophageal spasm. Gastroenterology 1974;66:1.
27. Campo S, Traube M. Lower esophageal sphincter dysfunction in diffuse esophageal spasm. Am J Gastroenterol 1989;84:928.
28. Pandolfino JE, Roman S, Carlson D, et al. Distal esophageal spasm in high-resolution esophageal pressure topography: defining clinical phenotypes. Gastroenterology 2011;141:469.
29. Spencer HL, Smith L, Riley SA. A questionnaire study to assess long-term outcome in patients with abnormal esophageal manometry. Dysphagia 2006;21:149.
30. Clouse RE, Lustman PJ, Eckert TC, et al. Low-dose trazodone for symptomatic patients with esophageal contraction abnormalities. A double-blind, placebo-controlled trial. Gastroenterology 1987;92:1027.

31. Cannon RO 3rd, Quyyumi AA, Mincemoyer R, et al. Imipramine in patients with chest pain despite normal coronary angiograms. N Engl J Med 1994;330:1411.
32. Agrawal A, Tutuian R, Hila A, et al. Successful use of phosphodiesterase type 5 inhibitors to control symptomatic esophageal hypercontractility: a case report. Dig Dis Sci 2005;50:2059.
33. Miller LS, Pullela SV, Parkman HP, et al. Treatment of chest pain in patients with noncardiac, nonreflux, nonachalasia spastic esophageal motor disorders using botulinum toxin injection into the gastroesophageal junction. Am J Gastroenterol 2002;97:1640.
34. Minami H, Isomoto H, Yamaguchi N, et al. Peroral esophageal myotomy (POEM) for diffuse esophageal spasm. Endoscopy 2014;46(S 01):E79–81.
35. Agrawal A, Hila A, Tutuian R, et al. Clinical relevance of the nutcracker esophagus: suggested revision of criteria for diagnosis. J Clin Gastroenterol 2006;40:504.
36. Korsapati H, Bhargava V, Mittal RK. Reversal of asynchrony between circular and longitudinal muscle contraction in nutcracker esophagus by atropine. Gastroenterology 2008;135:796.
37. Freidin N, Traube M, Mittal RK, et al. The hypertensive lower esophageal sphincter. Manometric and clinical aspects. Dig Dis Sci 1989;34:1063.
38. Cattau EL Jr, Castell DO, Johnson DA, et al. Diltiazem therapy for symptoms associated with nutcracker esophagus. Am J Gastroenterol 1991;86:272.
39. Vanuytsel T, Bisschops R, Farré R, et al. Botulinum toxin reduces Dysphagia in patients with nonachalasia primary esophageal motility disorders. Clin Gastroenterol Hepatol 2013;11:1115.
40. Patti MG, Gorodner MV, Galvani C, et al. Spectrum of esophageal motility disorders: implications for diagnosis and treatment. Arch Surg 2005;140(5):442–8.
41. Zamost BJ, Hirschberg J, Ippoliti AF, et al. Esophagitis in scleroderma. Prevalence and risk factors. Gastroenterology 1987;92:421.
42. Yarze JC, Varga J, Stampfl D, et al. Esophageal function in systemic sclerosis: a prospective evaluation of motility and acid reflux in 36 patients. Am J Gastroenterol 1993;88:870.
43. Poirier NC, Taillefer R, Topart P, et al. Antireflux operations in patients with scleroderma. Ann Thorac Surg 1994;58(1):66–72.
44. Watson DI, Jamieson GG, Bessell JR, et al. Laparoscopic fundoplication in patients with an aperistaltic esophagus and gastroesophageal reflux. Dis Esophagus 2006; 19(2):94–8.
45. Kent MS, Luketich JD, Irshad K, et al. Comparison of surgical approaches to recalcitrant gastroesophageal reflux disease in the patient with scleroderma. Ann Thorac Surg 2007;84(5):1710–5.
46. Hunter JG, Trus TL, Branum GD, et al. A physiologic approach to laparoscopic fundoplication for gastrointestinal reflux disease. Ann Surg 1996;223(6):673–87.
47. Tutuian R, Castell DO. Clarification of the esophageal function defect in patients with manometric ineffective esophageal motility: studies using combined impedance-manometry. Clin Gastroenterol Hepatol 2004;2:230.
48. Roman S, Lin Z, Kwiatek MA, et al. Weak peristalsis in esophageal pressure topography: classification and association with dysphagia. Am J Gastroenterol 2011;106:349–56.
49. Kauer WK, Peters JH, DeMeester TR, et al. A tailored approach to antireflux surgery. J Thorac Cardiovasc Surg 1995;110:141–7.
50. Horvath KD, Jobe BA, Herron DM, et al. Laparoscopic Toupet fundoplication is an inadequate procedure for patients with severe reflux disease. J Gastrointest Surg 1999;3(6):583–91.

51. Farrell TM, Archer SB, Galloway KD, et al. Heartburn is more likely to recur after Toupet fundoplication than Nissen fundoplication. Am Surg 2000;66(3):229–36.

52. Patti MG, Robinson T, Galvani C, et al. Total fundoplication is superior to partial fundoplication even when esophaegal peristalsis is weak. J Am Coll Surg 2004; 198:863–70.

53. Bell RC, Hanna P, Mills MR, et al. Patterns of success and failure with laparoscopic Toupet fundoplication. Surg Endosc 1999;13:1189–94.

54. Strate U, Emmerman A, Fibbe C, et al. Laparoscopic fundoplication: Nissen versus Toupet two-year outcome of a prospective randomized study of 200 patients regarding preoperative esophageal motility. Surg Endosc 2008;22: 21–30.

55. Rebecchi F, Giaccone C, Farinella E, et al. Randomized controlled trial of laparoscopic Heller myotomy plus Dor fundoplication versus Nissen fundoplication for achalasia: long-term results. Ann Surg 2008;248(6):1023–30.

56. Ilczyszyn A, Botha AJ. Feasibility of esophagogastric junction distensibility measurement during Nissen fundoplication. Dis Esophagus 2014;27(7):637–44.

57. Kwiatek MA, Kahrilas PJ, Soper NJ, et al. Esophagogastric junction distensibility after fundoplication assessed with a novel functional luminal imaging probe. J Gastrointest Surg 2010;14:268–76.

58. D'Journo XB, Ferraro P, Martin J, et al. Lower oesophageal sphincter dysfunction is part of the functional abnormality in epiphrenic diverticulum. Br J Surg 2009;96: 892–900.

59. Blom D, Peters JH, DeMeester TR, et al. Physiologic mechanism and preoperative prediction of new-onset dysphagia after laparoscopic Nissen fundoplication. J Gastrointest Surg 2002;6(1):22–7.

Approach to Patients with Esophageal Dysphagia

Udayakumar Navaneethan, MD, Steve Eubanks, MD*

KEYWORDS

- Dysphagia • Endoscopy • Manometry

KEY POINTS

- Patients present to a physician with complaints of difficulty swallowing, and the approach to evaluating these problems can be challenging for those who do not manage this complaint regularly.
- Dysphagia refers to difficulty with swallowing where there are problems with the transit of food from the mouth to the hypopharynx or through the esophagus.
- The most important step in assessing dysphagia is to determine whether it is oropharyngeal or esophageal in origin; potential causes and subsequent investigation and management can differ greatly.
- Numerous tools are available to aid with the determination of the cause of dysphagia and assist with the formulation of a logical treatment algorithm.

INTRODUCTION

Dysphagia refers to difficulty with swallowing where there are problems with the transit of food from the mouth to the hypopharynx or through the esophagus. Dysphagia can be classified based on the location and by the physiologic circumstances in which it occurs. Dysphagia is classified as oropharyngeal or esophageal dysphagia based on location.[1] In terms of physiology, dysphagia can be classified based on the transport of an ingested bolus. The transport depends on the consistency and size of the bolus, the caliber of the lumen, the integrity of peristaltic contraction, and whether there is deglutitive inhibition of both the upper and lower esophageal sphincter (LES). Structural dysphagia is caused by an oversized bolus or a narrow lumen; motor dysphagia is secondary to abnormalities of peristalsis or impaired deglutitive inhibition

Grant Support: None.

Conflict of Interest: None of the authors declared financial conflict of interest.

Center for Interventional Endoscopy, Florida Hospital Institute for Minimally Invasive Therapy, 601 E. Rollins Street, Orlando, FL 32803, USA

* Corresponding author. Institute for Surgical Advancement, Florida Hospital, 2415 North Orange Avenue, Suite 401, Orlando, FL 32804.

E-mail address: steve.eubanks.MD@flhosp.org

Surg Clin N Am 95 (2015) 483–489

Abbreviations	
CT	Computed tomography
EGD	Esophagogastroduodenoscopy
EUS	Endoscopic ultrasound
HRM	High-resolution manometry
LES	Lower esophageal sphincter

of the sphincters. The most important initial step in assessing dysphagia is to determine whether it is oropharyngeal or esophageal in origin, because their potential causes and subsequent investigation and management can differ greatly. Patients with oropharyngeal dysphagia present with symptoms of cough after swallowing and nasopharyngeal regurgitation.[1] It is seen commonly in patients with a history of head and neck surgery or radiation treatment, stroke, and other neurologic conditions, such as Parkinson's disease and motor neuron disease. This article provides an outline for approaching patients with esophageal dysphagia in terms of etiologies and clinical evaluation. The article discusses initially the physiology of esophageal swallowing, followed by pathophysiology and clinical evaluation of patients with various etiologies of esophageal dysphagia.

PHYSIOLOGY OF ESOPHAGEAL SWALLOWING

Swallowing begins with a voluntary (oral) phase that includes preparation during which food is masticated and mixed with saliva. Once the food is transferred to the esophagus through a complex physiologic transfer and relaxation of the upper esophageal sphincter, peristaltic contractions propel the food through the esophagus. The LES relaxes as the food enters the esophagus and remains relaxed until the peristaltic contraction has delivered the bolus into the stomach.[2] Peristaltic contractions elicited in response to a swallow are called primary peristalsis and involve sequenced inhibition followed by contraction of the musculature along the entire length of the esophagus. Local distention of the esophagus anywhere along its length activates secondary peristalsis that begins at the point of distention and proceeds distally. Tertiary esophageal contractions are nonperistaltic, disordered esophageal contractions. The distal esophagus and LES are composed of smooth muscle and are controlled by excitatory and inhibitory neurons within the esophageal myenteric plexus.[2] Peristalsis results from the patterned activation of inhibitory followed by excitatory ganglionic neurons, with progressive dominance of the inhibitory neurons distally. The function of the LES is supplemented by the right diaphragmatic crus, which acts as an external sphincter during inspiration, cough, or abdominal straining.[2]

PATHOPHYSIOLOGY AND ETIOLOGIES OF ESOPHAGEAL DYSPHAGIA

Solid food esophageal dysphagia becomes apparent when the esophageal lumen is narrowed to less than 13 mm; the normal diameter of the lumen varies from 2 to 3 cm. However, dysphagia can occur even with larger diameters when patients have motility disorders. The most common structural causes of dysphagia are Schatzki's rings, eosinophilic esophagitis, and peptic strictures. Disorders of motility could be secondary to abnormalities of peristalsis and/or deglutitive inhibition. In general, the etiologies of esophageal dysphagia can be divided broadly into either mechanical or dysmotility (**Box 1**). However, in a number of conditions, dysphagia could be mediated by both mechanical and dysmotility mechanisms.

Box 1
Etiologies of esophageal dysphagia

Mechanical causes

Benign strictures

- Peptic stricture
- Schatzki's ring
- Esophageal webs
- Anastomotic stricture
- Eosinophilic esophagitis
- Post fundoplication
- Radiation-induced strictures
- Postendoscopic mucosal resection
- Extrinsic compression from vascular compression (dysphagia lusorio)
- Extrinsic compression from benign lymph nodes or enlarged left atrium

Malignant strictures

- Esophageal adenocarcinoma
- Squamous cell cancer
- Extrinsic compression from malignant lymph nodes

Dysmotility

- Achalasia
- Hypotensive peristalsis
- Hypertensive peristalsis
- Nutcracker esophagus
- Diffuse esophageal spasm
- Functional obstruction

CLINICAL ASSESSMENT

The history and clinical assessment give clues to the etiologies of dysphagia and the evaluation required. Dysphagia to the type of food provides clues to the etiologies of dysphagia. Intermittent dysphagia that occurs only with solid food implies structural dysphagia, whereas constant dysphagia with both liquids and solids strongly suggests a motor abnormality.[2] Dysphagia that is progressive over the course of weeks to months raises concern for neoplasia. Episodic dysphagia to solids that is unchanged over years indicates a benign disease process such as a Schatzki's ring or eosinophilic esophagitis. Food impaction with a prolonged inability to pass an ingested bolus even with ingestion of liquid is typical of a structural dysphagia. Chest pain frequently accompanies dysphagia whether it is related to motor disorders, structural disorders, or reflux disease. A prolonged history of heartburn preceding the onset of dysphagia is suggestive of peptic stricture and, less commonly, esophageal adenocarcinoma. A history of head and neck surgery, ingestion of caustic agents or pills, previous radiation or chemotherapy, or associated mucocutaneous diseases may help to isolate the cause of dysphagia. With accompanying odynophagia, which usually is indicative of ulceration, infectious, or pill-induced esophagitis should be suspected. A strong history of allergy increases concerns for eosinophilic esophagitis.

CLINICAL INVESTIGATIONS

The initial clinical investigations depends on the suspected etiology. If mechanical causes, such as an obstructing mass lesion or stricture, are suspected, upper endoscopy is the initial investigation of choice. In contrast, if motility disorders such as achalasia are suspected, high-resolution manometry is the initial investigation. Radiographic evaluation with a barium swallow remains a useful investigation in some situations when upper endoscopy evaluation is normal.

Barium Swallow

The sensitivity of barium radiography for detecting esophageal strictures is greater than that of endoscopy, particularly for esophageal webs and rings, and remains the best initial evaluation strategy for dysphagia. The advantages are that it is noninvasive, can be done in patients who are poor candidates for endoscopic evaluation, and provides a good functional assessment of the esophagus. Barium swallow may also demonstrate anatomic abnormalities such as a stricture and Schatzki's ring.[3] The major drawback is that it is usually followed by endoscopic evaluation. A timed barium swallow is, however, used to follow up on treatment after achalasia as the height of the barium column at 1 minute after contrast ingestion 6 months after treatment was found to correlate with symptom scores.[3]

Upper Endoscopy

Upper esophagogastroduodenoscopy (EGD) is the first-choice investigation in patients with dysphagia, particularly with mechanical etiologies for dysphagia. It can diagnose intraluminal tumors, strictures and inflammatory disorders such as reflux disease, eosinophilic esophagitis, and pill-induced ulceration. In a systematic review of endoscopic findings in eosinophilic esophagitis, esophageal rings accounted for 44%; strictures, 21%; narrow-caliber esophagus, 9%; linear furrows, 48%; white plaques or exudates, 27%; pallor or decreased vasculature, 41%; and erosive esophagitis, 17%.[4] The endoscopic examination was normal in 17% of cases of eosinophilic esophagitis.[4] In patients who present for routine endoscopy for any indication, the prevalence of eosinophilic esophagitis is 6.5%, and in those undergoing an EGD for dysphagia, the prevalence is 10% to 15%.[5] In addition to the ability to take mucosal biopsies, EGD also has the opportunity of therapeutic potential with dilatation, which is useful for esophageal web, peptic stricture, anastomotic stricture, radiation-related stricture, and Schatzki's ring. In addition, it is a useful adjunct in the evaluation of underlying motility disorder. It may show the presence of a dilated esophagus, sigmoid esophagus with lack of contractions, and a tight LES, suggesting achalasia. Also, in evaluation of patients with achalasia, EGD is always performed to rule out pseudoachalasia secondary to tumors of the gastroesophageal junction and gastric cardia. Also, in achalasia patients who are unfit for surgical treatment, pneumatic balloon dilatation and botulinum toxin injection may offer alternative treatment. Recently, per oral endoscopic myotomy offers an exciting option in patients with achalasia.[6]

Manometry

Manometry is the most sensitive currently available technique to diagnose esophageal motility disorders.[7] High-resolution esophageal manometry (HRM) is a revolutionary step beyond conventional manometry, the traditional method of assessing esophageal motility. HRM has been developed with up to 36 recording points.[8] This enables pressure measurements of 1 cm or less apart along the entire esophagus. In HRM, the distal end of the catheter is passed into the gastric compartment below the LES and the catheter can provide recording from the stomach through the esophagus into the oropharynx.[8] During an HRM study, plots are generated, also known as "Clouse" plots. These plots are presented as a color spectrum on a plot of esophageal position (y-axis) against time (x-axis) produces a pressure topograph of swallowing generated by computer software during 10 wet (5 mL water) swallows.[8] HRM helps in the diagnosis of specific motility disorders; for example, the manometric finding of aperistalsis and incomplete LES relaxation without evidence of a mechanical obstruction solidifies the diagnosis of achalasia in the appropriate setting.[9]

Diagnostic Algorithm

In patients presenting with dysphagia, the initial evaluation includes EGD to rule out important etiologies such as cancer and stricture. In addition, evaluation for eosinophilic esophagitis needs to be performed with biopsies of the esophagus. Barium swallow evaluation can be performed in elderly patients who are not candidates for EGD. In patients with normal EGD and biopsies with dysphagia, HRM is required for evaluation.

Esophageal Cancer

The possibility of the cause for dysphagia being cancer of the esophagus is the greatest concern in the majority of patients who present with difficulty swallowing. In the United States, 18,000 people were diagnosed with esophageal cancer in 2014 and 15,000 patients died owing to esophageal cancer in the United States in 2014. The most common symptoms for patients who present with esophageal cancer are dysphagia (74%) and weight loss (57.3%).[10] The evaluation of the patient who is suspected or confirmed of having esophageal cancer can involve the following studies:

- Upper endoscopy
- Endoscopic biopsy
- Barium esophagram
- CT
- Endoscopic ultrasound (EUS)
- Bone scan
- Positron emission tomography

The patient with esophageal cancer presenting with dysphagia and weight loss usually describes difficulty swallowing solids, but often retains the ability to swallow liquids until the tumor is very advanced. The weight loss in esophageal cancer patients often exceeds what would be expected from the degree of dysphagia. Upper endoscopy is often the initial procedure or study performed in this patient population. Endoscopic evaluation allows direct visualization and simultaneous acquisition of tissue samples when indicated. The pattern of cell type of esophageal cancer is changing. In 2000, pathologic evaluation of esophageal cancers revealed squamous cell carcinoma in approximately 52% of patients and adenocarcinoma in 42% of patients.[10] Currently, The National Cancer Institute describes more than 50% of esophageal cancers as adenocarcinoma, primarily arising from Barrett's esophagus, and fewer than one-half of cancers as squamous cell carcinoma. The remaining tumors are usually sarcomas or small cell cancers. Benign gastrointestinal tumors such as gastrointestinal stromal tumors can be found within the esophagus. Endoscopy with biopsy is highly sensitive and specific for the diagnosis of esophageal cancer.

Box 2
Percentage of esophageal cancer patients by stage at time of diagnosis

Stage 1: 13.3%

Stage 2: 34.7%

Stage 3: 35.7%

Stage 4: 12.3%

Staging of esophageal cancer after establishing tissue diagnosis is necessary for planning treatment options and strategies. CT is used to evaluate the mass and involvement of surrounding structures. Additionally, CT can be very helpful in identifying metastatic tumors. EUS is being used with increasing frequency owing to the ability of this technology to define clearly the layers of the esophageal wall involved with the tumor. EUS is also highly sensitive in identifying adjacent nodal metastases and can guide needle biopsies of nodes suspected of containing metastatic disease. Positron emission tomography is used frequently to evaluate the patient for local and distant metastatic disease. Less frequently, nuclear medicine bone scans are used to evaluate the patient for bone metastases.

Esophageal cancer can be a highly lethal disease and the overall disease-free survival at 1 year after diagnosis is only 43%. Most patients are diagnosed with stage 2 (34.7%) or stage 3 (35.7%) disease (**Box 2**).[10]

SUMMARY

Patients frequently present to a physician with complaints of difficulty swallowing. The approach to evaluating systematically these problems can be challenging for those who do not manage this type of patient regularly. The potential for life-threatening malignancies is present and makes this evaluation a priority. Numerous excellent tools are available to aid with the determination of the cause of dysphagia and assist with the formulation of a logical treatment algorithm.

REFERENCES

1. Kuo P, Holloway RH, Nguyen NQ. Current and future techniques in the evaluation of dysphagia. J Gastroenterol Hepatol 2012;27(5):873–81.
2. Patel D, Vaezi MF. Normal esophageal physiology and laryngopharyngeal reflux. Otolaryngol Clin North Am 2013;46(6):1023–41.
3. Andersson M, Lundell L, Kostic S, et al. Evaluation of the response to treatment in patients with idiopathic achalasia by the timed barium esophagogram: results from a randomized clinical trial. Dis Esophagus 2009;22:264–73.
4. Kim HP, Vance RB, Shaheen NJ, et al. The prevalence and diagnostic utility of endoscopic features of eosinophilic esophagitis: a meta-analysis. Clin Gastroenterol Hepatol 2012;10(9):988–96.
5. Peery AF, Cao H, Dominik R, et al. Variable reliability of endoscopic findings with white-light and narrow-band imaging for patients with suspected eosinophilic esophagitis. Clin Gastroenterol Hepatol 2011;9:475–80.
6. Familiari P, Gigante G, Marchese M, et al. Peroral endoscopic myotomy for esophageal achalasia: outcomes of the first 100 patients with short-term follow-up. Ann Surg 2014. [Epub ahead of print].

7. Bogte A, Bredenoord AJ, Oors J, et al. Reproducibility of esophageal high-resolution manometry. Neurogastroenterol Motil 2011;23:e271–6.
8. Rice TW, Shay SS. A primer of high-resolution esophageal manometry. Semin Thorac Cardiovasc Surg 2011;23(3):181–90.
9. Vaezi MF, Pandolfino JE, Vela MF. ACG clinical guideline: diagnosis and management of achalasia. Am J Gastroenterol 2013;108(8):1238–49.
10. Daly JM, Fry WA, Little AG, et al. Esophageal cancer: results of an ACS patient care survey. J Am Coll Surg 2000;190(5):562–72.

Benign Esophageal Tumors

Cindy Ha, MD[a], James Regan, MD[a], Ibrahim Bulent Cetindag, MD[a],
Aman Ali, MD[b], John D. Mellinger, MD[a],*

KEYWORDS

- Leiomyoma • Gastrointestinal stromal tumor • Mediastinal cyst

KEY POINTS

- Endoscopic evaluation including endoscopic ultrasonography is foundational to the evaluation of benign and indeterminate esophageal pathology.
- Leiomyomas have distinctive distributions, behavior, and entailed therapeutic significance in pediatric patients.
- Immunohistochemical analysis is an important adjunctive diagnostic tool in distinguishing noncarcinomatous tumors of the esophagus.
- Symptomatic lesions and those with rapid change in size dictate surgical management.
- Endoscopic, thoracoscopic, and laparoscopic techniques including enucleation are widely used in the management of benign tumors of the esophagus.

INTRODUCTION

Unlike esophageal carcinoma, benign esophageal tumors and cysts are rare. Multiple autopsy series have been performed in the past, and although the specific results vary, the overall incidence is less than 1%. In addition, benign tumors account for less than 5% of all surgically resected esophageal tumors.[1] Nevertheless, the past century has shown an increasing trend in the incidence of these lesions, most likely a reflection of improving diagnostic methods,[2] and continued advancements in the understanding of their natural history and management. Benign esophageal tumors are often asymptomatic and typically require only close surveillance. If surgery is indicated because of symptoms or diagnostic uncertainty, many of these tumors can be successfully resected with excellent long-term outcomes. Because these lesions are rare, the general or gastrointestinal (GI) surgeon should have a strong foundation in their diagnosis and treatment.

[a] Department of Surgery, Division of General Surgery at SIU, Southern Illinois University School of Medicine, 701 North First Street, Springfield, IL 62794, USA; [b] Department of Internal Medicine, Division of Gastroenterology, Southern Illinois University School of Medicine, 701 North First Street, Springfield, IL 62794, USA
* Corresponding author. PO Box 19638, 701 North First Street, Springfield, IL 62794.
E-mail address: jmellinger@siumed.edu

Surg Clin N Am 95 (2015) 491–514
http://dx.doi.org/10.1016/j.suc.2015.02.005   surgical.theclinics.com

HISTORY

The first documented record of a benign esophageal tumor was in 1559 by Sussius. The tumor was discovered on autopsy, located in the distal esophagus, and has been cited as a leiomyoma, although histologic confirmation is lacking.[3] In 1763, Dallas-Monro performed one of the first treatments of a benign esophageal tumor when he excised a pedunculated esophageal mass using a snare from a 64-year-old man who had regurgitated the mass into his mouth. The first successful surgical treatment of a benign esophageal tumor is generally credited to Sauerbach, who performed a partial esophagectomy with esophagogastrostomy in 1932 for a myoma, most likely a leiomyoma. One year later, Oshawa performed the first open enucleation of an esophageal leiomyoma, and in 1937, Churchill performed the first open enucleation of a benign esophageal tumor in the United States for what was initially described as a neurofibroma but later reclassified as a leiomyoma.

According to Storey and Adams[4] in their case report and review of leiomyoma of the esophagus, only 16 documented surgical cases were found up until 1948, but between then and time of their publication in 1956, they found an additional 94 cases described, including 4 cases of their own. Since then, there have been many more recorded surgeries for benign esophageal tumors, and within the past 2 decades, there has been a shift toward minimally invasive approaches, specifically via thoracoscopy and endoscopy.

INCIDENCE

Several autopsy series and medical literature reviews have been performed in the past, searching for the true incidence of benign esophageal neoplasms. In 1932, Patterson[5] reported a total of 62 benign esophageal tumors during a 215-year period from 1717 to 1932. In 1944, Moersch[6] found 44 benign tumors and cysts in 7459 autopsy examinations, for an incidence of 0.59%. Plachta[7] in 1962 reviewed 19,982 postmortem examinations and found a total of 505 esophageal neoplasms, 90 of which were benign, resulting in an overall incidence of 0.45% with approximately 18% of all esophageal tumors being benign. In 1968, Attah and Hajdu[8] found 26 benign tumors among 15,454 autopsies during a 30-year period, for an incidence of 0.16%. Allowing for some variation among these studies, the overall incidence is cumulatively documented as less than 1%.[1] By way of comparison, malignant esophageal carcinoma is approximately 50 times more common.[9] The mean age of presentation for benign lesions is between the third and fifth decade of life, much younger than the mean age of presentation for esophageal carcinoma, and studies suggest a slight male predominance with an average ratio of 2:1.[1]

Unlike other benign tumors, esophageal duplications and cysts are more common in children. Accordingly, although such lesions are estimated to comprise only 0.5% to 3.3% of all benign esophageal masses in adults, they account for approximately 12% of all mediastinal tumors in the pediatric population. Between 25% and 35% of all esophageal duplications first become manifest in adults, and of these, most present in adults younger than 50 years.[10]

CLINICAL FEATURES

Benign esophageal tumors are generally slow-growing masses, and they may remain stable without any change in size for many years. At least 50% of benign esophageal masses are asymptomatic,[7] and they are frequently diagnosed incidentally on imaging or endoscopy performed for other reasons.[2] Choong and Meyers[1] broadly categorized the clinical presentations of benign esophageal neoplasms into 5 groups: asymptomatic, obstruction from intraluminal growth, compression of adjacent tissue by extraluminal tumor, regurgitation of a pedunculated tumor, and ulceration with bleeding.

The most common presenting symptom is dysphagia, and the degree of severity varies between patients. Because of the compliance of the esophagus, symptoms often occur late in the disease process as the lesions grow enough to cause luminal obstruction or compression. Typically, a size of 5 cm or more correlates with the likelihood of such symptoms developing.

The next most common symptoms are pain, usually retrosternal or epigastric in location, and pyrosis. Obstructive symptoms more commonly occur with intraluminal tumors,[1] and rarely, these tumors can present with ulceration,[11] bleeding, or regurgitation. Circumferential or annular involvement has been described, causing luminal narrowing and obstruction,[11] but this is an uncommon presentation.[1]

Respiratory symptoms may occur as well. Storey and Adams[4] found that 10 of the 110 reviewed patients presented with predominately respiratory symptoms, which were thought to be the result of tracheal or bronchial compression by the tumor. Presenting respiratory complaints are more common in the pediatric population.

In contrast to patients with malignant esophageal carcinomas, patients with benign tumors often present with multiple symptoms of long duration. Seremetis and colleagues[12] in their analysis of 838 cases of esophageal leiomyoma found that 30% of symptomatic patients reported a symptom duration of more than 5 years; another 30%, 2 to 5 years; and the remaining 40%, an average of 11 months.

DIAGNOSIS

Frequently, the diagnosis of a benign esophageal tumor or cyst is made incidentally on imaging or endoscopy performed for other indications. A plain chest radiograph may reveal a posterior and/or middle mediastinal, paraesophageal mass. However, the sensitivity and specificity of a plain radiograph is low, and the mass must reach a significant size before it becomes apparent on a chest radiograph.[4]

A contrast swallow study is most likely the best initial test to obtain in the evaluation of a symptomatic patient. Esophagography is usually performed in a biphasic manner with upright double-contrast views with high-density barium suspension and prone single-contrast views with low-density barium suspension. The former allows for evaluation of the mucosa, and the latter facilitates evaluation of any areas of luminal narrowing. Benign esophageal tumors usually are manifest as mobile lesions with smooth contours. Occasionally, altered peristalsis is seen with intraluminal tumors.[13]

Computed tomography (CT) of the chest is helpful in the evaluation of extraesophageal tumors and exclusion of other mediastinal masses that could lead to similar clinical presentations. The relationships between the esophageal tumor and surrounding tissues are also better defined with CT, which may be invaluable in preoperative planning when indicated by symptoms or diagnostic uncertainty.[14]

Endoscopy and endoscopic ultrasound (EUS) imaging are mandatory in the evaluation of a symptomatic esophageal tumor. In addition to excluding malignant carcinomas, endoscopy allows for visualization of the mucosa and biopsy of intraluminal and submucosal tumors. Although intramural tumors are not visualized on endoscopy, it is essential to confirm an intact mucosa if an intramural tumor is suspected. EUS imaging provides visualization of the esophageal layers and defines which layers are involved with the tumor, which is invaluable in perioperative planning and surveillance. In addition, EUS imaging can reveal certain unique sonographic characteristics that can aid in the diagnosis of the tumor. Lack of enlarged lymph nodes, smaller size, homogeneous echo pattern, and smooth borders favor a benign lesion on EUS imaging.[2] EUS imaging also allows needle biopsy of these lesions and any associated pathology including lymph nodes, which is more often diagnostic than simple endoluminal biopsy for lesions beyond the confines of the mucosa.[14]

MANAGEMENT

In the past, surgical resection was recommended for most esophageal neoplasms, including benign ones. However, recent advances have shown that most benign esophageal tumors are slow growing,[15] and with the exception of esophageal gastrointestinal stromal tumors (GISTs) and adenomas, malignant transformation is rare.[16] Accordingly, many of these lesions can be followed with serial studies if asymptomatic.[14] Historically, if surgery was indicated, an open approach was advocated. However, in the past 2 decades there has been an increasing shift toward minimally invasive techniques with endoscopic, laparoscopic, or thoracoscopic resections.[17] These methods are discussed in greater detail as they apply to each individual type of lesion in the following sections.

CLASSIFICATION

Benign esophageal tumors can be classified in several ways, and various classification schemes have been proposed in the past based on esophageal layer of origin, histologic cell type, and location as well as clinical appearance. Many of the histologic tumor types can occur in multiple and varying layers of the wall. Rice[2] described the 5 discrete esophageal layers seen on EUS imaging, specifically the superficial mucosa, deep mucosa, submucosa, muscularis propria, and paraesophageal tissue. As a way of characterizing layer of origin and relationship to adjacent structures, EUS imaging has become a practically essential tool in the diagnosis and characterization of these benign esophageal tumors. Having weighed all these variables, classification by location is probably the most practical method, primarily because it dictates the treatment strategy. A summary of a location-based classification scheme is given in **Box 1**.

Box 1
Classification of benign esophageal tumors

Intramural

Leiomyoma

Gastrointestinal stromal tumor

Schwannoma

Intraluminal

Epithelial polyps (adenomatous and inflammatory)

Lipomatous polyps

Fibrovascular polyps

Papilloma

Hemangioma

Granular cell tumor

Extraesophageal

Duplications and cysts

INTRAMURAL TUMORS
Leiomyoma

Leiomyoma is a benign smooth muscle tumor found throughout the GI tract, and although only 10% of all GI leiomyomas are located in the esophagus,[11] they are the most common benign esophageal masses, accounting for approximately two-thirds of all benign esophageal tumors.[14] Morgagni provided the first description of a GI leiomyoma in 1761.[4]

Many autopsy reviews have been performed to assess the incidence of benign esophageal tumors as documented earlier, and in regards to leiomyomas specifically, the general incidence ranges from 0.006% to 0.1%.[9] The incidence of clinically significant leiomyomas is much lower, as at least half of these lesions are asymptomatic and diagnosed incidentally. There has been an increase in incidence during the past few decades because of improved and more widespread use of endoscopy.[2]

Leiomyomas can arise from smooth muscle in the muscularis propria or muscularis mucosae, but the latter is much less commonly encountered, presenting as an intraluminal polypoid lesion in 7% of documented cases based on a review by Hatch and colleagues.[15] Most lesions arise from the muscularis propria, with 80% being found in intramural and 7% in extraesophageal positions. Most are solitary and involve a localized area of the esophageal wall. Less than 2.4% of documented cases reported multiple tumors, and 10% to 13% were annular with circumferential involvement.[14]

Anatomically, leiomyoma is found most often in the middle and distal thirds of the esophagus, which reflects the increasing proportion of smooth muscle as opposed to striated muscle within the esophageal wall. In their review of 838 cases, Seremetis and colleagues[12] found that 56% were found in the distal third, 33% in the middle third, and 11% in the upper third. Furthermore, approximately 6.8% also involved the gastroesophageal junction and/or proximal stomach.

These benign esophageal smooth muscle tumors can occur at any age, but more than 80% are found between the second and sixth decades, with the peak time of presentation between ages 30 and 50 years. It is also more commonly seen in adult men, with an overall 2:1 male to female ratio.[14] The natural history of the esophageal leiomyoma reflects an overall slow, indolent progression, and malignant transformation is extremely rare. There have only been 4 documented cases in the past of progression to leiomyosarcoma, and each case was heralded by a preceding change in size.[12,14,15]

Esophageal leiomyoma has rarely been found in the pediatric population.[11] In contradistinction to adults, leiomyomas in the pediatric population are twice as common in girls. Furthermore, 91% of cases show multiple tumors and/or diffuse involvement, with 35% involving the entire length of the esophagus. Individuals with this more diffuse form of involvement typically require more aggressive surgical management strategies, as outlined further in the discussion.[18]

Leiomyoma has been associated with a variety of other benign esophageal conditions such as achalasia, other dysmotility disorders, esophageal diverticulum, and gastroesophageal reflux. The most commonly associated condition is hiatal hernia, found in 4.5% to 23% of patients with leiomyoma.[14]

In the past, leiomyoma was considered apart of a spectrum of mesenchymal tumors, which also included GISTs. However, studies have shown that these 2 tumors are distinct entities in regards to ultrastructure, histology, and genetic and immunohistochemical markers.[16,19]

In regards to gross appearance, leiomyomas are firm, rubbery, well-encapsulated masses with smooth surfaces. They range from white, gray, tan, or yellow in color and often have a whorled appearance on cut section.[12] Although shapes vary, smaller ones tend to be oval or spherical and larger ones, horseshoe or dumbbell-like in shape. Most are small in size as well, likely reflecting the more slow-growing natural history, with approximately 50% less than 5 cm and 93% less than 15 cm.[14] On histologic examination, leiomyomas are characteristically composed of uniform spindle cells arranged in fascicles or whorls with eosinophilic cytoplasm and surrounding hypovascular connective tissue, few to no mitotic figures, bland cigar-ended nuclei, minimal to no cellular atypia, and overall hypocellularity.[12,14,16]

The description of GISTs in regards to gross, histologic, and immunohistochemical characteristics are discussed in more detail in a separate section, but in brief comparison for the sake of review of leiomyomas, GISTs grossly appear soft with fish flesh–like consistency and histologically appear overall basophilic with high cellularity and increased mitotic figures and cellular atypia. The histologic features in turn reflect the higher malignant potential and more aggressive nature of GISTs vis-à-vis leiomyomas.[16,19]

Although gross appearance and histology can help differentiate leiomyoma from GIST, the definitive foundation for distinguishing between these 2 entities lies in 4 immunohistochemical markers. Leiomyoma is typically positive for desmin and smooth muscle antigen (SMA) and negative for CD117 and CD34. By way of contrast, GISTs are uniformly positive for CD117 and almost uniformly positive for CD34, and usually negative for desmin and SMA. The most specific of these markers is CD117, which corresponds to the c-kit protein.[16]

These histopathologic and immunohistochemical characteristics are essential to differentiate leiomyoma from GIST, which in turn becomes important in defining management and surveillance strategies.

Approximately 50% of leiomyomas are asymptomatic and incidentally diagnosed, which likely reflects the smaller average size of these masses. Although not absolute, the presence of symptoms seems to trend directly with the increase in size, with symptoms usually presenting once the leiomyoma reaches a dimension of 5 cm.[1] Overall, symptoms tend to be vague and nonspecific in nature and develop over a longer duration than in the case of malignant esophageal lesions. Seremetis and colleagues[12] found that 30% of reviewed cases reported symptoms for more than 5 years and another 30% for 2 to 5 years; of the remaining 40%, the average length of symptom duration was 11 months. In addition, most present with multiple symptoms rather than 1 predominant one.[3]

The most common initial symptoms are dysphagia and/or chest pain. The pain is located usually in the epigastrium and/or retrosternal region and described as a pressurelike pain. The level of the dysphagia and pain vary widely, but in general, these symptoms are less severe and present less acutely compared with esophageal carcinomas.[15] Other frequently encountered symptoms include pyrosis, mild and gradual weight loss (rarely more than 20 lb [9.1 kg]), and nausea.[12] Respiratory symptoms such as dyspnea, recurrent respiratory infections, and cough can occur as well but are uncommon, occurring in approximately 10% of cases.[3] Hemorrhage and ulceration rarely occur with esophageal leiomyomas and constitute an indication for removal.[15]

In regards to the pediatric population, esophageal leiomyomas are more often symptomatic in contrast to adults. In addition, although dysphagia is still the most common presenting symptom in children, unlike in adults, the second most common symptom in pediatric patients is dyspnea, with respiratory symptoms in general being more often encountered.[18]

It is important to distinguish leiomyoma from leiomyomatosis, a benign condition characterized by diffuse smooth muscle proliferation. In leiomyomatosis, there is typically involvement of muscularis propria and muscularis mucosae along the entire length of the esophagus. Most patients, approximately 95%, are symptomatic, and it is often associated with Alport syndrome or other smooth muscle hypertrophy disorders affecting multiple organs.[20]

Although not particularly sensitive or specific, plain chest radiographs are often the first diagnostic modalities to suggest the presence of leiomyoma, leading to its incidental diagnosis. These lesions can be missed if they are small, but if large enough, an esophageal leiomyoma may appear as a smooth, round hyperdense mass in the posterior mediastinum.[3]

Because of its high sensitivity and noninvasive nature, barium swallow study is the best initial diagnostic test. Leiomyoma classically is seen as a smooth, well-defined filling defect with approximately half of the submucosal mass protruding into the lumen as a convex mass and the other half within the esophageal wall. It is often half-moon or crescent shaped and characteristically forms right or slight obtuse angles with the adjacent esophageal wall when seen on lateral view. The mass is usually mobile and nonobstructing, rarely presenting with proximal esophageal dilatation. Over the mass itself, flattened mucosal folds are classically described.[14]

In addition to barium swallow, endoscopic evaluation is mandatory (**Fig. 1**). Although leiomyomas, in the absence of ulceration, would be characterized by normal overlying mucosa and as such would not be well visualized by endoscopy, it is necessary to rule out mucosal abnormalities, which would point toward another cause. The presence and location of the tumor should also be identified.[12] The 4 characteristic endoscopic findings of leiomyoma according to Postlethwait are (1) intact, normal overlying mucosa; (2) tumor projecting into the lumen at varying degrees; (3) tumor mobility with overlying mucosa sliding easily over the mass itself; and (4) possible luminal narrowing but rarely any findings of stenosis or obstruction.[21]

If leiomyoma is suspected, blind endoscopic biopsy is not recommended as it increases the risk for perioperative complications and rarely obtains adequate tissue for diagnosis because of the submucosal location. In regards to the former, endoscopic biopsies increase the risk for adhesions to the mucosa during healing and as a result may complicate surgical enucleation, increasing the risk for violation of the mucosa at the time of resection via that technique.[22]

EUS imaging is emerging as an essential test in the diagnosis and management of leiomyoma. Although esophagoscopy is limited to partial mucosal visualization, EUS imaging allows evaluation of all esophageal layers. As described by Rice[2] and

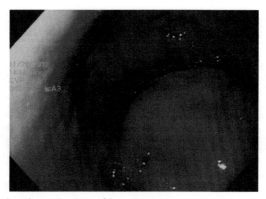

Fig. 1. Endoluminal endoscopic view of leiomyoma.

mentioned earlier, there are 5 alternating hyperechoic and hypoechoic layers visualized on EUS imaging, which in turn represent the mucosal, deep mucosal, submucosal, muscularis propria, and surrounding connective tissue layers, respectively. In the evaluation of an esophageal mass, EUS imaging provides the ability to determine the layer of origin as well as the ability to evaluate for other features such as size, borders, regional lymphadenopathy, echoic pattern, and local invasion.

On EUS imaging, leiomyoma appears as a well-circumscribed, homogenous, hypoechoic mass with smooth borders, arising from the third submucosal layer. There is no regional lymphadenopathy. Findings of size greater than 4 cm, irregular borders, invasion into other layers, and/or regional lymphadenopathy are atypical[14] and would require further workup to rule out malignancy, such as endoscopic biopsy,[22] fine-needle aspiration (FNA) via EUS imaging, and/or surgical enucleation or resection to rule out other causes.[14]

EUS-FNA may be used in conjunction with EUS imaging to obtain cytology and possibly more definitive diagnosis of leiomyoma (**Fig. 2**).[14] Cytology would allow for immunohistochemical analysis as well, which as described earlier, would help differentiate leiomyoma from GIST and leiomyosarcoma. Although EUS-FNA has not been proved more accurate than EUS imaging alone in terms of esophageal submucosal tumors specifically, it has been proved to improve diagnostic accuracy for similar gastric and duodenal tumors, and, accordingly, is worthy of consideration if more definitive diagnosis is needed.[23]

CT may also be performed to evaluate a possible esophageal leiomyoma with an estimated sensitivity of 91%. It is most helpful in evaluating for invasion, the presence of extrinsic compression, and anatomic relationships to nearby structures.[14] Leiomyoma classically appears as a smooth, well-demarcated, round or lobulated mass with homogenously low or isoattenuation. CT scanning does not typically differentiate cystic from solid masses and is therefore limited in its utility for evaluation of intramural pathology.[13]

The treatment of symptomatic leiomyoma is surgical enucleation, either via an open or a thoracoscopic approach (**Fig. 3**) or via laparoscopy for lesions in the distal esophagus or gastroesophageal junction area.[22] The management of asymptomatic leiomyoma, however, is more debatable as suggested by the natural history studies outlined earlier. In the past, the recommendation was to excise every esophageal leiomyoma diagnosed.[3,15] However, it has been demonstrated that leiomyoma rarely progresses to malignant leiomyosarcoma and often remains stable in size for years.[1]

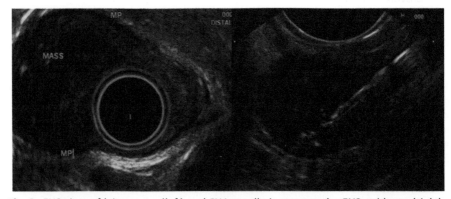

Fig. 2. EUS view of leiomyoma (*left*) and FNA needle in same under EUS guidance (*right*).

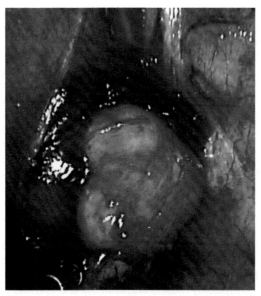

Fig. 3. Esophageal leiomyoma undergoing thoracoscopic enucleation. (*Courtesy of* Stephen R. Hazelrigg, MD, Department of Surgery, Southern Illinois University School of Medicine, IL.)

In general, the indications for surgery for leiomyoma is the presence of symptoms; size greater than 4 cm[14]; atypical findings on studies concerning for malignancy such as the presence of irregular borders, regional lymphadenopathy, heterogenous echoic pattern, or mucosal abnormalities; ulceration; and increase in size.[22] If the leiomyoma is small and asymptomatic, it may be followed with surveillance endoscopy and EUS imaging with or without chest CT every 6 to 12 months and perhaps at longer intervals if stability is demonstrated over time along with continuing asymptomatic clinical status.[14]

The technique for surgical removal of leiomyoma is enucleation via an open or a minimally invasive approach. In the past, thoracotomy or laparotomy was the standard approach.[9] The first documented thoracoscopic enucleation was by Everitt in 1992,[22] and since then, there has been a shift toward minimally invasive techniques. Multiple studies have been performed comparing open and minimally invasive approaches, and the overall mortality is not significantly different between the 2 approaches.[24–26] Minimally invasive techniques are associated with decreased postoperative respiratory complications, shorter hospital stays, and improved postoperative pain control and hence have become more standard as skills and instrumentation appropriate for such strategies have evolved.[25,26]

For the open technique, the approach depends on the location of the tumor. A right thoracotomy would be indicated to reach tumors of the upper two-thirds of the esophagus and left thoracotomy for those of the lower one-third and of intrathoracic location. For tumors of the intra-abdominal portion of the esophagus, including those involving the gastroesophageal junction, laparoscopy or laparotomy may be indicated. Intraoperative endoscopy and ultrasonography can be used to facilitate identification of the tumor and also to evaluate for possible intraoperative mucosal injury.[17]

The specific techniques in regards to right or left thoracoscopy or laparoscopy are generally the same with minimally invasive techniques. The placement of the trocars depends on the location of the lesion, and as in most minimally invasive strategies, the lesion should be in the base of a baseball diamond trocar configuration with the camera on the opposite corner of the diamond and working ports at the other angles of the same. Single lung ventilation is crucial for exposure of the mediastinum if a thoracoscopic approach is used.[25,26]

Regardless of open or minimally invasive technique, the key principles regarding the surgical enucleation of leiomyoma are largely the same. A longitudinal myotomy is created just over the tumor itself, taking care to stay over its apex, and after splitting the muscular coat, the tumor is visualized, often as a well-circumscribed, avascular mass. Blunt dissection is used to separate the tumor from the mucosa, often with the placement of a traction suture in the mass to facilitate the process, with the goal of avoiding violation of the mucosa itself.[22] This procedure can usually be accomplished without difficulty, noting that the risk of mucosal injury may be increased if preoperative endoscopic biopsy was performed.[17] If there are dense adhesions between the tumor and mucosa, possible malignancy must be considered as well, in which case frozen section may be indicated, recognizing that it may or may not be conclusive.[27]

After completing enucleation of the tumor, the presence of mucosal injuries can be evaluated with the use of intraoperative endoscopy and insufflation, and any injuries should be repaired with interrupted absorbable sutures.[17] Finally, it is recommended to reapproximate the myotomy muscle edges at the end to avoid possible postoperative mucosal bulging, diverticulum formation, and associated dysphagia and/or gastroesophageal reflux disease (GERD) symptoms.[9,17,22,24,25]

Variations of surgical enucleation include the balloon push-out method, a thoracoscopic approach with assistance of a balloon-mounted endoscope to promote intraluminal expulsion of the tumor from the esophageal wall,[14] and robotic-assisted thoracoscopic enucleation.[27,28]

Up to 10% of esophageal leiomyomas may require esophagectomy. In general, the indications for esophagectomy are size greater than 8 to 10 cm, annular morphology, multiple or diffuse involvement, extensive damage and/or ulceration to the mucosa, or presence of or suspicion for leiomyosarcoma.[12] Esophagectomy is more commonly required in the pediatric population because of the increased incidence of multiple tumors and diffuse esophageal involvement as detailed earlier.[18]

The mortality associated with open esophagectomy is 10.5% in adults[22] and up to 21% in children[18] and is primarily related to the risk of anastomotic leak and associated sepsis as well as pulmonary complications. The mortality of open enucleation is approximately 1.3%. There have been no reported deaths with patients treated with minimally invasive enucleation.[22]

Most patients treated with enucleation report complete resolution of their symptoms. According to a retrospective review by Jiang and colleagues[24] of 40 cases of thoracoscopic enucleation of leiomyoma, all patients had complete resolution of their symptoms at a mean follow-up of 27 months. In addition, there have been no documented cases of recurrence of leiomyoma after surgical removal. Postoperative complications are uncommon but include esophageal leak due to mucosal injury and GERD. The development of postoperative GERD is most likely due to a disturbance of esophageal motility or lower esophageal sphincter function and may require future fundoplication; however, it is overall uncommon and, as such, routine fundoplication with enucleation is not recommended.[17]

Endoscopic excision of leiomyoma is possible. This strategy may be especially appropriate for the occasional leiomyoma of muscularis mucosal origin with an intraluminal or polypoid growth pattern. In general, pedunculated lesions of this type are removed via endoscopic snare techniques. Endoscopic mucosal resection (EMR) has also become more popular in recent years for a variety of mucosal and submucosal pathologic conditions. As pertains to leiomyomas, submucosal saline injection followed by cap-fitted endoscopic snaring typical of EMR methodology has been described for more wide-based yet smaller lesions up to 2 cm in size. Ethanol injection also has been used as a tool for facilitating lesion necrosis and involution, yet the experience in the United States is limited.[9,14] Finally, endoscopic submucosal dissection (ESD) techniques continue to evolve and may become a more prevalent option for enucleation via an endoluminal approach in years to come, particularly again for lesions originating from the muscularis mucosa.

Gastrointestinal Stromal Tumor

The second most common esophageal mesenchymal tumor is the GIST. Even though these lesions have malignant potential, many behave in a benign manner, and these lesions are thought to be worthy of discussion for several reasons, including their similarities to other mesenchymal benign tumors, as well as the fact that GISTs must be distinguished from other lesions to make appropriate treatment decisions. Less than 5% of GISTs are found in the esophagus compared with 60% in the stomach and 30% in the small intestine.[19]

Based on the finding of shared expression of CD117 and CD34, GISTs are thought to arise from the interstitial cells of Cajal, also known as the GI pacemaker cells, and/or the intestinal mesenchymal precursor cells.

Most of these tumors present between the fifth and seventh decades of life. In a review of 17 esophageal GISTs by Miettinen and colleagues, the median age of presentation was 63 years, with a range from 49 to 75 years.[19] These tumors are rarely found before the age of 40 years, and the diagnosis of a GIST in a younger patient may suggest a lesion of particularly malignant potential. Like leiomyomas, approximately half are asymptomatic. Of the remaining, the most common presenting symptom is dysphagia followed by chest discomfort. Other less common symptoms include cough, gradual mild weight loss, and GI bleeding.

Similar to most other benign esophageal tumors, GISTs of the esophagus are most often located in the distal third and may extend to involve the gastroesophageal junction.[16,27] Sizes are widely variable. In a series by Miettinen of 17 esophageal GISTs, most were less than 10 cm, with a median size of 8 cm and range from 2.6 to 25 cm.[19]

The characteristic histologic findings include overall basophilic appearance with high cellularity and mild-to-no nuclear pleomorphism on hematoxylin-eosin staining. Like gastric GISTs, approximately 70% to 80% of esophageal GISTs are spindle cell tumors and the rest, predominately epithelioid tumors. The spindle cell form can present histologically with growth of tumors cells in solid sheets or in myxoid, pseudo-organoid, palisading, or perivascular collar patterns. Coagulation necrosis may be seen as well, but lymphatic or vascular or diffuse mucosal invasion is uncommon. Mitotic figures are more often found in GISTs than in leiomyomas, where they are quite rare. However, mitotic activity can still vary widely among GISTs and plays a key role in predicting malignant potential, as described in more detail later in discussion.[16]

As mentioned in the leiomyoma section, GISTs previously were classified alongside leiomyoma, schwannoma, and other mesenchymal tumors, but recent studies and discoveries have shown GISTs to be distinct from these other mesenchymal tumors. Although gross and histologic features may help differentiate GISTs from other similar tumors, the best method of distinction is immunohistochemical testing. The most reliable marker is the expression of c-kit protein, CD117, which is uniformly seen in GISTs. In addition, the vast majority also express CD34. In turn, GISTs are almost never positive for desmin, and most do not stain positive for α-smooth muscle actin

(SMA) either. Most studies show an approximately 20% to 40% frequency of SMA positivity in all GISTs throughout the GI tract, and the expression is usually partial and focal in comparison with the diffuse reactivity seen in leiomyomas.[16] Furthermore, GISTs are negative for S-100 as well in comparison with schwannomas.[19] These markers are invaluable in distinguishing these lesions and guiding decisions regarding management that are linked to underlying histology and the associated potential for future malignant behavior, which is significantly higher for GISTs.[16]

Because GISTs are also intramural esophageal tumors, the diagnostic workup is similar to that of leiomyoma. Typical workup includes a contrast swallow study, EGD, and EUS imaging, and findings are usually similar to leiomyoma, which makes distinguishing between the 2 tumors difficult based solely on such criteria.

Overall, approximately 70% of all GISTs are benign. In the past, these tumors were classified as benign or malignant based on mitotic activity and size, but studies have shown that prediction and classification of GISTs into those with benign versus malignant behavior can be challenging.[29] As a result, the National Institutes of Health (NIH) developed a classification scheme for GISTs in general, categorizing these tumors into 4 categories of risk for recurrence and metastasis, specifically very low risk, low risk, intermediate risk, and high risk, based on mitotic activity and size (**Table 1**).[30]

Although the NIH classification can provide some guidance in distinguishing low- and high-risk GISTs in regards to malignant potential, small size and/or low mitotic activity does not guarantee benign behavior. Other favorable prognostic factors include gastric location, low proliferation index, absence of infiltration to adjacent organs, DNA diploidy in G2 peak on flow cytometry, and possibly female gender and younger age.[19] In regards to esophageal GISTs in particular, mitotic index and size are not proven prognostic factors, possibly in part due to the low incidence.[31] Esophageal GISTs are more commonly aggressive and malignant histologically. Miettinen and colleagues reported in their series of 17 esophageal GISTs a mortality rate of 59% with a median survival of 27 months. One disease-associated death occurred in a patient with a mitotic rate less than 5 mitoses per 50 high-power field (HPF), again underlining the inconsistent relationship between malignant behavior and mitotic rate.[17]

Although it is important to differentiate GIST from leiomyoma for the reasons outlined, it is often difficult because the findings of the typical diagnostic studies of contrast swallow, EGD, and EUS imaging frequently overlap between the 2 entities. Occasionally, mucosal changes may be seen with GISTs in a manner less common with leiomyomas, which rarely are associated with such findings as mentioned previously. The appearance of ulceration, Barrett esophagus, and/or esophagitis accordingly calls for further investigation to rule out GIST as well as other possible malignant tumors such as carcinoma. However, mucosal changes are still uncommon.

Table 1 Risk classification for GIST tumors	
Classification	**Size and/or Mitotic Activity**
Very low risk	<2 cm and <5 mitoses/50 HPF
Low risk	2–5 cm and <5 mitoses/50 HPF
Intermediate risk	<5 cm and 6–10 mitoses/50 HPF 5–10 cm and <5 mitoses/50 HPF
High risk	>5 cm and >5 mitoses/50 HPF >10 cm and mitotic rate any size and >10 mitoses/50 HPF

Abbreviation: HPF, high-power field.

Consequently, the addition of a PET scan[29] and/or FNA via EUS imaging may provide further assistance in distinguishing between GISTs and leiomyomas.[31]

GISTs are PET-avid, especially malignant GISTs, in comparison with leiomyomas.[29] Furthermore, FNA may be performed under EUS guidance and provide adequate tissue for immunohistochemical testing for CD117, CD34, and other markers. Blum and colleagues[27] recommended addition of EUS-FNA for any intramural esophageal tumor larger than 2 cm, demonstrating positive growth on serial surveillance examination and/or manifesting increased PET scan activity.

Although initially small GISTs may be observed with serial examinations similar to leiomyoma, once the actual diagnosis of GIST has been made, the management changes and usually entails a combination of medical and surgical treatments, specifically with complete resection of the mass.[23]

The management of GISTs has significantly changed in recent years because of introduction of imatinib, a monoclonal antibody inhibiting the tyrosine-kinase c-kit protein. Imatinib use is indicated for unresectable, recurrent, or residual GISTs and, in turn, can be used as primary, adjuvant, or neoadjuvant treatment. Its addition has led to a significant increase in median survival of patients with advanced GIST from approximately 20 to 60 months. Adjuvant imatinib is recommended for most patients for 2 years, including those with residual disease after resection or larger primary tumors. Serial CT and/or PET scans can help track disease response, which may be manifest as a decrease in tumor attenuation more so than size and decrease in maximum standard uptake value on PET.[32]

Along with the use of imatinib, complete surgical excision is recommended whenever possible and is still associated with the best chance for survival. Although the standard of surgical treatment is complete excision,[23,27,32] the optimal extent of surgery with regards to margin sizes and approaches has not yet been well defined[23]; however, negative margins without lymphadenectomy is generally considered an adequate resection.[27] Enucleation may be performed via open or minimally invasive approaches for smaller tumors of low malignant potential.[23] In general, an open approach may be preferred in the setting of known preoperative diagnosis of GIST because of the poor integrity of the tumor and high frequency of adhesions to the mucosa or submucosa,[27] but personal surgical experience may also play a role in determining the approach in such settings.

For larger tumors, esophagectomy with gastric tube reconstruction is recommended. The specific size threshold for enucleation versus esophagectomy has also not been well established. Blum and colleagues[27] recommended esophagectomy for GISTs greater than 2 cm, whereas Lee and colleagues[23] reported safe excision via enculeation of tumors up to 5 cm in size. The concurrent findings of mucosal and/or muscular invasion, involvement of the gastroesophageal junction, and other features relating to risk of malignant behavior as outlined play a role in determining the best approach and extent of resection. The techniques of enucleation and esophagectomy otherwise are similar to those described for leiomyomas. In comparison with leiomyoma, it is frequently difficult to assess adequacy of the resection intraoperatively because of the occasional presence of adhesions to surrounding layers blurring anatomic planes and the unreliability of frozen section to assess adequate margins. The adequacy of resection can only be assessed with immunohistochemical staining, which determines the presence or absence of tumors cells along the excised borders.

In the past, esophageal GISTs have been associated with poor prognosis with high mortality and recurrence rates. Blum and colleagues[27] cited only a 14% 5-year survival rate, but the addition of imatinib has significantly changed the outcomes and prognoses. Shingare and colleagues[33] in a series of 7 patients, all treated with imatinib and 3 with surgical excision, found no disease progression or metastasis in all patients at the end of mean follow-up of 26 months. The availability of newer-generation tyrosine kinase inhibitors for patients not responding to imatinib, such as gefitinib, erlotinib, and sunitinib, offers hope for alternative therapies focused on underlying tumor biology with these lesions.

Schwannoma

Schwannoma is the least common esophageal mesenchymal tumor. In general, they are uncommonly found in the GI tract, and of these, most occur in the stomach.[33] Esophageal schwannoma is extremely rare, with less than 30 reported cases in the literature.[34]

These submucosal tumors arise from the Schwann cells of the neural plexus within the GI tract wall, and although they can occur at any age, they most commonly present during middle age, between 50 and 60 years.[35] In a literature review of 19 reported cases, Murase and colleagues[37] reported a median age of 54 years, with a range from 10 to 79 years. In addition, there is a mild female predominance, with reported male to female ratios ranging from 1:1.6 and 1:2.8.

Unlike other benign esophageal tumors, schwannomas are located most frequently in the upper esophagus, specifically the cervical and upper thoracic regions. Size varies widely, ranging from less than 0.5 cm to up to 15 to 16 cm. Similar to leiomyoma and GIST, schwannoma is often asymptomatic, and if symptomatic, the most common presenting symptoms are dysphagia and chest discomfort.[36]

Grossly, these tumors are yellow-white to tan and appear rubbery and/or firm with glistening, smooth surfaces. They may appear trabeculated without necrosis or hemorrhage on cut surface. Histologically, schwannomas feature peripheral lymphoid cuffs composed of lymphoid follicles, moderate cellularity, and broad bundles, interlacing fascicles, or whorls of elongated cells.[37] Additional histologic characteristics also include nuclear palisading, intermixing collagen fibers, nuclear pleomorphism with evenly distributed chromatin, and inflammatory cell infiltrates composed of plasma cells and lymphocytes. The presence of the distinctive peripheral lymphoid cuff ranges from complete to partial between tumors, and may be missed depending on sectioning, but when seen, is pathognomonic for schwannoma.[36,37]

The diagnostic workup for schwannoma is similar to that of leiomyoma and GIST, consisting of contrast swallow study, EGD, and EUS imaging. CT and PET scans can also be added for further details, as mentioned previously.[36] Schwannomas characteristically appear homogenous on postenhanced CT images.[34] However, the findings from these diagnostic tests for schwannoma usually overlap with those of other submucosal tumors, including GIST, and immunohistochemical testing is required for definitive diagnosis. Adding EUS-FNA or proceeding to surgical excision may provide adequate tissue for such testing, and schwannomas characteristically express S-100 protein as well as vimentin and glial fibrillary acidic protein. On the other hand, they are negative for CD117, CD34, desmin, and SMA, thus allowing for differentiation from GISTs and leiomyomas.[16,38,39]

The management of schwannomas is similar to that of leiomyomas. Smaller, asymptomatic ones may be observed with serial examinations.[38] Indications for excision include larger size (generally >2 cm), the presence of symptoms, and/or the findings of growth on serial examinations. Schwannomas less than 2 cm may be safely excised endoscopically.[36] Larger ones may be enucleated through thoracotomy or thoracoscopy.[34,35,39]

There is a malignant potential associated with schwannomas as well with 3 to 4 reported cases of malignant schwannoma in the literature. The malignancy criteria are histologic and based on mitotic activity, cellularity, nuclear atypia, and presence of tumor necrosis. Of these, mitotic rate is the most reliable. The presence of 5 or more mitotic figures per 50 HPF correlates most strongly with malignancy. In the setting of malignant disease, complete surgical excision is necessary, and although some studies suggest enucleation may be adequate for smaller tumors with intact mucosa and absent local invasion, the standard is still esophagectomy.[39]

Granular Cell Tumor

Granular cell tumors (GCTs), historically known as granular cell myoblastomas, were first described by Abrikossoff in the 1920s. They are soft-tissue neoplasms that have a neural origin located in the submucosa. The exact cell type that they originate from is thought to be a Schwann cell because of staining characteristics; however, there is still some debate.

GCTs are mostly benign, but it is reported that 1% to 2% of cases are malignant.[40] GCTs are found in many different tissues, with approximately 1% to 8% located in the GI tract and around one-third of these localized to the esophagus.[41–43] Most of these are found in the distal esophagus.

GCTs are usually asymptomatic and found incidentally during radiological evaluation or endoscopy. When symptomatic they tend to be larger.[44] GCTs present similar to leiomyomas. The most common symptom accordingly is dysphagia; however, they may present with chest pain, cough, nausea, or gastroesophageal reflux. GCTs are often found on contrast radiography or during endoscopy. On endoscopy they appear as pale yellow wide-based polypoid lesions with intact thin mucosa protruding into the lumen. EUS imaging is useful in that it can help determine the size, location, and invading layer of the tumor. The tumor looks hypoechoic and is surrounded with hypoechoic mucosa. Definitive diagnosis can be difficult, and tissue is typically required. Tissue is usually obtained during endoscopy with multiple biopsies taken from the same site to reach the submucosal position. Histologic evaluation and immunostaining are performed to help differentiate malignant from benign tumors.

At present, there is no consensus on the treatment. But if the tumor is determined as benign, there are no instances of malignant transformation reported. However, there is 1% to 3% malignancy rate, and if the malignancy is suspected, resection is indicated. It has been suggested that symptomatic tumors, tumors larger then 10 mm, rapidly growing lesions, and those with histologic features concerning for malignancy be resected.[44,45] Conversely, small, asymptomatic tumors may be biopsied and followed up.[46,47] Historically, surgical treatment when dictated has been a transthoracic approach. However, EMR (**Fig. 4**) has been successful for lesions that do not extend beyond the submuscosal layer.[48–56]

Inflammatory Pseudotumor

Inflammatory pseudotumors are generally localized masses found in the distal esophagus. They arise from the mucosal layer and often appear as pedunculated lesions. It is thought that they originate from underlying injury such as mechanical injury or from ulceration as a result of chronic reflux. Infection with Epstein-Barr virus has been suggested as a cause, as has autoimmune disorders. These lesions can be mistaken for malignancy, so it is important to biopsy them when found for histologic characterization.

Histology of inflammatory pseudotumors show inflammatory changes and are composed of mostly fibroblasts, inflammatory cells, and blood vessels. Once these lesions are determined to not be a malignancy or other pathology mandating other

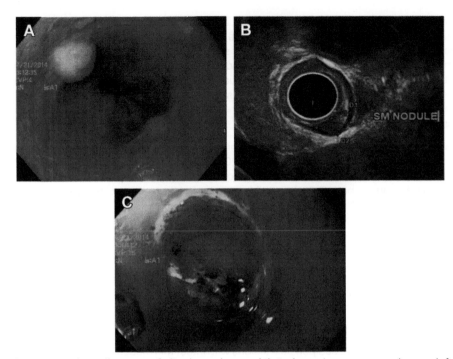

Fig. 4. Granular cell tumor of distal esophagus. (*A*) Endoscopic appearance (*upper left panel*); (*B*) EUS appearance (*upper right panel*); (*C*) after EMR using cap fitted endoscopic band and snare technique (*lower left panel*).

intervention, no specific treatment is required. If chronic reflux is suspected as the cause, treatment of reflux is suggested.

Hemangioma

Hemangiomas are benign vascular tumors that arise from the submucosal layer in the esophagus as a localized hypertrophy of blood vessels. They are benign tumors and represent approximately 3% of all benign tumors of the esophagus.[7] Given their rarity there are no data regarding their demographics. They can be found in the distal esophagus and can present as a solitary lesion or as multiple lesions in association with Rendu-Osler-Weber syndrome. As with other benign tumors of the esophagus, they are often asymptomatic. When symptomatic, their most common symptoms are dysphagia and hematemesis. Hematemesis is often the result of mucosal ulceration overlying the lesion and, given the vascular nature of the lesion, can be minimal or life threatening.

These tumors can be evaluated by several different techniques. On barium esophagography they appear as well-defined submucosal lesions. Endoscopy is often used, and they appear as bluish, polypoid submucosal lesions that are compressible. As opposed to some of the other submucosal lesions mentioned earlier, CT with contrast is particularly useful in confirming a diagnosis and delineating further characteristics.[57] MRI as well as radionuclide study or angiography may also be useful. EUS imaging has started to play an increasing role as it provides further characterization of the lesion including confirming the absence of continuity with major blood vessels.[58,59] Finally, a tissue biopsy may allow a tissue diagnosis; however, this should generally be avoided because of concern for inducing hemorrhage. If a bluish submucosal lesion is found on endoscopy, contrast-enhanced CT scan, radionuclide study, or angiography can establish the diagnosis. Generally, observation of asymptomatic lesions with no occult blood loss is an acceptable option, and signs of ongoing active or otherwise unexplained occult blood loss dictates intervention.

For symptomatic lesions several options have been reported. More recently, hemangiomas have been treated with endoscopic resection, sclerotherapy, radiation, laser fulguration, and video-assisted thoracoscopic resection.[60–63] However, both esophagectomy and tumor enucleation have been performed as well. Given their rarity and an increasing number of options described in their management, a multidisciplinary treatment discussion for symptomatic or bleeding lesions would seem appropriate.

Adenoma

Adenomatous polyps of the esophagus are the result of a benign neoplastic proliferation of columnar cells. They often occur in the distal esophagus and may share the same dysplastic characteristics as colonic adenomas. In the esophagus they have also been found to be associated with Barrett esophagus.[64,65] These polyps may harbor high-grade dysplasia or carcinoma or progress into the same over time. As such, it is recommended that they be removed endoscopically or rigorously sampled and ablated if documented as benign. If high-grade dysplasia or cancer is found, then aggressive surgical resection has historically been advised. EMR may be used for smaller lesions, recognizing that increasingly large lesions are being approached with techniques such as EMR and ESD after careful histologic and EUS evaluation, when appropriate. For sessile or wide-based lesions, aggressive sampling and excisional therapy treatment is indicated, with surgical resection still representing an appropriate consideration for patients of acceptable risk status who exhibit foci of invasive disease or high-grade dysplasia. When associated with Barrett esophagus, focal lesional treatment endoscopically with management of underlying GERD is appropriate, but presence of dysplasia or high-risk markers dictates mucosal ablative therapy.

Papilloma

Squamous papillomas of the esophagus are extremely rare. Their incidence was found to be 0.01% on an autopsy series and 0.07% in an endoscopy series.[66,67] They are more common in older individuals. The exact cause is unknown; however, it is thought that their development is related to chronic gastroesophageal reflux or infection with human papilloma virus or possibly a combination of the two. These lesions tend to be small and solitary and are found most often in the distal esophagus.[66] Rarely, multiple papillomas can be found, which may be associated with a rare condition known as esophageal papillomatosis.[68]

The lesions are generally asymptomatic and identified incidentally on endoscopy. Rarely, they may cause dysphagia. They are generally small, less than 1 cm, solitary, sessile projections that are generally pink and appear fleshy on endoscopy. Often they can be confused with squamous carcinoma, so it is imperative that they be biopsied. EUS imaging may be performed to determine the noninvasive nature of the lesion, but once diagnosed by biopsy, further workup is not indicated. There has only been one case of malignant transformation of an esophageal papilloma.[69] Resection of a papilloma is indicated if it is symptomatic due to obstruction, if it has atypical histologic features, or if malignancy cannot be ruled out. Endoscopic resection (EMR) is the treatment of choice. However, if this is not possible or cancer is still a concern after resection, then an esophagotomy with local resection can be performed.

Fibrovascular Polyp

Fibrovascular polyps are the most common benign intraluminal tumor of the esophagus. They are mostly located in the upper esophagus, generally located distal to the cricopharyngeus in the posterior midline above the confluence of the longitudinal layer of esophageal muscle called Lamier triangle. These lesions are the product of submucosal thickening that progresses to polypoid formation. They can be long because of peristalsis and its effect on the lesion once it develops.[70] They may have spectacular presentations, such as regurgitation from the mouth or even causing sudden death due to asphyxia.[11] It is most likely the aforementioned first case of resection of an esophageal tumor by Dallas-Monro was of this type, since the description was of a regurgitated, pedunculated tumor.

Contrast esophagography shows a large sausagelike elongated tumor.[11] CT and MRI may demonstrate heterogenous attenuation based on the relative amount of adipose and fibrous tissue.[71] Endoscopy demonstrates a fleshy, sausagelike elongated lesion typically arising from the postcricopharyngeal, posterior location outlined earlier.[70]

Once diagnosed, removal is recommended because of the risk for fatal airway complications. The resection planning is developed by information obtained by endoscopy and EUS imaging. The vascularity of the stalk, location, and size dictate the method of resection.[52] Smaller lesions are easily removed endoscopically with either direct snare or EMR techniques. It is recommended to have airway control during endoscopic procedures performed for this pathologic condition to minimize the risk of airway complications during the procedure. Larger lesions or those with abundant blood flow in the stalk demonstrated on EUS imaging require longitudinal esophagotomy on the opposite side of the tumor origin. The tumor stalk is ligated and resected, followed by 2-layer closure of the esophagotomy.[72]

EXTRAESOPHAGEAL TUMORS
Cysts and Duplications

Cysts and duplications are not neoplasms but malformations of the esophagus. They can cause symptoms similar to those of the lesions already discussed by creating mass effects and collectively constitute the second most common tumorlike condition of the esophagus. They can originate not only from the foregut itself but also from developmental aberrations of the trachea that may manifest with dysphagia, hemorrhage, and infection. Other cystic lesions besides congenital developmental cysts and duplications can include inclusion and neuroenteric cysts.

Histologically, esophageal duplication cysts have muscular and epithelial layers and an intramural component. Bronchogenic cysts originate from lung primordia and typically have cartilage in them. Inclusion cysts conversely have similar epithelial lining as esophageal duplications, yet there is no muscle or cartilage. The neuroenteric cysts are malformations resulting from aberrant separation of the foregut from the primitive spinal column. They are posterior in location and often associated with other spinal abnormalities such as spina bifida.[10]

Presenting symptoms in younger patients can include dysphagia or airway symptoms such as wheezing and stridor. In older patients, these lesions may present with infection, dysphagia, chest pain, hemorrhage, fistulization, and malignant transformation.[70]

Diagnosis is made by a combination of esophagography (**Fig. 5**), endoscopy and EUS imaging, and CT (**Fig. 6**) or MRI. These lesions are generally not biopsied because the resulting scar tissue from these biopsies may make future resection more challenging. If a smooth lesion is seen on endoscopy and EUS imaging documents the fluid-filled nature of the lesion (**Fig. 7**), a cross-sectional imaging study is typically obtained next to

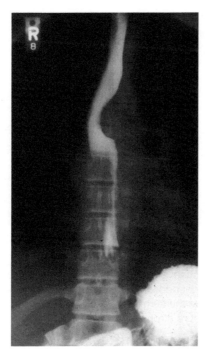

Fig. 5. Extrinsic compression of esophagus due to adjacent cystic lesion on barium study. (*Courtesy of* Stephen R. Hazelrigg, MD, Department of Surgery, Southern Illinois University School of Medicine, IL.)

further delineate the characteristics and extent of the pathology for operative planning purposes. On cross-sectional imaging, the fluid-filled nature of the lesion is typically confirmed, although previous infections can make this determination difficult because the attenuation of the fluid is thicker in such cysts. In those situations, the findings on EUS imaging are used in a complimentary manner for establishing the diagnosis. As for all posterior mediastinal tumors, if the cyst appears to be neuroenteric, an MRI and neurosurgical consultation may be appropriate in preoperative planning.

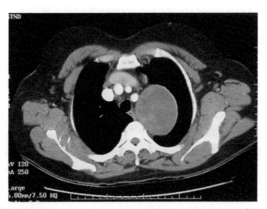

Fig. 6. Posterior mediastinal cyst compressing esophagus. (*Courtesy of* Stephen R. Hazelrigg, MD, Department of Surgery, Southern Illinois University School of Medicine, IL.)

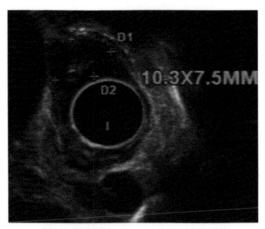

Fig. 7. Radial EUS image of intramural duplication cyst of esophagus.

Once diagnosed, resection is recommended, and thoracoscopy is typically successful with intraoperative endoscopic assistance.[73] A history of previous biopsies and/or infection may make the surgical resection challenging, and in such instances, thoracotomy should be more strongly considered.

SUMMARY

Given the rarity of benign esophageal tumors, the clinician must have a thorough grasp of their causes, behaviors, and respective management strategies. Many of these lesions may be safely observed if they are asymptomatic and stable on serial assessment. Symptomatic and larger or growing lesions require more careful characterization by EUS imaging, FNA, and cross-sectional imaging to guide therapeutic decision making. A familiarity with related medical conditions such as GERD and Barrett esophagus, with the distinctive patterns of disease characterizing pediatric and adult patient groups, and with the biologic complexities characterizing behavior and treatment of pathologies such as GISTs, is a requisite cognitive skill set for the managing provider. Removal of symptomatic lesions can be approached increasingly by minimally invasive methods and with some pathologies with advancing endoluminal resective techniques. Surgeons managing these patients should either have the current skills necessary for their management, including skills in minimally invasive thoracoscopic and laparoscopic surgery as well as therapeutic endoscopy and EUS imaging, or participate in multidisciplinary treatment teams that include individuals with these skills. With appropriate characterization of the pathologic condition, these lesions are increasingly able to be appropriately managed with techniques that can optimize outcomes and limit both short- and long-term morbidity and risk for the patient.

REFERENCES

1. Choong CK, Meyers BF. Benign esophageal tumors: introduction, incidence, classification, and clinical features. Semin Thorac Cardiovasc Surg 2003;15: 3–8 No. 1. WB Saunders.
2. Rice TW. Benign esophageal tumors: esophagoscopy and endoscopic esophageal ultrasound. Semin Thorac Cardiovasc Surg 2003;15:20–6 No. 1. WB Saunders.

3. Watson RR, O'Connor TM, Weisel W. Solid benign tumors of the esophagus. Ann Thorac Surg 1967;4(1):80–91.
4. Storey CF, Adams WC Jr. Leiomyoma of the esophagus: a report of four cases and review of the surgical literature. Am J Surg 1956;91(1):3–23.
5. Patterson EJ. Benign neoplasms of the esophagus: report of a case of myxofibroma. Ann Otol Rhinol Laryngol 1932;41(3):942–50.
6. Moersch HJ. Benign tumor of the esophagus. Ann Otol Rhinol Laryngol 1944;53: 800–17.
7. Plachta A. Benign tumors of the esophagus. Review of literature and report of 99 cases. Am J Gastroenterol 1962;38:639–52.
8. Attah EB, Hajdu SI. Benign and malignant tumors of the esophagus at autopsy. J Thorac Cardiovasc Surg 1968;55(3):396.
9. Mutrie CJ, Donahue DM, Wain JC, et al. Esophageal leiomyoma: a 40-year experience. Ann Thorac Surg 2005;79(4):1122–5.
10. Arbona JL, Fazzi JG, Mayoral J. Congenital esophageal cysts: case report and review of literature. Am J Gastroenterol 1984;79(3):177–82.
11. Levine MS, Buck JL, Pantongrag-Brown L, et al. Fibrovascular polyps of the esophagus: clinical, radiographic, and pathologic findings in 16 patients. AJR Am J Roentgenol 1996;166:781–7.
12. Seremetis MG, Lyons WS, deGuzman VC, et al. Leiomyomata of the esophagus. An analysis of 838 cases. Cancer 1976;38:2166–77.
13. Levine MS. Benign tumors of the esophagus: radiologic evaluation. Semin Thorac Cardiovasc Surg 2003;15:9–19 No. 1. WB Saunders.
14. Lee LS, Singhal S, Brinster CJ, et al. Current management of esophageal leiomyoma. J Am Coll Surg 2004;198:136–46.
15. Hatch GF III, George F, Hatch KF, et al. Tumors of the esophagus. World J Surg 2000;24:401–11.
16. Miettinen M, Sarlomo-Rikala M, Sobin LH, et al. Esophageal stromal tumors: a clinicopathologic, immunohistochemical, and molecular genetic study of 17 cases and comparison with esophageal leiomyomas and leiomyosarcomas. Am J Surg Pathol 2000;24:211–22.
17. Kent M, d'Amato T, Nordman C, et al. Minimally invasive resection of benign esophageal tumors. J Thorac Cardiovasc Surg 2007;134:176–81.
18. Bourque MD, Spigland N, Bensoussan AL, et al. Esophageal leiomyoma in children: two case reports and review of the literature. J Pediatr Surg 1989;24: 1103–7.
19. Miettinen M, Lasota J. Gastrointestinal stromal tumors–definition, clinical, histological, immunohistochemical, and molecular genetic features and differential diagnosis. Virchows Arch 2001;438:1–12.
20. Calabrese C, Fabbri A, Fusaroli P, et al. Diffuse esophageal leiomyomatosis: case report and review. Gastrointest Endosc 2002;55:590–3.
21. Postlethwait RW. Benign tumors and cysts of the esophagus. Surg Clin North Am 1983;63:925–31.
22. Samphire J, Nafteux P, Luketich J. Minimally invasive techniques for resection of benign esophageal tumors. Semin Thorac Cardiovasc Surg 2003;15:35–43 No. 1. WB Saunders.
23. Lee HJ, Park SI, Kim DK, et al. Surgical resection of esophageal gastrointestinal stromal tumors. Ann Thorac Surg 2009;87:1569–71.
24. Jiang G, Zhao H, Yang F, et al. Thoracoscopic enucleation of esophageal leiomyoma: a retrospective study on 40 cases. Dis Esophagus 2009;22: 279–83.

25. Von Rahden BH, Stein HJ, Feussner H, et al. Enucleation of submucosal tumors of the esophagus: minimally invasive versus open approach. Surg Endosc 2004;18: 924–30.
26. Zaninotto G, Portale G, Costantini M, et al. Minimally invasive enucleation of esophageal leiomyoma. Surg Endosc 2006;20:1904–8.
27. Blum MG, Bilimoria KY, Wayne JD, et al. Surgical considerations for the management and resection of esophageal gastrointestinal stromal tumors. Ann Thorac Surg 2007;84:1717–23.
28. Bodner JC, Zitt M, Ott H, et al. Robotic-assisted thoracoscopic surgery (RATS) for benign and malignant esophageal tumors. Ann Thorac Surg 2005;80:1202–6.
29. Chang WC, Tzao C, Shen DH, et al. Gastrointestinal stromal tumor (GIST) of the esophagus detected by positron emission tomography/computed tomography. Dig Dis Sci 2005;50:1315–8.
30. Joensuu H. Risk stratification of patients diagnosed with gastrointestinal stromal tumor. Hum Pathol 2008;39:1411–9.
31. Emory TS, Sobin LH, Lukes L, et al. Prognosis of gastrointestinal smooth-muscle (stromal) tumors: dependence on anatomic site. Am J Surg Pathol 1999;23: 82–7.
32. Portale G, Zaninotto G, Costantini M, et al. Esophageal GIST: case report of surgical enucleation and update on current diagnostic and therapeutic options. Int J Surg Pathol 2007;15:393–6.
33. Shinagare AB, Zukotynski KA, Krajewski KM, et al. Esophageal gastrointestinal stromal tumor: report of 7 patients. Cancer Imaging 2012;12:100–8.
34. Kwon MS, Lee SS, Ahn GH. Schwannomas of the gastrointestinal tract: clinicopathological features of 12 cases including a case of esophageal tumor compared with those of gastrointestinal stromal tumors and leiomyomas of the gastrointestinal tract. Pathol Res Pract 2002;198:605–13.
35. Yoon HY, Kim CB, Lee YH, et al. An obstructing large schwannoma in the esophagus. J Gastrointest Surg 2008;12:761–3.
36. Kobayashi N, Kikuchi S, Shimao H, et al. Benign esophageal schwannoma: report of a case. Surg Today 2000;30:526–9.
37. Murase K, Hino A, Ozeki Y, et al. Malignant schwannoma of the esophagus with lymph node metastasis: literature review of schwannoma of the esophagus. J Gastroenterol 2001;36:772–7.
38. Iwata H, Kataoka M, Yamakawa Y, et al. Esophageal schwannoma. Ann Thorac Surg 1993;56:376–7.
39. Hou YY, Tan YS, Xu JF, et al. Schwannoma of the gastrointestinal tract: a clinicopathological, immunohistochemical and ultrastructural study of 33 cases. Histopathology 2006;48:536–45.
40. Fanburg-smith JC, Meis-Kindblom JM, Fante R, et al. Malignant granular cell tumor of soft tissue: diagnostic criteria and clinicopathologic correlation. Am J Surg Pathol 1998;22:779–94.
41. Lack EE, Worsham GF, Callihan MD, et al. Granular cell tumor: a clinicopathlogic study of 110 patients. J Surg Oncol 1980;13:301–16.
42. McSwain GR, Colpitt R, Kreutner A, et al. Granular cell myoblastoma. Surg Gynecol Obstet 1980;150:703–10.
43. Johnston J, Helwig EB. Granular cell tumors of the gastrointestinal tract and perineal region: a study of 74 cases. Dig Dis Sci 1981;26:807–16.
44. Coutinho DS, Soga J, Yoshikawa T, et al. Granular cell tumors or the esophagus: a report of two cases and review of the literature. Am J Gastroenterol 1985;80:758.

45. Percinel S, Savas B, Yilmaz G, et al. Granular cell tumor of the esophagus: report of 5 cases and review of diagnostic and therapeutic techniques. Dis Esophagus 2007;20:435–43.
46. Voskuil J, Van Dijk MM, Wagenaar SS, et al. Occurrence of esophageal granular cell tumors in the Netherlands between 1988 and 1994. Dig Dis Sci 2001;24: 1610–4.
47. Mineo TC, Biancari F, Francioni, et al. Conservative approach to granular cell tumor of the esophagus: three case reports. Scand Cardiovasc J 1995;29:141–4.
48. Hyun JH, Jeen YT, Chu HJ, et al. Endoscopic resection of submucosal tumor of the esophagus: result in 62 patients. Endoscopy 1997;29:165–70.
49. Fujiwara Y, Watanabe T, Hamasaki N, et al. Endoscopic resection of two granular cell tumours of the oesophagus. Eur J Gastroenterol Hepatol 1999;11:1413–6.
50. Fotiadis C, Manolis EN, Troupis TG, et al. Endoscopic resection of a large granular cell tumor of the esophagus. J Surg Oncol 2000;75:277–9.
51. van der Peet DL, Berends FJ, Klinkengerg-Knol EC, et al. Endoscopic treatment of benign esophageal tumors: case report of three patients. Surg Endosc 2001; 15:1489.
52. Kinney T, Waxman I. Treatment of benign esophageal tumors by endoscopic techniques. Semin Thorac Cardiovasc Surg 2003;15:27–34.
53. Wehrmann T, Martchenko K, Nakamura M, et al. Endoscopic resection of submucosal esophageal tumors: a prospective case series. Endoscopy 2004;36:802–7.
54. Bataglia G, Rampado S, Bocus P, et al. Single-band mucosectomy of granular cell tumor of the esophagus: safe and easy technique. Surg Endosc 2006;20: 1296–8.
55. Zhong N, Katzka DA, Smyrk TC, et al. Endoscopic diagnosis and resection of esophageal granular cell tumors. Dis Esophagus 2011;24:438–543.
56. Kahng DH, Kim GH, Park DY, et al. Endoscopic resection of granular cell tumors in the gastrointestinal tract: a single center experience. Surg Endosc 2013;27: 3228–36.
57. Taylor FH, Fowler FC, Betsill WL, et al. Hemangioma of the esophagus. Ann Thorac Surg 1996;61:726.
58. Tominaga K, Arakawa T, Ando K, et al. Oesophageal cavernous haemangioma diagnosed histologically, not by endoscopic procedures. J Gastroenterol Hepatol 2000;15:215–9.
59. Cantero D, Yoshida T, Ito M, et al. Esophageal hemangioma:endoscopic diagnosis and treatment. Endoscopy 1994;26:250–3.
60. Yoshikane H, Suzuki T, Yoshioka N, et al. Hemangioma of the esophagus. Endoscopic imaging and endoscopic resection. Endoscopy 1995;27:267.
61. Shigemitsu K, Naomoto Y, Yamatsuji T, et al. Esophageal hemangioma successfully treated by fulguration using potassium titanyl phosphate/yttrium aluminum garnet (KTP/YAG) laser: a case report. Dis Esophagus 2000;13:161.
62. Aoki T, Okagawa K, Uemura Y, et al. Successful treatment of an esophageal hemangioma by endoscopic injection sclerotherapy: report of a case. Surg Today 1997;27:450.
63. Ramo OJ, Salo JA, Bardini R, et al. Treatment of a submucosal hemangioma of the esophagus using simultaneous video-assisted thoracoscopy and esophagoscopy: Description of a new minimally invasive technique. Endoscopy 1997;29: S27–8.
64. Lee RG. Adenomas arising in Barrett's esophagus. Am J Clin Pathol 1986;85:629–32.
65. McDonald GB, Brand DL, Thorning DR. Multiple adenomatous neoplasms arising in columnar-lined (Barrett's) esophagus. Gastroenterology 1977;72:1317–21.

66. Weitzer S, Hentel W. Squamous papilloma of esophagus. Case report and review of the literature. Am J Gastroenterol 1968;50:391.
67. Mosca S, Manes G, Onaco R, et al. Squamous papilloma of the esophagus: long-term follow up. J Gastroenterol Hepatol 2001;16:857–61.
68. Sandvik AK, Aase S, Kvberg KH, et al. Papillomatosis of the esophagus. J Clin Gastroenterol 1996;22:35–7.
69. Van Cutsem E, Geboes K, Vantrappen G, et al. Malignant degeneration of esophageal squamous papilloma associated with the human papillomavirus. Gastroenterology 1992;103:1119.
70. Pitichote H, Ferguson MK. Minimally invasive treatment of benign esophageal tumors. Surgical management of benign esophageal disorders. Springer-Verlag; 2014. p. 181–99.
71. Ascenti G, Racchiusa S, Mazziotti S, et al. Giant fibrovascular polyp of the esophagus: CT and MR findings. Abdom Imaging 1999;24(2):109–10.
72. Solerio D, Gasparri G, Ruffini E, et al. Giant fibrovascular polyp of the esophagus. Dis Esophagus 2005;18(6):410–2.
73. Hirose S, Clifton MS, Bratton B, et al. Thoracoscopic resection of foregut duplication cysts. J Laparoendosc Adv Surg Tech A 2006;16(5):526–9.

Physiology and Pathogenesis of Gastroesophageal Reflux Disease

CrossMark

Dean J. Mikami, MD[a], Kenric M. Murayama, MD[b],*

KEYWORDS

- Gastroesophageal reflux disease • GERD • Heartburn • Pathology of GERD
- Pathogenesis of GERD

KEY POINTS

- Gastroesophageal reflux disease (GERD) represents a wide range of pathologic conditions that are poorly understood.
- Reflux of gastric acid most commonly presents as heartburn, but GERD can also be associated with bile (alkaline) reflux, gastric or esophageal distention, and motility disorders.
- Pain associated with gastroesophageal reflux is secondary to the stimulation and activation of mucosal chemoreceptors by acid; the lower esophageal sphincter (LES) plays a vital role in the frequency and severity of GERD.
- Development of Barrett esophagus is believed to be due to repeated and uncontrolled acid exposure of the distal esophagus resulting in metaplasia, which can progress to dysplasia of the epithelium of the distal esophagus.

INTRODUCTION: NATURE OF THE PROBLEM

GERD is a common problem treated by primary care physicians. It is estimated that up to 20% of Americans experience symptomatic GERD weekly and that an even higher percentage of people have heartburn monthly.[1] The cost of managing a disease of this prevalence is substantial, with estimates of direct and indirect costs exceeding $14 billion in the United States, 60% of which is accounted for by medication costs.[2] Although the physiology and pathogenesis of GERD are poorly understood, heartburn, the most common symptom, occurs in most patients and is thought to be due to the stimulation and activation of mucosal chemoreceptors in the distal esophagus.[3] The

[a] Center for Minimally Invasive Surgery, Division of Gastrointestinal Surgery, The Ohio State University Wexner Medical Center, N717 Doan Hall, 410 West 10th Avenue, Columbus, OH 43210, USA; [b] Department of Surgery, Abington Memorial Hospital, 1245 Highland Avenue, Price Building, Suite 604, Abington, PA 19001, USA
* Corresponding author. Department of Surgery, Abington Memorial Hospital, 1245 Highland Avenue, Price Building, Suite 604, Abington, PA 19001.
E-mail address: kmurayama@abingtonhealth.org

Surg Clin N Am 95 (2015) 515–525
http://dx.doi.org/10.1016/j.suc.2015.02.006
0039-6109/15/$ – see front matter © 2015 Elsevier Inc. All rights reserved.

pain associated with heartburn is usually due to gastric acid present in the esophagus, but it can also be due to bile salt irritation of the esophagus, esophageal distention, and motility disorders of the distal esophagus.[4] There has been an alarming increase in the prevalence of GERD in the United States over the past 2 decades, and although the cause is likely multifactorial and our understanding of GERD has improved, 2 factors that seem to have contributed most are the obesity epidemic and improvements in diagnostic techniques, with the routine use of endoscopy becoming more commonplace.[5,6]

The wide range of symptoms from mild to severe heartburn with or without acid exposure in combination with the multifactorial nature of GERD makes understanding this disease challenging. GERD and its associated symptoms occur as the end product of a collection of anatomic and/or physiologic abnormalities. Under normal circumstances, the intra-abdominal pressure is positive, whereas the intrathoracic pressure is negative, a physical principle that should promote reflux of gastric contents into the esophagus. Not surprisingly, small amounts of reflux occur throughout the day in everyone, but pathologic GERD is prevented by the normal anatomy and physiology of the esophagus, LES, diaphragm muscles at the hiatus, and the stomach. In general, pathologic reflux is most commonly a consequence of the breakdown of the normal reflux barrier of the LES, but it can also result from factors that increase the pressure gradient between the abdomen and thorax (eg, morbid obesity and pregnancy) or dysmotility of the esophagus, hiatus musculature, and/or the stomach. This article examines the physiology of GERD and the pathologic conditions resulting from it.

PHYSIOLOGY OF THE DISTAL ESOPHAGUS

The distal esophagus and LES are dynamic and interrelated (**Fig. 1**). The antireflux mechanism of the esophagus consists of the LES, the angle of His, and the muscle fibers of the diaphragm. The LES is 2 to 4 cm in length of the distal esophagus and is composed of tonically contracted circular smooth muscle located within the diaphragm hiatus.[7,8] Gastroesophageal reflux occurs when there is inappropriate relaxation of the LES permitting gastric acid to enter the distal esophagus, stimulating the chemoreceptors and causing irritation, leading to the manifestation of symptoms. In addition, several drugs can alter the LES tone (**Table 1**) and affect the natural defenses of the esophagus to induce heartburn; however, more commonly, many different foods can trigger heartburn (**Box 1**). As mentioned, other key contributors to reflux in addition to the drugs and foods listed are factors that increase intra-abdominal pressure, overcoming the antireflux barrier, such as pregnancy or obesity.[9]

The LES is a circular muscle layer of the distal esophagus that generates a resting pressure higher than the intra-abdominal pressure.[7] The LES resting pressure is normally sufficient to prevent reflux of gastric contents into the esophagus thereby preventing symptomatic heartburn, but during times of increased abdominal pressure (ie, Valsalva maneuver, lifting, Trendelenburg position, and pregnancy) other mechanisms aid in preventing reflux.[10] The left and right crural muscles of the diaphragm constitute the second mechanism of defense to protect the esophagus from reflux. The crural muscles and the LES are anatomically connected by the phrenoesophageal ligament (**Fig. 2**) and give the esophagus 2 distinct but interactive mechanisms to prevent reflux of stomach contents into the esophagus.[11]

Swallowing is a complex physiologic process that results in the propulsion of the food bolus from the pharynx into the esophagus and then into the stomach. This process can be started consciously or reflexively by stimulation of areas of the mouth or pharynx. Pharyngeal activity during swallowing stimulates the esophageal phase and

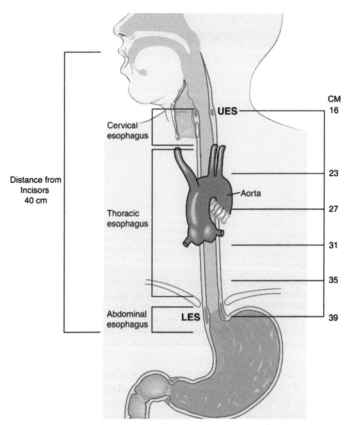

Fig. 1. Schematic view of the esophagus. The esophagus is approximately 40 cm from the incisors to the bottom of the LES. UES, upper esophageal sphincter. (*From* Patel D, Vaezi MF. Normal esophageal physiology and laryngoesophageal reflux. Otolaryngol Clin North Am 2013;46:1025; with permission.)

Table 1		
Effect of drugs on the lower esophageal sphincter tone		
Increase	**Decrease**	**No Change**
Metoclopramide	Atropine	Propranolol
Domperidone	Glycopyrrolate	Oxprenolol
Prochlorperazine	Dopamine	Cimetidine
Cyclizine	Sodium nitroprusside	Ranitidine
Edrophonium	Ganglion blockers	Atracurium
Neostigmine	Thiopental	?Nitrous oxide
Succinylcholine	Tricyclic antidepressants	
Pancuronium	β-Adrenergic stimulants	
Metoprolol	Halothane	
α-Adrenergic stimulants	Enflurane opioids	
Antacids	?Nitrous oxide	
	Propofol	

? indicates possibly.
Data from Sharma VK. Role of endoscopy in GERD. Gastroenterol Clin North Am 2014;43(1): 39–46.

Box 1
Foods that are commonly associated with heartburn

Alcohol, particularly red wine

Black pepper

Garlic

Raw onions

Spicy foods

Chocolate

Citrus fruits

Coffee

Tea

Soda

Peppermint

Tomatoes

Data from Kahrilas PJ, Shaheen NJ, Vaezi MF, et al. American Gastroenterological Association Medical Position Statement on the management of gastroesophageal reflux disease. Gastroenterology 2008;135:1383–91; and Vaezi MF. The Esophagus: Anatomy, Physiology, and Diseases. In: Flint PW, Haughey BH, Lund VJ, et al., editors. Cummings Otolaryngology: Head and Neck Surgery. 5th edition. Philadelphia: Mosby Elsevier; 2010. p. 953–80.

---

because of the helical arrangement of the circular smooth muscle, the esophageal body functions as a "worm drive" propulsive pump. The esophageal phase of swallowing moves food from the esophagus into the stomach and accomplishes this against a pressure gradient of 12 mm at rest (−6 mm Hg pressure in the thoracic cavity and +6 mm Hg pressure in the abdominal cavity).[11] The upper esophageal sphincter (UES) closes rapidly after the initiation of a swallow, and the contraction that follows relaxation of the UES proceeds down the esophagus as a peristaltic wave.[11] When present, defects in primary and secondary peristalsis contribute to GERD, so understanding the physiology in a patient with GERD is essential.

The symptoms resulting from GERD are because of mucosal injury and are directly related to the frequency of reflux events, the duration of mucosal acidification, and the

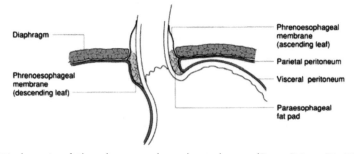

Fig. 2. Attachments of the phrenoesophageal membrane. (*From* Peters JH, Watson TJ, DeMeester TR. Esophagus: anatomy, physiology and gastroesophageal reflux disease. In: Greenfield LJ, editor. Surgery: scientific principles and practice. 3rd edition. Philadelphia: Lippincott Williams and Wilkins; 2001. p. 660; with permission.)

caustic potency of the refluxate.[12] The esophageal mucosa in normal individuals exists in a milieu that constantly fluctuates between damaging and protective forces. The main mechanism that leads to most physiologic reflux events is termed transient lower esophageal sphincter relaxations (TLESRs).[13] TLESRs are the normal gastric venting mechanism of the stomach, and a normal TLESR event is activated by different stimuli such as distension of the stomach. In patients with GERD there is an increased percentage of TLESRs predisposing to symptomatic heartburn. The main relaxation is mediated through the vagus nerve, which inhibits the crural fibers of the diaphragm (**Fig. 3**).[14–16] The overexaggeration of this phenomenon is seen in patients with a hiatal hernia and can contribute to significant heartburn symptoms.

HIATAL HERNIA

There are 4 types of hiatal hernias (**Fig. 4**). Type 1 hiatal hernias are called sliding hiatal hernias with upward migration of the LES. Type 2 hiatal hernias are called paraesophageal hiatal hernias and have a normal gastroesophageal junction (GEJ) location below the diaphragmatic hiatus with migration of gastric fundus through the hiatus. Type 3 hiatal hernias represent a combination of type 1 and 2 hernias with both the GEJ and gastric fundus migrating through the diaphragmatic hiatus. The last and rarest is the type 4 hiatal hernia, which involves herniation of other abdominal organs such as the colon or the spleen. The most common type of hiatal hernia is type 1, which is seen in 90% of patients with a hiatal hernia.[15] The disruption of the crural muscle and the phrenoesophageal ligament secondary to the hiatal hernia creates a proximal pouch in the distal esophagus. This pouch has been termed an acid pocket and can cause an increased environment for acid exposure.[16] Development of a hiatal hernia is

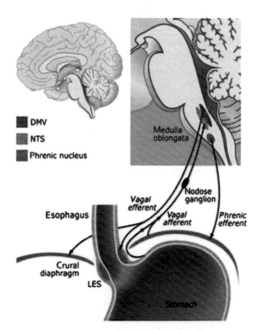

Fig. 3. Neural pathway involved in TLESRs. DMV, dorsal motor nucleus of the vagus nerve; NTS, nucleus of the solitary tract. (*From* Boeckxstaens GE, Rohof WO. Pathophysiology of gastroesophageal reflux disease. Gastroenterol Clin North Am 2014;43(1):17; with permission.)

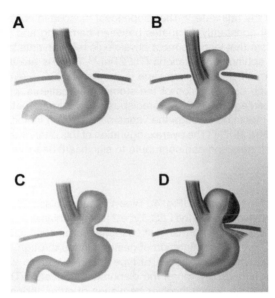

Fig. 4. Types of hiatal hernias. (*A*) Type I (sliding hiatal hernia); (*B*) type II (paraesophageal hernia). (*C*) type III (mixed type); (*D*) type IV (complex with other organs in hernia). (*From* Laparoscopic paraesophageal hernia repair. In: Jones DB, Maithel SK, Schneider BE, editors. Atlas of minimally invasive surgery. 1st edition. Woodbury (CT): Cine-Med, Inc; 2006. p. 129; with permission.)

poorly understood but is more common in obese patients,[17] and a hiatal hernia greater than 2 cm is associated with a greater incidence of erosive esophagitis and Barrett esophagus. Repeated shortening of the esophagus as a result of swallowing or retching and loss of elasticity of the phrenoesophageal ligaments are thought to be primary contributors to the formation of a hiatal hernia.

Hiatal hernias disrupt the normal anatomic and physiologic mechanisms of the LES and TLESRs. There is a reduction in LES length and pressure and alterations of esophageal peristalsis that can result in increased acid exposure at the distal esophagus contributing to mucosal injury.[15] In sliding hiatal hernias (type I), there is a circumferential weakness of the phrenoesophageal ligament leading to migration of the esophagogastric junction in a craniad direction into the lower mediastinum. Type II (paraesophageal) hernias result from local weakness of the phrenoesophageal ligament laterally resulting in migration of the fundus into the lower mediastinum.[18]

GASTRIC FUNCTION

The third and often overlooked component of GERD is the contribution of gastric function. Delay in gastric emptying can cause prolonged gastric retention of food, which in turn increases the propensity for GERD. With this phenomenon, there is an increase in the gastroesophageal pressure gradient, gastric volume, and the volume of potential refluxate.[16] Normal peristaltic movement in the stomach is important for the clearance and propulsion of liquids and solids toward the pylorus. Patients with gastroparesis often feel bloated and full because of the resultant poor emptying of the stomach, and this may lead to heartburn symptoms. It is important to distinguish between gastroparesis and gastric outlet obstruction because the treatment algorithm is different for both groups and a preoperative upper endoscopy should be done in the workup of these patients.[19] Gastric outlet obstruction can be caused by ulcer disease, large gastric polyps, or cancer, and the subsequent poor gastric emptying can lead to gastric distention pressures that overcome the LES closing pressure and result in GERD. Gastric emptying studies should be carried out in any patient with a history of abdominal bloating before antireflux surgery or a preoperative esophageal manometry that is incongruous with the diagnosis of GERD. A scintigraphy test of a solid-phase meal rather than a liquid meal is the gold standard for the diagnosis of gastroparesis.[20] Gastric emptying of liquids may seem normal even in patients with advanced gastroparesis, and gastroparesis is seen more often in patients with GERD than in those without GERD.[21]

TREATMENT OPTIONS

While the surgical treatment of GERD is comprehensively addressed in the remainder of this article, it is essential to remember that nonsurgical therapy is the mainstay of initial treatment. However, several published trials have supported the premise that surgery results in similar resolution of GERD symptoms as medical therapy. In a recent study by Rossetti and colleagues[22] comparing medical versus surgical therapy for GERD in 301 patients, there was not a significant improvement of quality of life scores (36-Item Short Form Health Survey and Health Related Quality of Life) in the medical versus the surgical group at 1 year in patients with documented acid reflux.

In the LOTUS (Long-Term Usage of Esomprazole versus Surgery) trial, one of the largest prospective randomized trials, 554 patients with documented GERD were randomly assigned to receive either esomeprazole (20–40 mg/d) or laparoscopic antireflux surgery. The conclusion from this multicenter trial was that both medical and surgical antireflux therapies result in most patients remaining in symptom remission at 5 years.[23]

The long-term use of proton pump inhibitors has been shown to increase the risk of hip fractures, community-acquired pneumonia, diarrhea, and drug interactions especially in patients taking clopidogrel.[24] Patients with refractory GERD despite high-dose protein pump inhibitor therapy remain a treatment dilemma, and a pH study is indicated to provide clarity regarding whether symptoms are related to acid reflux. Talaie and colleagues[25] studied 48 patients with refractory GERD, and they had a mean DeMeester score of 10.06 (standard deviation = 10.48). The study demonstrated that most of patients with refractory GERD did not have acid reflux. Patients with refractory heartburn should undergo impedance pH monitoring while on acid suppressive therapy to best clarify the relationship between symptoms and acid or nonacid reflux. Patients with acid or nonacid reflux that either fails or does not respond to medical therapy may benefit from an antireflux operation. Unfortunately, unlike acid reflux for which there is effective medical therapy, options are limited for patients with nonacid reflux and antireflux surgery may be the best option.

SPECIAL CIRCUMSTANCES
Barrett Esophagus

Barrett esophagus is the most feared consequence of longstanding GERD because there is a small but real risk of conversion to adenocarcinoma. The progression to Barrett esophagus (metaplastic columnar mucosa) from the normal esophageal stratified squamous epithelium is seen with repeated and untreated acid exposure of the distal esophagus. The prevalence of Barrett esophagus varies between studies, but it has been estimated that 5.6% of the adult population in the United States has the disease.[26] The risk of developing esophageal adenocarcinoma in patients with non-dysplastic Barrett esophagus is only 0.1% to 0.3% per year, but male sex and the presence of long-segment Barrett esophagus increases this risk. The standard workup of a patient suspected of having Barrett esophagus starts with a standard esophagogastroduodenoscopy and a systematic biopsy protocol with the finding of columnar epithelium proximal to the GEJ. Esophageal biopsies should demonstrate intestinal metaplasia with the presence of goblet cells to make the diagnosis of Barrett esophagus. The proximal extent of the columnar metaplasia above the GEJ determines whether there is long-segment (≥3 cm) or short-segment (<3 cm) Barrett esophagus.[26] To prevent the progression to Barrett esophagus, the 3 main pathophysiologic causes of GERD (ie, dysfunctional esophageal motility, a weakened LES, and impaired gastric emptying) discussed previously need to be evaluated and treated if present. Interestingly, routine screening of patients with GERD symptoms may have a low yield because most patients with short-segment Barrett esophagus have no GERD symptoms and up to 40% of patients with esophageal adenocarcinoma have no history of symptomatic GERD. The rate of progression to adenocarcinoma is estimated to be approximately 6% per year if high-grade dysplasia is present. Traditionally, esophagectomy was the recommended treatment for patients with high-grade dysplasia, but more recently endoscopic resection and ablation have become more commonplace to eradicate dysplasia. The mainstay of treatment is the use of proton pump inhibitors and modulation of the proinflammatory mechanisms. Antireflux surgery for Barrett esophagus has been shown to be equally effective in the LOTUS trial.[27] The current recommendation for patients with low-grade dysplasia is endoscopic surveillance at 6- to 12-month intervals or endoscopic ablative therapy. Patients with nondysplastic metaplasia should undergo routine surveillance, but currently ablation therapy is not indicated.[26]

Upright Versus Supine Reflux

Upright versus supine GERD symptoms differ in presentation, pathophysiology, and management options. Patients who have upright reflux generally reflux during the day, whereas those who have supine reflux generally have GERD symptoms at night.[28] Relaxation pressure, distal latency, and distal contractility are significantly lower in the upright position when compared with supine.[29] In general, patients with supine reflux tend to have weakness of the LES, can have bipositional GERD (upright and supine), and tend to have more severe GERD. Patients with upright daytime GERD tend to have reflux primarily because of the TLESRs discussed earlier and, generally, have less severe disease. Interestingly, TLESRs are decreased in the supine position, so patients with normal LES function tend not to reflux in the supine position; however, if the LES is defective as in patients with supine reflux, TLESRs are a nonfactor.[28]

Extraesophageal Manifestations of gastroesophageal reflux disease

Some of the more common extraesophageal complications of GERD include aspiration pneumonia, reflux-induced asthma, reflux cough syndrome, and laryngitis.[30] Asthma, chronic cough, and laryngitis have been shown to have a direct correlation with GERD, whereas aspiration pneumonias are usually multifactorial.[31] The usual management is medical therapy with the mainstay of treatment being proton pump inhibitors. Antireflux surgery should be offered if medical therapy is ineffective, if patients cannot or will not take medications, or if complications of reflux worsen in spite of adequate medical therapy (ie, volume regurgitation and aspiration). Unfortunately, treatment outcomes and benefits for these extraesophageal manifestations of GERD are less predictable than for heartburn or esophagitis symptoms.

Laryngopharyngeal reflux (LPR) is an extraesophageal variant of GERD, because the main symptomatic region involves the larynx and the pharynx. Heartburn and regurgitation are the hallmark symptoms of GERD in contrast to the symptoms of LPR, which often include hoarseness, chronic cough, sore throat, globus pharyngeus ("lump in the throat"), and frequent throat clearing. Recognition of LPR as an extraesophageal variant of GERD has increased, and approximately 10% of all otolaryngology clinic patients overall and 50% of patients with voice complaints have been diagnosed with LPR.[32]

Eosinophilic Esophagitis

Eosinophilic esophagitis (EOE) is a chronic, immune-antigen-mediated disease recognized with increasing frequency that is often confused with GERD. This disease is characterized by symptoms of esophageal dysfunction clinically and by eosinophil-predominant inflammation on endoscopic biopsy. EOE can cause dysphagia and food impaction in both adults and children, and the diagnosis requires an esophageal biopsy of the esophageal epithelium with 15 or more eosinophils per high-power field (HPF).[33] Eosinophils are not present in normal mucosa, but eosinophilic infiltration can occur from various diseases, such as GERD, eosinophilic gastroenteritis, collagen vascular disease, achalasia, and parasitic infections. Eosinophils can be observed in the mucosa in small numbers ($\leq$4 per HPF) in GERD, but the characteristic appearance of EOE such as longitudinal furrows is not seen in GERD.[34] The importance of EOE in the discussion of GERD is that it occurs with increasing frequency and patients with EOE are often treated for GERD and fall into the category of patients with "GERD unresponsive to medical therapy." Therefore, any patient who is refractory to medical therapy who has dysphagia should be evaluated for EOE.

SUMMARY

GERD remains one of the most common gastrointestinal problems. The heartburn a patient feels is related to multiple factors of which fluctuations in LES pressures is the most important. The diagnosis, treatment, and follow-up of these patients with GERD are significant burdens to our health care system, as is evident from the fact that some of the most costly and commonly prescribed medications in the United States are proton pump inhibitors. There are many options to treat GERD including medical and surgical options, but it is unlikely that one option will be best for every patient. More studies are being conducted in this field to improve understanding of this complex disease process.

REFERENCES

1. Peery AF, Dellon ES, Lund J, et al. Burden of gastrointestinal disease in the United States: 2012 update. Gastroenterology 2012;143:1179–87.
2. Richter JE. The many manifestations of gastroesophageal reflux disease: presentation, evaluation, and treatment. Gastroenterol Clin North Am 2007;36:577–99.
3. DeVault KR. Symptoms of Esophageal Disease. In: Feldman M, Friedman LS, Brandt LJ, editors. Sleisenger and Fordtran's Gastrointestinal and Liver Disease. 9th edition. Philadelphia: Saunders Elsevier; 2010. p. 173–82.
4. Rodriguez-Stanley S, Robinson M, Earnest DL, et al. Esophageal hypersensitivity may be a major cause of heartburn. Am J Gastroenterol 1999;94:628–31.
5. El-Serag HB. Time trends of gastroesophageal reflux disease: a systematic review. Clin Gastroenterol Hepatol 2007;5:17–26.

6. Sharma VK. Role of endoscopy in GERD. Gastroenterol Clin North Am 2014; 43(1):39–46.
7. Mittal RK, Balaban DH. The esophagogastric junction. N Engl J Med 1997;336: 924–32.
8. Tantawy H, Myslajek T. Diseases of the Gastrointestinal System. In: Hines RL, Marschall KE, editors. Stoelting's Anesthesia and Co-Exising Disease. 6th edition. Philadelphia: Elsevier Saunders; 2012. p. 287–304.
9. Kahrilas PJ, Shaheen NJ, Vaezi MF, et al. American Gastroenterological Association medical position statement on the management of gastroesophageal reflux disease. Gastroenterology 2008;135:1383–91.
10. Mittal RK. The crural diaphragm, an external lower esophageal sphincter: a definitive study. Gastroenterology 1993;105:1565–7.
11. Peters JH, Watson TJ, DeMeester TR. Esophagus: anatomy, physiology and gastroesophageal reflux disease. In: Greenfield LJ, editor. Surgery: scientific principles and practice. 3rd edition. Philadelphia: Lippincott Williams and Wilkins; 2001. p. 659–92.
12. Barham CP, Gotley DC, Mills A, et al. Precipitating causes of acid reflux episodes in ambulant patients with gastro-oesophageal reflux disease. Gut 1995;36:505.
13. Iwakiri K, Hayashi Y, Kotoyori M, et al. Transient lower esophageal sphincter relaxations (TLESRs) are the major mechanism of gastroesophageal reflux but are not the cause of reflux disease. Dig Dis Sci 2005;50(6):1072–7.
14. Page AJ, Blackshaw LA. An in vitro study of the properties of vagal afferent fibres innervating the ferret oesophagus and stomach. J Physiol 1998;512(Pt 3):907–16.
15. Gordon C, Kang JY, Neild PJ, et al. The role of the hiatus hernia in gastro-oesophageal reflux disease. Aliment Pharmacol Ther 2004;20:719–32.
16. Boeckxstaens GE, Rohof WO. Pathophysiology of gastroesophageal reflux disease. Gastroenterol Clin North Am 2014;43(1):15–25.
17. Schoenfeld PS. Medical or surgical therapy for GERD. Gastroenterology 2011; 141:1938–45.
18. Fuchs KH, Babic B, Breithaupt W, et al. EAES recommendations for the management of gastroesophageal reflux disease. Surg Endosc 2014;28:1753–73.
19. Arruda SL, Silva Oliveira ML, Figueiredo E. Correlation between hiatus hernia, gastroesophageal reflux disease and body mass index in an obese population. Surg Obes Relat Dis 2010;6(3):S39.
20. Fass R, McCallum RW, Parkman HP. Treatment challenges in the management of gastroparesis-related GERD. Gastroenterol Hepatol 2009;5(10 Suppl 18): 4–16.
21. Penagini R, Bravi I. The role of delayed gastric emptying and impaired oesophageal body motility. Best Pract Res Clin Gastroenterol 2010;24:831–45.
22. Rossetti G, Limongelli P, Cimmino M, et al. Outcome of medical and surgical therapy of GERD: predictive role of quality of life scores and instrumental evaluation. Int J Surg 2014;12(S1):S112–6.
23. Galmiche JP, Hatlebakk J, Attwood S, et al. Laparoscopic antireflux surgery vs esomeprazole treatment for chronic GERD. JAMA 2011;305(19):1969–77.
24. Caestecker J, Cram M. Hiatus hernia and gastro-oesophageal reflux disease. Medicine 2011;39(3):132–6.
25. Talaie R, Forootan M, Donboli K, et al. 24-hour ambulatory pH-metry in patients with refractory heartburn: a prospective study. J Gastrointestin Liver Dis 2009; 18(1):11–5.
26. Spechler SJ, Souza RF. Barrett's esophagus. N Engl J Med 2014;371:836–45.

27. Fiocca R, Mastracci L, Attwood SE, et al. Gastric exocrine and endocrine cell morphology under prolonged acid inhibition therapy: results of a 5-year follow-up in the LOTUS trial. Aliment Pharmacol Ther 2012;36(10):959–71.
28. Meining A, Fackler A, Tzavella K, et al. Lower esophageal sphincter pressure in patients with gastroesophageal reflux diseases and posture and time patterns. Dis Esophagus 2004;17:155–8.
29. Zhang X, Xiang X, Tu L, et al. Esophageal motility in the supine and upright positions for liquid and solid swallows through high-resolution manometry. J Neurogastroenterol Motil 2013;19(4):467–72.
30. Parasa S, Sharma P. Complications of gastro-oesophageal reflux disease. Best Pract Res Clin Gastroenterol 2013;27(3):433–42.
31. Bansal A, Kahrilas PJ. Treatment of GERD complications (Barrett's, peptic stricture) and extra-oesophageal syndromes. Best Pract Res Clin Gastroenterol 2010;24(6):961–8.
32. Patel D, Vaezi MF. Normal esophageal physiology and laryngopharyngeal reflux. Otolaryngol Clin North Am 2013;46:1023–41.
33. Kern E, Lin D, Larson A, et al. Prospective assessment of the diagnostic utility of esophageal brushings in adults with eosinophilic esophagitis. Dis Esophagus 2014. [E-pub ahead of print].
34. Park H. An overview of eosinophilic esophagitis. Gut Liver 2014;8(6):590–7.

Surgical Treatment of Gastroesophageal Reflux Disease

Robert B. Yates, MD[a],*, Brant K. Oelschlager, MD[b]

KEYWORDS

- Gastroesophageal reflux disease • Laparoscopic antireflux surgery • Hiatal hernia
- Fundoplication

KEY POINTS

- Gastroesophageal reflux disease is abnormal distal esophageal acid exposure that results in bothersome symptoms. It is caused by the failure of endogenous antireflux barriers, including the lower esophageal sphincter and esophageal clearance mechanisms.
- Appropriate preoperative patient evaluation increases the likelihood that gastroesophageal reflux disease–related symptoms will improve after laparoscopic antireflux surgery.
- In patients that have a clinical history suggestive of gastroesophageal reflux disease, diagnostic testing should include ambulatory pH monitoring, esophageal manometry, esophagogastroduodenoscopy, and upper gastrointestinal series.
- Correct construction of the fundoplication reduces the risk of postoperative dysphagia caused by an inappropriately tight fundoplication, posterior herniation of gastric fundus, and slipped fundoplication.
- Recurrent symptoms of gastroesophageal reflux disease should be evaluated with esophageal manometry and ambulatory pH testing.
- Reoperative antireflux surgery should be performed by experienced gastroesophageal surgeons.

INTRODUCTION

Gastroesophageal reflux disease (GERD) is the most common benign medical condition of the stomach and esophagus. GERD is defined by abnormal distal esophageal acid exposure that is associated with patient symptoms. Most patients who present to their primary medical doctor with typical GERD symptoms (ie, heartburn and regurgitation) never undergo formal diagnostic evaluation and are effectively managed with nonoperative therapy, specifically proton pump inhibitors (PPIs). PPIs are so effective at decreasing

[a] Department of General Surgery, Center for Videoendoscopic Surgery, University of Washington, 1959 NE Pacific Street, Box 356410/Suite BB-487, Seattle, WA 98195, USA; [b] Division of General Surgery, Department of Surgery, Center for Esophageal and Gastric Surgery, University of Washington, 1959 NE Pacific Street, Box 356410/Suite BB-487, Seattle, WA 98195, USA
* Corresponding author.
E-mail address: rby2@uw.edu

Surg Clin N Am 95 (2015) 527–553
http://dx.doi.org/10.1016/j.suc.2015.02.007
0039-6109/15/$ – see front matter © 2015 Elsevier Inc. All rights reserved.

Abbreviations	
BOS	Bronchiolitis obliterans syndrome
EGD	Esophagogastroduodenoscopy
FEV$_1$	Forced expiratory volume in 1 second
GEJ	Gastroesophageal junction
GER	Gastroesophageal reflux
GERD	Gastroesophageal reflux disease
IPF	Idiopathic pulmonary fibrosis
LARS	Laparoscopic antireflux surgery
LES	Lower esophageal sphincter
PEH	Paraesophageal hernia
PPI	Proton pump inhibitor
UGI	Upper gastrointestinal series

gastric acid production that they provide some improvement in typical GERD-related symptoms in nearly all patients with GERD. Consequently, an empirical trial of PPI therapy has become viewed as both diagnostic and therapeutic for patients that present with typical GERD symptoms. Moreover, improvement in GERD symptoms with the initiation of PPI therapy is considered a predictor of good response to antireflux surgery.

In patients that experience persistent, life-limiting symptoms despite maximal PPI therapy, a formal diagnostic evaluation should be completed. This evaluation includes ambulatory esophageal pH monitoring, esophageal manometry, upper gastrointestinal series (UGI), and esophagogastroduodenoscopy (EGD). For patients who exhibit elevated distal esophageal acid exposure and life-limiting symptoms despite maximal medical therapy, antireflux surgery should be strongly considered. Importantly, patients that experience no improvement in their symptoms with PPI use may not have GERD; surgeons must carefully consider alternative causes before offering surgical treatment. Endoscopic evidence of severe esophageal injury (eg, ulcerations, peptic strictures, and Barrett esophagus) can be considered evidence of gastroesophageal reflux (GER); however, these findings should not be considered an indication for operative therapy by themselves.

The application of laparoscopy to antireflux surgery has decreased perioperative morbidity, hospital length of stay, and cost compared with open operations. Conceptually, laparoscopic antireflux surgery (LARS) is straightforward; however, the correct construction of a fundoplication requires significant operative experience and skills in complex laparoscopy. In patients who present with late complications of antireflux surgery, including recurrent GERD and dysphagia, reoperative antireflux surgery can be effectively performed. Compared with first-time operations, however, reoperative antireflux surgery is technically more challenging, associated with a higher risk for perioperative complications, and results in less durable symptom improvement. Therefore, compared with first-time antireflux surgery, surgeons should have a higher threshold for offering patients reoperation; reoperations should be performed by experienced, high-volume gastroesophageal surgeons.

The purpose of this article is to review the surgical management of GERD, including relevant preoperative and postoperative patient care, operative technique, and the common complications of LARS and their management.

RELEVANT ANATOMY, PHYSIOLOGY, AND PATHOPHYSIOLOGY

Endogenous antireflux mechanisms include the lower esophageal sphincter (LES) and spontaneous esophageal clearance. GERD results from the failure of these endogenous antireflux mechanisms.

The LES has the primary role of preventing reflux of gastric contents into the esophagus. Rather than a distinct anatomic structure, the LES is a zone of high pressure located just cephalad to the gastroesophageal junction (GEJ). The LES can be identified during esophageal manometric evaluation.

The LES is made up of 4 anatomic structures (**Box 1**):

1. The *intrinsic musculature of the distal esophagus* is in a state of tonic contraction. With the initiation of a swallow, these muscle fibers relax and then return to a state of tonic contraction.
2. *Sling fibers of the gastric cardia* are at the same anatomic depth as the circular muscle fibers of the esophagus but are oriented diagonally from the cardia-fundus junction to the lesser curve of the stomach (**Fig. 1**). The sling fibers contribute significantly to the high-pressure zone of the LES.
3. The *crura of the diaphragm* surround the esophagus as it passes through the esophageal hiatus. During inspiration, when intrathoracic pressure decreases relative to intra-abdominal pressure, the anteroposterior diameter of the crural opening is decreased, compressing the esophagus and increasing the measured pressure at the LES.
4. With the GEJ firmly anchored in the abdominal cavity, increased *intra-abdominal pressure* is transmitted to the GEJ, which increases the pressure on the distal esophagus and prevents reflux of gastric contents.

GER occurs when intragastric pressure is greater than the high-pressure zone of the distal esophagus and can develop under two conditions: (1) the LES resting pressure is too low (ie, hypotensive LES) and (2) the LES relaxes in the absence of peristaltic contraction of the esophagus (ie, spontaneous LES relaxation).[1] Small changes in this high-pressure zone can compromise its effectiveness, and GER is a normal physiologic process that occurs even in the setting of a normal LES. Importantly, the distinction between physiologic reflux (ie, GER) and pathologic reflux (ie, GERD) hinges on the total amount of esophageal acid exposure, patient symptoms, and the presence of mucosal damage of the esophagus.

GERD is often associated with a hiatal hernia. Although any type of hiatal hernia may give rise to an incompetent LES, the most common is the type I hiatal hernia, also called a sliding hiatal hernia (**Fig. 2**). A type I hernia is present when the GEJ is not maintained in the abdominal cavity by the phrenoesophageal ligament, a continuation of the endoabdominal peritoneum that reflects onto the esophagus at the hiatus. Thus, the cardia migrates back and forth between the posterior mediastinum and peritoneal cavity. The presence of a small sliding hernia does not necessarily imply an incompetent cardia. Although a patient with typical symptoms of GERD may be found to have a hiatal or paraesophageal hernia (PEH), these hernias are neither necessary nor sufficient to make the diagnosis of GERD; the presence of such a hernia does not constitute an indication for operative correction. In fact, many patients with hiatal hernias do not have symptoms and do not require treatment.

Box 1
The anatomic components of the LES

1. Intrinsic musculature of the distal esophagus

2. Sling fibers of the gastric cardia

3. Diaphragmatic crura at the esophageal hiatus

4. Intra-abdominal pressure exerted on the gastroesophageal junction

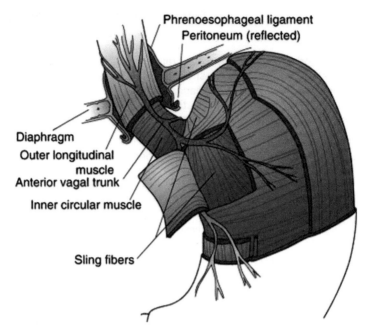

Fig. 1. The muscle layers at the GEJ. The intrinsic muscle of the esophagus, diaphragm, and sling fibers contribute to the LES pressure. The sling fibers of the cardia are located at the same depth as the circular muscle fibers of the esophagus. (*From* Oelschlager BK, Eubanks TR, Pellegrini CA. Hiatal hernis and gastroesophageal reflux disease. In: Townsend CM, Beauchamp RD, Evers MB, et al, editors. Sabiston Textbook of Surgery. 19th edition. Philadelphia: Elsevier; 2012; with permission.)

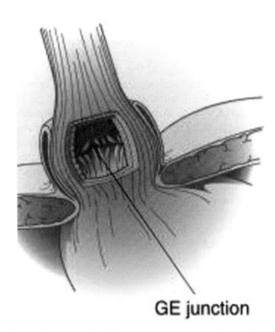

Fig. 2. Type I, or sliding, hiatal hernia. GE, gastroesophageal. (*From* Oelschlager BK, Eubanks TR, Pellegrini CA. Hiatal hernis and gastroesophageal reflux disease. In: Townsend CM, Beauchamp RD, Evers MB, et al, editors. Sabiston Textbook of Surgery. 19th edition. Philadelphia: Elsevier; 2012; with permission.)

CLINICAL PRESENTATION OF GASTROESOPHAGEAL REFLUX DISEASE
Typical Symptoms of Gastroesophageal Reflux Disease

The prevalence of symptoms among 1000 patients with GERD is presented in **Table 1**. Heartburn, regurgitation, and water brash are the 3 typical esophageal symptoms of GERD. Heartburn is very specific to GERD and described as epigastric and/or retrosternal caustic or stinging sensation. Typically, it does not radiate to the back and is not described as a pressure sensation, both of which are more characteristic of pancreatitis and acute coronary syndrome, respectively. It is important to ask patients about their symptoms in detail to differentiate typical heartburn from symptoms of peptic ulcer disease, cholelithiasis, or coronary artery disease.

The presence of regurgitation often indicates progression of GERD. In severe cases, patients will be unable to bend over without experiencing an episode of regurgitation. Regurgitation of gastric contents to the oropharynx and mouth can produce a sour taste that patients will describe as either acid or bile. This phenomenon is referred to as water brash. In patients that report regurgitation as a frequent symptom, it is important to distinguish between regurgitation of undigested and digested food. Regurgitation of undigested food is not common in GERD and suggests the presence of a different pathologic process, such as an esophageal diverticulum or achalasia.

Extraesophageal Symptoms of Gastroesophageal Reflux Disease

Extraesophageal symptoms of GERD arise from the respiratory tract and include both laryngeal and pulmonary symptoms (**Box 2**). Two mechanisms may lead to extraesophageal symptoms of GERD.[2] First, proximal esophageal reflux and microaspiration of gastroduodenal contents cause direct caustic injury to the larynx and lower respiratory tract; this is probably the most common mechanism. Second, distal esophageal acid exposure triggers a vagal nerve reflex that results in bronchospasm and cough. The latter mechanism is caused by the common vagal innervation of the trachea and esophagus.

Unlike typical GERD symptoms (ie, heartburn and regurgitation), extraesophageal symptoms of reflux are not specific to GERD. Before performing LARS, it is necessary to determine whether a patient's extraesophageal symptoms are caused by abnormal GER or a primary laryngeal-bronchial-pulmonary cause. This endeavor can be challenging. A lack of response of extraesophageal symptoms to a trial of PPI therapy

Table 1
Prevalence of symptoms occurring more than once per week among 1000 patients with GERD

Symptom	Prevalence (%)
Heartburn	80
Regurgitation	54
Abdominal pain	29
Cough	27
Dysphagia for solids	23
Hoarseness	21
Belching	15
Bloating	15
Aspiration	14
Wheezing	7
Globus	4

Box 2
Extraesophageal symptoms of GERD

Laryngeal symptoms of reflux

1. Hoarseness/dysphonia

2. Throat clearing

3. Throat pain

4. Globus

5. Choking

6. Postnasal drip

7. Laryngeal and tracheal stenosis

8. Laryngospasm

9. Contact ulcers

Pulmonary symptoms of reflux

1. Cough

2. Shortness of breath

3. Wheezing

4. Pulmonary disease (idiopathic pulmonary fibrosis, chronic bronchitis, asthma, and others)

---

cannot reliably refute GERD as the cause of extraesophageal symptoms. Although PPI therapy can improve or completely resolve *typical* GERD symptoms, patients with *extraesophageal symptoms* experience a variable response to medical treatment.[3–5] This variability may be explained by recent evidence that suggests acid is not the only underlying caustic agent that results in laryngeal and pulmonary injury.[6–8] PPI therapy will suppress gastric acid production; but microaspiration of nonacid refluxate, which contains caustic bile salts and pepsin, can cause ongoing injury and symptoms. Therefore, in patients with extraesophageal symptoms of GERD, a mechanical barrier to reflux (ie, esophagogastric fundoplication) may be necessary to prevent ongoing laryngeal-tracheal-bronchial injury.

In patients that present with abnormal GER and bothersome extraesophageal symptoms, a thorough evaluation must be completed to rule out a primary disorder of their upper or lower respiratory tract. This evaluation should be completed whether or not typical GERD symptoms are also present. At the University of Washington Center for Esophageal and Gastric Surgery, the authors frequently refer patients with extraesophageal symptoms to an otolaryngologist and/or a pulmonologist to determine if a nongastrointestinal condition is present. If nonreflux causes of the extraesophageal symptoms are not identified, then proceeding with an antireflux operation is acceptable. The authors counsel these patients that there is a 70% likelihood of improvement in extraesophageal symptoms following LARS.[9] If a patient's laryngeal or pulmonary symptoms are not caused by abnormal GER, an antireflux operation is not performed.

Pulmonary Disease, Gastroesophageal Reflux Disease, and Antireflux Surgery

Increasing evidence suggests GERD is a contributing factor to the pathophysiology of several pulmonary diseases.[10,11] In their extensive review, Bowrey and colleagues[12] examined medical and surgical antireflux therapy in patients with GERD and asthma.

In these patients, the use of antisecretory medications was associated with improved respiratory symptoms in only 25% to 50% of patients with GERD-induced asthma. Furthermore, less than 15% of these patients experienced objective improvement in pulmonary function. One explanation for these results is that most of these studies lasted 3 months or less, which is potentially too short to see any improvement in pulmonary function. Additionally, in several trials, gastric acid secretion was incompletely blocked by acid suppression therapy, and patients experienced ongoing GERD.

In patients with asthma and GERD, antireflux surgery seems to be more effective than medical therapy at managing pulmonary symptoms. Antireflux surgery is associated with improvement in respiratory symptoms in nearly 90% of children and 70% of adults with asthma and GERD. Several randomized trials have compared histamine-2 receptor antagonists and antireflux surgery in the management of GERD-associated asthma. Compared with patients treated with antisecretory medications, patients treated with antireflux surgery were more likely to experience relief of asthma symptoms, discontinue systemic steroid therapy, and improve peak expiratory flow rate.

Idiopathic pulmonary fibrosis (IPF) is a severe, chronic, and progressive lung disease that generally results in death within 5 years of diagnosis. Recently, the pathophysiology of IPF has been shown to hinge on alveolar epithelial injury followed by abnormal tissue remodeling. Proximal esophageal reflux and microaspiration of acid and nonacid gastric contents has been implicated as one possible cause of alveolar epithelial injury that can lead to IPF.

The incidence of GERD in patients with IPF has been reported to be between 35% and 94%.[13–16] Importantly, typical symptoms of GERD are not sensitive for abnormal reflux in patients with IPF; many patients with IPF do not experience any heartburn, regurgitation, or acid brash.[17] Consequently, the threshold to test for GERD in patients with IPF should be low; several authors have recommended ambulatory pH monitoring in all patients with IPF.[18,19] Several studies have demonstrated that the severity of reflux measured by ambulatory pH monitoring does not seem to be associated with the severity of pulmonary disease in patients with IPF.[20] Therefore, a mildly abnormal pH study does not mean that GERD is playing a minor role in a patient's IPF.

Several studies have investigated the effect of GERD treatment on pulmonary function and survival in patients with IPF. In reviewing the charts of 204 patients with IPF, Lee and colleagues[21] used logistic regression to show that both acid suppression therapy and history of Nissen fundoplication were associated with longer survival and slower pulmonary decline. As previously stated, nonacid reflux has been implicated in both extraesophageal symptoms of reflux as well as IPF. Although PPI use suppresses gastric acid production, it does not prevent reflux of nonacid gastroduodenal contents. In 18 patients with IPF, Kilduff and colleagues[22] demonstrated PPI use was associated with fewer episodes of acid reflux on pH monitoring; however, these patients experienced no change in reported cough severity and were found to have persistent and significant nonacid reflux on esophageal impedance testing. Therefore, in patients with IPF with significant GERD, the argument could be made that a mechanical barrier to both acid and nonacid reflux (ie, LARS) is more appropriate than PPI therapy.

Although very little literature exists on LARS in patients with IPF, it seems to be safe, provide effective control of distal esophageal acid exposure, and may mitigate decline in pulmonary function. Raghu and colleagues[23] published their experience with LARS in one patient with IPF and GERD. During 72 months of follow-up, they demonstrated stabilization of forced vital capacity, diffusion capacity of the lung to carbon monoxide, room air oxygen saturation, and exercise capacity on 6-minute walk test. Although this represents a single case report, these results are profound, given that most patients with IPF would have experienced rapid deterioration in lung function over the study time period.

Linden and colleagues[24] performed LARS on 19 patients with chronic lung disease (14 with IPF) and GERD. No patient deaths occurred within 30 days of the operation. When the 14 patients with IPF who underwent LARS were compared with non-GERD matched controls, there was a significant decrease in supplemental oxygen requirement for patients that underwent LARS. However, no other objective measurements of lung function differed between the groups at a mean follow-up of 15 months. These patients did not undergo postoperative pH monitoring; therefore, potentially ongoing, yet unidentified, reflux could explain these results. At the time of this publication, a National Institutes of Health–funded multicenter prospectively randomized trial in patients with IPF and GERD is comparing LARS with PPI therapy. The results of this study may profoundly impact the management of these patients.

Survival after lung transplant is limited by the function of the transplanted lungs, and bronchiolitis obliterans syndrome (BOS) is a major contributing factor to allograft dysfunction. At 5 years after transplant, BOS can affect up to 80% of lung transplant patients; by 3 years after transplant, it accounts for up to 30% of all deaths.[25] There is increasing evidence that GERD may contribute to BOS. GERD is found in as many as 75% of patients after lung transplant, and it is now viewed as a modifiable risk factor for allograft deterioration. Consequently, it is becoming more common for lung transplant patients to be evaluated for GERD and undergo LARS.

Lung transplant patients are a high operative risk group. Compared with a matched cohort of patients without pulmonary disease undergoing elective LARS, they have a higher overall comorbidity burden and higher rates of diabetes mellitus and chronic renal disease; and pulmonary allografts do not function as well as healthy native lungs.[26] A single-center study found pulmonary transplant patients undergoing LARS have a longer postoperative length of stay (2.89 vs 0.71 days) and higher readmission rate (25% vs 3%) compared with the general population.[27] In a nationwide study using propensity-matched controls without a history of lung transplant, Kilic and colleagues[26] found that lung transplant patients undergoing antireflux surgery had similar rates of postoperative mortality as well as overall and individual morbidity (cardiac, pulmonary, renal, wound, hollow viscous injury). Similar to single-center studies, hospital length of stay and estimated costs of care were higher in lung transplant patients.

In lung transplant patients with GERD, LARS is associated with improved objective measurement of allograft function. Hoppo and colleagues[28] retrospectively reviewed their experience with LARS in 22 lung transplant patients with GERD. After LARS, 91% of patients experienced significant improvement in forced expiratory volume in 1 second (FEV_1). In 12 patients that had decreasing FEV_1 before LARS, 11 patients experienced a reversal of this trend after LARS. Additionally, following LARS, there were fewer episodes of pneumonia and rejection.

DIAGNOSTIC PROCEDURES

Frequently, the diagnosis of GERD is made clinically based on the presence of typical GERD symptoms and improvement in those symptoms with PPI therapy. However, when patients are referred to a surgeon for antireflux surgery, 4 tests are helpful to establish the diagnosis and, thus, should strongly be considered (**Box 3**): (1) Ambulatory pH monitoring confirms the presence of elevated distal esophageal acid exposure. (2) Esophageal manometry identifies esophageal motility disorders that may affect the type of antireflux operation performed. (3) EGD can identify the competence

---

Box 3
Four key diagnostic tests in the evaluation of GERD

1. Ambulatory pH monitoring

2. Esophageal manometry

3. Esophagogastroduodenoscopy

4. Upper gastrointestinal series (esophagram)

---

of the antireflux valve and gastroesophageal mucosal changes (eg, erosive esophagitis and Barrett esophagus). (4) UGI provides the surgeon detailed anatomy of the esophagus and stomach, including the presence of hiatal and PEH.

ADDITIONAL PREOPERATIVE CONSIDERATIONS
Dysphagia

Occasionally, patients with GERD will experience dysphagia. The causes of dysphagia are listed in **Box 4**. In patients with GERD, reflux-associated peptic strictures are pathognomonic for long-standing reflux and develop from the chronic mucosal inflammation that occurs with GERD. When strictures result in significant dysphagia, patients can experience weight loss and protein/calorie malnutrition. Additionally, strictures can be associated with esophageal shortening, which makes obtaining adequate intra-abdominal esophageal length at the time of operation more difficult (see section on Intraoperative Management of Short Esophagus). Since the widespread adoption of PPI therapy in patients with reflux, peptic strictures are much less common.

In patients with peptic strictures, it can be challenging to document GERD on ambulatory pH monitoring because the presence of a tight stricture may prevent reflux of acid, resulting in a false-negative pH study. In patients with typical GERD symptoms and a peptic stricture, it is reasonable to forego ambulatory pH monitoring because the presence of a peptic stricture is considered pathognomonic for severe GER. If pH monitoring is performed, it is ideally completed after dilation of the

---

Box 4
Causes of dysphagia in patients undergoing evaluation for GERD

Esophageal obstruction

1. Peptic strictures

2. Schatzki ring

3. Malignant neoplasm

4. Benign neoplasm

5. Foreign body

Esophageal motility disorders

1. Diffuse esophageal spasm

2. Hypercontractile (nutcracker) esophagus

3. Ineffective esophageal motility

4. Achalasia

---

stricture to increase the validity of the test. Importantly, because they are associated with long-standing GER, peptic strictures should be biopsied to rule out intestinal metaplasia, dysplasia, and malignancy.

Most peptic strictures are effectively treated with dilation and PPI therapy. Successful dilation can be performed with either a balloon dilator or Savary dilator, and no strong data exist to support the superiority of one dilation technique over another. Refractory peptic strictures are defined as strictures that recur after dilation despite PPI therapy. Although rare, refractory strictures can pose significant challenge to surgeons and gastroenterologists. In these patients, LARS should be strongly considered. For patients who are unfit for or do not wish to undergo an operation, steroid injections of the stricture have been shown to result in fewer dilations.[29]

A second common cause of dysphagia in patients with GERD is a Schatzki ring. Similar to peptic strictures, these are located in the distal esophagus. However, Schatzki rings are submucosal fibrotic bands (as opposed to mucosal strictures). Typically, peptic strictures and Schatzki rings can be differentiated on endoscopy. Both should be dilated to relieve obstruction; but Schatzki rings develop in the submucosal space, so in the absence of other endoscopically identified mucosal abnormalities, biopsies do not need to be performed. Furthermore, Schatzki rings are not pathognomonic for GERD, so abnormal distal esophageal acid exposure must be documented on ambulatory pH monitoring to confirm the presence of abnormal GER before performing LARS.

In patients who present with dysphagia and GERD, other causes of dysphagia must be excluded, including tumors, diverticula, and esophageal motor disorders. Although these conditions are much less common than peptic strictures and Schatzki rings, they require dramatically different treatments. In patients that report simultaneous onset of dysphagia to liquids and solids, one must have a high suspicion for a neuromuscular or autoimmune disorder as the cause. Finally, it is important to recognize that some patients with GERD report dysphagia without any anatomic or physiologic abnormality. The authors have found that such patients typically experience improvement in dysphagia following LARS.

Obesity

Obesity is a significant risk factor for the development of GERD. Compared with patients of normal weight, obese patients have increased intra-abdominal pressure, decreased LES pressure, and more frequent transient LES relaxations.[30] Obese patients with GERD present a particular challenge to surgeons. Although it is clear that LARS can be performed safely in obese patients, the literature is mixed on the ability of LARS to provide long-term control of GERD-related symptoms.[30–33] In appropriately selected patients, laparoscopic Roux-en-Y gastric bypass is the most durable method of weight loss and control of obesity-related comorbidities, including GERD.[31,32] In severely obese patients with GERD, serious consideration should be given to performing a laparoscopic Roux-en-Y gastric bypass instead of a fundoplication. Ultimately, the decision to pursue gastric bypass instead of fundoplication must include a careful balance of the patients' interest in bariatric surgery, presence of other medical comorbidities, and availability of a surgeon to perform the operation.

Partial Versus Complete Fundoplication

Antireflux operations include partial posterior (180° and 270°), partial anterior (90° and 180°), and 360° esophagogastric fundoplications. In antireflux surgery, there has been a long-standing debate over which fundoplication provides superior control of GERD symptoms while mitigating postoperative side effects (eg, dysphagia and gas-bloat). Furthermore, studies have attempted to determine whether the type of fundoplication performed should be tailored to the patients' preoperative esophageal motility and symptoms.

In patients with GERD and esophageal dysmotility, it has been suggested that partial fundoplication should be performed because of concern that a Nissen fundoplication will lead to greater postoperative dysphagia. Booth and colleagues[34] completed a randomized controlled trial to compare laparoscopic Nissen fundoplication with Toupet fundoplication in patients who were stratified based on preoperative manometry. At 1 year postoperatively, there were no differences between the Nissen and Toupet groups for heartburn and regurgitation. Dysphagia was more frequent in patients that underwent Nissen fundoplication. However, when a Nissen fundoplication was constructed, patients with normal and impaired esophageal motility experienced similar rates of postoperative dysphagia. Similarly, the authors have shown that a Nissen fundoplication can be performed in patients with ineffective esophageal motility without an increase in development of dysphagia.[35]

Fein and Seyfried[36] reviewed 9 randomized trials that evaluated laparoscopic anterior, partial posterior, and total fundoplications in the management of GERD. Anterior fundoplication was associated with greater risk of recurrent GERD symptoms. Nissen was associated with increased postoperative dysphagia, but these patients required minimal treatment and no reoperations. In the randomized trials reviewed, no difference in gas-bloat symptoms was seen between Nissen and Toupet fundoplication. However, Nissen was associated with more gas-bloat in nonrandomized trials.

Shan and colleagues[37] reviewed 32 studies, including 9 randomized controlled trials, that compared laparoscopic Nissen fundoplication with laparoscopic Toupet fundoplication. No differences were noted between the groups concerning patient satisfaction with the operation or perioperative morbidity and mortality. In 24 studies that assessed postoperative dysphagia, no difference was noted between fundoplication types when esophageal motility was normal. However, in patients with abnormal esophageal motility, laparoscopic Nissen fundoplication was associated with greater rates of dysphagia. An additional analysis was performed that compared rates of dysphagia in patients with normal motility who underwent a Nissen and patients with abnormal motility who underwent a Toupet. In this comparison, the patients who underwent a Nissen fundoplication reported more dysphagia. Finally, this meta-analysis found increased rates of postoperative gas-bloat and an inability to belch in patients that underwent Nissen. This review would suggest that Toupet fundoplication is the treatment of choice, leading to effective GERD symptom control and less postoperative side effects.

As evidenced earlier, despite numerous randomized clinical trials and 2 meta-analyses, there still remains conflicting evidence regarding which fundoplication provides the most durable control of reflux and the best side-effect profile. The reason for this is likely the heterogeneity of these studies in terms of patient characteristics, patient selection, and operative technique. For example, in the studies evaluated by Fein and Seyfried,[36] there were 4 different bougie sizes used (34 F to 60 F); fixation of the stomach to the esophagus and hiatus was inconsistent among surgeons; and division of the short gastric vessels was not always performed. Currently, the only consistent finding in these studies is that anterior fundoplications provide less durable control of GERD than posterior partial and total fundoplications. Otherwise, surgeons should perform the fundoplication that they are most comfortable performing and not tailor the fundoplication type to esophageal dysmotility.

OPERATIVE TECHNIQUE

The authors perform all laparoscopic antireflux operations with patients in the low lithotomy position. This position provides the surgeon improved ergonomics by standing between the patients' legs; the assistant stands at the patients' left. Additionally, patients are placed in steep reverse Trendelenburg position, which allows for an unobstructed view of the esophageal hiatus. Patients are appropriately padded to prevent pressure ulcers and neuropathies. Preoperative antibiotics are administered to reduce the risk of surgical site infection, and subcutaneous heparin and sequential compression devices are used to reduce the risk of venous thromboembolic events.

Access to the abdomen is obtained using a Veress needle at Palmer's point in the left upper quadrant of the abdomen. Three additional trocars and a Nathanson liver retractor are placed. The surgeon operates through the two most cephalad ports, and the assistant operates through the two caudad ports. The liver retractor is placed in the subxiphoid region, just left of the midline (**Fig. 3**).

The authors begin the dissection at the left crus by dividing the phrenogastric membrane and then enter the lesser sac at the level of the inferior edge of the spleen. Doing so allows for early ligation of the short gastric vessels and mobilization of the gastric fundus (**Fig. 4**). After the fundus is mobilized, the left phrenoesophageal membrane is divided to expose the length of the left crus (**Fig. 5**).

Right crural dissection is then performed. The gastrohepatic ligament is divided, and the right phrenoesophageal membrane is opened to expose the right crus. A retroesophageal window is created. Care is taken to preserve the anterior and posterior vagi during this mobilization. A Penrose drain is placed around the esophagus to facilitate the posterior mediastinal dissection and assist with creation of the fundoplication.

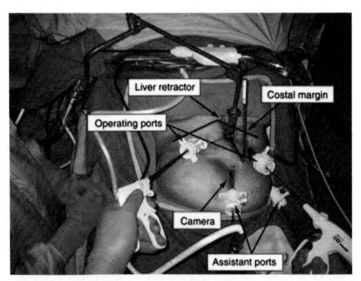

Fig. 3. Port placement for LARS. The surgeon operates through the 2 cephalad ports, and the assistant operates through the 2 caudad ports. A Nathanson liver retractor is placed in the subxiphoid location. (*From* Oelschlager BK, Eubanks TR, Pellegrini CA. Hiatal hernis and gastroesophageal reflux disease. In: Townsend CM, Beauchamp RD, Evers MB, et al, editors. Sabiston Textbook of Surgery. 19th edition. Philadelphia: Elsevier; 2012; with permission.)

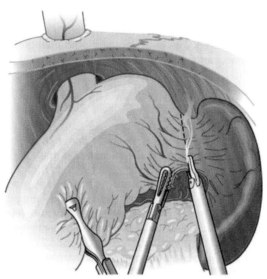

Fig. 4. In the left crus approach to the esophageal hiatus, the fundus of the stomach is mobilized early during the operation to provide early visualization of the spleen, which helps prevent splenic injury. (*From* Oelschlager BK, Eubanks TR, Pellegrini CA. Hiatal hernis and gastroesophageal reflux disease. In: Townsend CM, Beauchamp RD, Evers MB, et al, editors. Sabiston Textbook of Surgery. 19th edition. Philadelphia: Elsevier; 2012; with permission.)

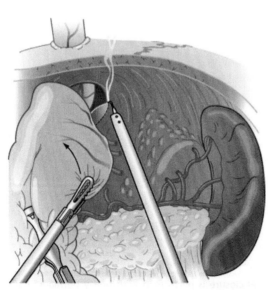

Fig. 5. After the fundus has been mobilized, the phrenoesophageal membrane is incised at the left crus, taking care to avoid injury to the esophagus and posterior vagus. (*From* Oelschlager BK, Eubanks TR, Pellegrini CA. Hiatal hernis and gastroesophageal reflux disease. In: Townsend CM, Beauchamp RD, Evers MB, et al, editors. Sabiston Textbook of Surgery. 19th edition. Philadelphia: Elsevier; 2012; with permission.)

The esophagus is mobilized in the posterior mediastinum to obtain a minimum of 3 cm of intra-abdominal esophagus. Then, the crura are approximated posteriorly with permanent sutures. The esophagus should maintain a straight orientation without angulation, and a 52-F bougie should easily pass beyond the esophageal hiatus and into the stomach (**Fig. 6**). At this point, the fundoplication is created.

Creation of a 360° Fundoplication

When performing a Nissen fundoplication, the most common technical failure is incorrect construction of the fundoplication. The description that follows clearly explains the authors' method of performing a correct, effective, and reproducible Nissen. During creation of the fundoplication, it is necessary to maintain appropriate orientation of the gastric fundus. To do this, the posterior aspect of the fundus is marked with a suture 3 cm distal to the GEJ and 2 cm off the greater curvature (**Fig. 7**). The posterior fundus is then passed behind the esophagus from the patients' left to right. The anterior fundus on the left side of the esophagus is then grasped 2 cm from the greater curvature and 3 cm from the GEJ, and both portions of the fundus are positioned on the anterior aspect of the esophagus. As demonstrated in **Fig. 8**, it is of paramount importance that the two points at which the fundus is grasped are equidistant from the greater curvature. Creation of the fundoplication in this manner decreases the chance of constructing the fundoplication with the body of the stomach, which creates a redundant posterior aspect of the wrap that can impinge on the distal esophagus and cause dysphagia. Using 3 or 4 interrupted permanent sutures, the fundoplication is created to a length of 2.5 to 3.0 cm. Similar to the crural repair, the completed fundoplication should allow the easy passage of a 52-F bougie. After removal of the bougie, the wrap is anchored to the esophagus and crura (**Fig. 8**, inset) to help prevent herniation into the mediastinum and slipping of the fundoplication over the body of the stomach. The suture line of the fundoplication should lie parallel to the right-anterior aspect esophagus.

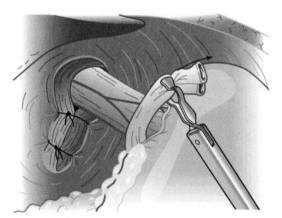

Fig. 6. Posterior crural closure is performed with heavy permanent suture taking care to incorporate the peritoneum into the closure. The exposure is facilitated by displacement of the esophagus anteriorly and to the left using the Penrose drain. (*From* Oelschlager BK, Eubanks TR, Pellegrini CA. Hiatal hernis and gastroesophageal reflux disease. In: Townsend CM, Beauchamp RD, Evers MB, et al, editors. Sabiston Textbook of Surgery. 19th edition. Philadelphia: Elsevier; 2012; with permission.)

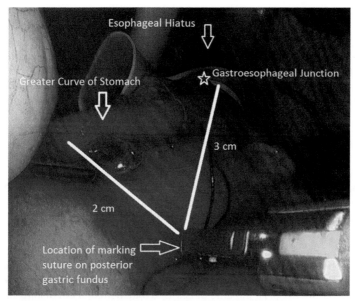

Fig. 7. With the greater curvature of the stomach rotated to the patients right, the posterior stomach is exposed. The authors place a marking stitch on the posterior fundus located 3 cm from the GEJ and 2 cm from the greater curvature to facilitate the creation of a geometrically appropriate Nissen fundoplication.

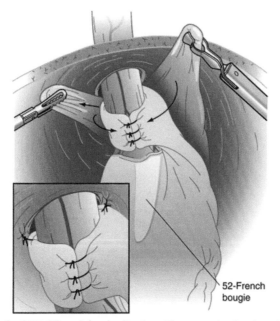

Fig. 8. Creation of a 360° (Nissen) fundoplication. The posterior (patients' *right*) and anterior (patients' *left*) gastric fundus are grasped by the surgeon 3 cm from the GEJ and 2 cm from the greater curvature. The fundoplication is then created over a 52-F bougie and anchored to the diaphragm using permanent sutures (*inset*). (*From* Oelschlager BK, Eubanks TR, Pellegrini CA. Hiatal hernis and gastroesophageal reflux disease. In: Townsend CM, Beauchamp RD, Evers MB, et al, editors. Sabiston Textbook of Surgery. 19th edition. Philadelphia: Elsevier; 2012; with permission.)

Creation of a Partial Fundoplication

There are several types of partial fundoplications. The most commonly performed is the Toupet fundoplication. In this operation, the gastric and esophageal dissections, as well as the repair of the crura, are the same as for a 360° fundoplication. Additionally, the fundoplication must be created with the fundus, and not the body, of the stomach. The key difference is that the stomach is positioned 180° to 270° (compared with 360°) around the posterior aspect of the esophagus (**Fig. 9**). On both sides of the esophagus, the most cephalad sutures of the fundoplication incorporate the fundus, crus, and esophagus; the remaining sutures anchor the fundus to either the crura or the esophagus.

If an anterior fundoplication is to be performed (eg, Thal or Dor), there is no need to disrupt the posterior attachments of the esophagus; the fundus is folded over the anterior aspect of the esophagus and anchored to the hiatus and esophagus (**Fig. 10**).

Intraoperative Management of Short Esophagus

Normal esophageal length exists when the GEJ rests at or below the esophageal hiatus. As the GEJ becomes displaced cephalad to the esophageal hiatus, the esophagus effectively shortens. At the time of LARS, a minimum of 3 cm of intra-abdominal esophagus should be obtained. When the GEJ is mildly displaced cephalad to the GEJ, adequate intra-abdominal esophageal length can be obtained with distal esophageal mobilization in the posterior mediastinum. However, if the GEJ migrates high into the posterior mediastinum, as occurs with a large hiatal or PEH, the effective length of the esophagus can decrease significantly. Furthermore, this process causes adhesions to develop between the esophagus and the mediastinum, which anchor the

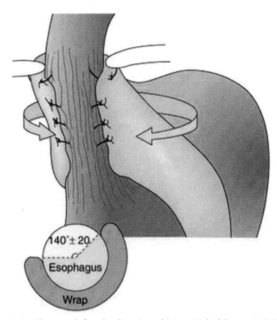

Fig. 9. Partial posterior (Toupet) fundoplication. (*From* Oelschlager BK, Eubanks TR, Pellegrini CA. Hiatal hernis and gastroesophageal reflux disease. In: Townsend CM, Beauchamp RD, Evers MB, et al, editors. Sabiston Textbook of Surgery. 19th edition. Philadelphia: Elsevier; 2012; with permission.)

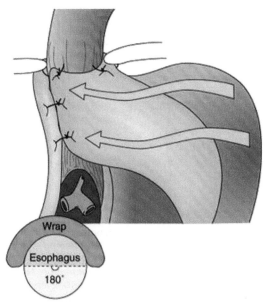

Fig. 10. Partial anterior (Dor) fundoplication. (*From* Oelschlager BK, Eubanks TR, Pellegrini CA. Hiatal hernis and gastroesophageal reflux disease. In: Townsend CM, Beauchamp RD, Evers MB, et al, editors. Sabiston Textbook of Surgery. 19th edition. Philadelphia: Elsevier; 2012; with permission.)

contracted esophagus in the chest. When this occurs, extensive mobilization of the esophagus must be undertaken, sometimes to the level of the inferior pulmonary veins. However, even in the case of large hiatal or PEHS, usually mediastinal dissection alone can return the GEJ to the abdominal cavity.

In some cases, adequate esophageal length cannot be obtained despite extensive mediastinal mobilization of the esophagus. In these rare cases, a unilateral vagotomy provides an additional 1 to 2 cm of esophageal length; division of both vagi typically yields 3 to 4 cm of additional esophagus. Many surgeons hesitate to electively transect the vagi because of concern for patients developing postoperative delayed gastric emptying. However, the authors have shown this not to be the case. In the authors' study of 102 patients who underwent reoperative LARS (*n* = 50) or PEH repair (*n* = 52), they performed a vagotomy in 30 patients (29%) to increase intra-abdominal esophageal length following extensive mediastinal mobilization.[38] Compared with patients that did not undergo vagotomy, patients that underwent vagotomy reported similar severity of abdominal pain, bloating, diarrhea, and early satiety.

Finally, if adequate intra-abdominal esophageal length cannot be accomplished with the aforementioned techniques, a Collis gastroplasty may be performed. A double-staple technique may be used to create the neoesophagus (**Fig. 11**). However, it should be emphasized that in only a very small number of patients have the authors found this technique necessary.

Robotic Antireflux Surgery

In 2000, the Food and Drug Administration approved the da Vinci Surgical System (Intuitive Surgical, Sunnyvale, CA) for general laparoscopic surgery. Touted for providing surgeons with improved manual dexterity, visualization, and ergonomics over traditional laparoscopic surgical equipment, robotic surgery has been widely

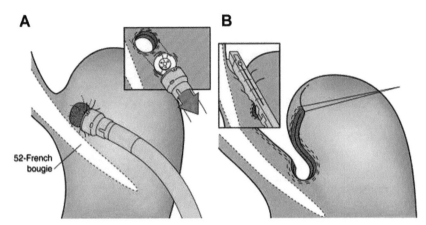

Fig. 11. Double-staple technique for esophageal lengthening. (*A*) A circular stapling and cutting device is used to create a through-and-through opening of the cardia-fundus junction. (*B*) A linear stapling and cutting device is then used to transect the remaining stomach toward the GEJ. (*From* Oelschlager BK, Eubanks TR, Pellegrini CA. Hiatal hernis and gastroesophageal reflux disease. In: Townsend CM, Beauchamp RD, Evers MB, et al, editors. Sabiston Textbook of Surgery. 19th edition. Philadelphia: Elsevier; 2012; with permission.)

advertised and applied to a variety of surgical fields. Markar and colleagues[39] completed a meta-analysis of prospective randomized trials comparing robotic Nissen fundoplication with laparoscopic Nissen fundoplication. They reviewed 6 trials for 3 primary outcome measures (postoperative dysphagia, requirement for reoperation, and mortality) and 4 secondary outcome measures (operative time, operative complications, hospital length of stay, and cost). There were no differences in clinical outcomes between patients that underwent robotic versus laparoscopic Nissen fundoplication. However, both cost of the operation and operative time were greater for robotic Nissen fundoplication. Importantly, none of these studies evaluated postoperative improvement in GERD symptoms, recurrence of GERD symptoms, or normalization of distal esophageal acid exposure. Although it seems robotic Nissen fundoplication is safe, there are no studies that support its clinical superiority over laparoscopy. Furthermore, robotic Nissen fundoplication costs more and takes longer to perform than laparoscopic Nissen fundoplication.

POSTOPERATIVE CARE AND RECOVERY

Except when the patients' comorbid medical conditions dictate otherwise, postoperatively patients are admitted to a general surgical floor without cardiac or pulmonary monitoring. Patients are given a clear-liquid diet the evening of the operation and are advanced to a full-liquid diet on postoperative day 1. Discharge requirements include tolerance of a diet to maintain hydration and nutrition, adequate pain control on oral analgesics, and ability to void without a Foley catheter. After discharge from the hospital, patients can slowly introduce soft foods into their diet; they should expect to resume a diet without limitations in about 4 to 6 weeks.

OPERATIVE COMPLICATIONS AND SIDE EFFECTS OF ANTIREFLUX SURGERY

LARS is a safe operation when performed by experienced surgeons. Mortality rates at 30 days postoperatively are far less than 1%.[40] Rates of general complications vary according to surgeon, technique, and extent of patient follow-up. Since 1993, using the National Inpatient Database, the rate of complications following LARS has fluctuated between 4.7% and 8.3%.[41–43]

These complications are typically minor; not related specifically to LARS; and include urinary retention, wound infection, venous thrombosis, and ileus. Complications that are specific to antireflux surgery include pneumothorax, gastric/esophageal injury, splenic/liver injury, and bleeding. Additionally, LARS can result in postoperative side effects, including bloating and dysphagia. Complications in 400 patients that have undergone LARS at the University of Washington are listed in **Table 2**.

Operative Complications

Pneumothorax
Although pneumothorax is one of the most common intraoperative complications, it is reported to occur in only approximately 2% of patients.[44] Although postoperative chest radiographs are not obtained in all patients, pneumothorax should rarely be missed, as intraoperative identification of pleural violation should be identified. The pleural violation results in intrathoracic infusion of carbon dioxide, which is absorbed rapidly. Because no underlying lung injury exists, the lung will re-expand without incident. When violation of the pleura is identified intraoperatively, the pleural should be closed with a suture, and a postoperative radiograph should be obtained. If a pneumothorax is identified on this radiograph, patients may be maintained on oxygen therapy to facilitate its resolution. Unless patients experience shortness of breath or persistent oxygen therapy to maintain hemoglobin oxygenation saturation, no further radiographs are obtained.

Gastric and esophageal injuries
Gastric and esophageal injuries have been reported to occur in approximately 1% of patients undergoing LARS.[44–46] Typically, these injuries result from overaggressive manipulation of these organs or at the time the bougie is passed into the stomach. Injuries are more likely to occur in reoperative cases and should be rare during initial operations. If identified at the time of operation, repair of these injuries can be performed with suture or stapler without sequelae. If the injury is not identified intraoperatively, patients will likely need a second operation to repair the viscus, unless the leak is small and contained.

Table 2
Complications in 400 laparoscopic antireflux procedures at the University of Washington

Complication	No. of Patients (%)
Postoperative ileus	28 (7)
Pneumothorax	13 (3)
Urinary retention	9 (2)
Dysphagia	9 (2)
Other minor complications	8 (2)
Liver trauma	2 (0.5)
Acute herniation	1 (0.25)
Perforated viscus	1 (0.25)
Death	1 (0.25)
Total:	**72 (17.25)**

Splenic/liver injuries and bleeding

The incidence of splenic parenchymal injury that results in bleeding is about 2.3% in population-based studies, and major liver injury is rarely reported.[47] Although splenic bleeding is relatively uncommon, in rare cases, it can require splenectomy. Most commonly, splenic parenchymal injury occurs during mobilization of the fundus and greater curvature of the stomach. For this reason, the authors prefer to begin laparoscopic Nissen fundoplication with the left crus approach. Dividing the phrenogastric ligament and the short gastric vessels early in the operation provides a direct view of the short gastric vessels and the spleen. Care must be taken during mobilization of the fundus to avoid excessive traction on the splenogastric ligament.

A second type of injury that can occur to the spleen is a partial splenic infarction. This injury typically occurs during transection of the short gastric vessels and inadvertent coagulation of superior pole branch of the main splenic artery.[48] Partial splenic infarction rarely causes any symptoms. Finally, lacerations and subcapsular hematomas of the left lateral section of the liver can be avoided by carefully retracting it out of the operative field using a fixed retractor.

Side Effects

Bloating

The normal swallowing of air is the main factor leading to gastric distention, and the physiologic mechanism for venting this air is belching. Gastric belching occurs via vagal nerve–mediated transient LES relaxation. Following antireflux surgery, patients experience fewer transient LES relaxations[49] and, therefore, decreased belching. Consequently, patients can experience abdominal bloating. Kessing and colleagues[50] investigated the impact of gas-related symptoms on the objective and subjective outcomes of both Nissen and Toupet fundoplications. They demonstrated that preoperative belching and air swallowing was not predictive of postoperative gas-related symptoms, including bloating. They concluded that gas-related symptoms are, in part, caused by gastrointestinal hypersensitivity to gaseous distention. In this study, all patients experienced postoperative normalization of esophageal acid exposure. However, these investigators found that patients who developed postoperative gas symptoms were less satisfied with LARS when compared with patients who did not experience these symptoms.

During the early postoperative period, patients who report persistent nausea or demonstrate inadequate intake of a liquid diet should undergo an abdominal radiograph. If significant gastric distention is identified, a nasogastric tube can safely be placed to decompress the stomach for 24 hours. Few patients require further intervention for gastric bloating.

Dysphagia

It is expected that patients will experience mild, temporary dysphagia during the first 2 to 4 weeks postoperatively. This dysphagia is thought to be a result of postoperative edema at the fundoplication and esophageal hiatus. In most of these patients, this dysphagia spontaneously resolves. A second, but less common, cause of dysphagia is a hematoma of the stomach and/or esophageal wall that develops during the placement of the sutures to create the fundoplication. Although this may create more severe dysphagia, typically it resolves in several days. In both these situations, surgeons should ensure that patients can maintain their nutrition and hydration on a liquid or soft diet; however, additional interventions are rarely needed.

If severe dysphagia exists and patients cannot tolerate liquids, a UGI should be obtained to ensure no anatomic abnormality exists, such as an early hiatal hernia.

Assuming there is no early recurrent hiatal hernia, and patients can tolerate liquids, patience should be used for 3 months. If patients cannot maintain hydration, or dysphagia persists beyond 3 months, a UGI should be obtained to ensure that there is no anatomic abnormality that could explain the dysphagia. If the UGI demonstrates an appropriate positioned fundoplication below the diaphragm, an EGD with empirical dilation of the GEJ may provide relief.

CLINICAL OUTCOMES OF ANTIREFLUX SURGERY

The results of antireflux surgery can be measured by relief of symptoms, improvement in esophageal acid exposure, operative complications, and failures. Several randomized trials with long-term follow-up have compared medical and surgical therapy for GERD (**Table 3**). Spechler and colleagues[51] found that surgical therapy results in good symptom control after a 10-year follow-up. Although they reported 62% of patients in the surgical group were taking antisecretory medications at the long-term follow-up, the indications for this medication use were not necessarily GERD; reflux symptoms did not change significantly when these patients stopped taking these medications.

Lundell and colleagues[52] randomized patients with erosive esophagitis into surgical or medical therapy. Treatment failure was defined as moderate or severe symptoms of heartburn, regurgitation, dysphagia and/or odynophagia, recommencement of PPI therapy, reoperation, or grade 2 esophagitis. At the 7-year follow-up, fewer treatment failures were seen in patients managed with fundoplication than omeprazole (33% vs 53%, $P = .002$). In patients who did not respond to the initial dose of omeprazole,

Table 3			
Randomized controlled trials comparing surgery and medical therapies for GERD			
Study, Year	**Study Groups**	**Follow-up (y)**	**Outcome**
Grant et al,[57] 2008	PPI, $n = 179$ ARS, $n = 178$	1	Reflux score: PPI, 73; ARS, 85; $P<.05$
Lundell et al,[53] 2009	Omeprazole, $n = 71$ ARS, $n = 53$	12	Treatment failure: Omeprazole, 55%; ARS, 47%; $P = .022$
Lundell et al,[52] 2007	Omeprazole, $n = 119$ ARS, $n = 99$	7	Treatment failure: Omeprazole, 53%; ARS, 33%; $P = .002$
Mahon et al,[58] 2005	PPI, $n = 108$ ARS, $n = 109$	1	12-mo GI well-being score: PPI, 35; ARS, 37; $P = .003$ 3-mo DeMeester score: PPI, 17.7; ARS, 8.6; $P<.001$ 3-mo % time pH <4: PPI, 3.8; ARS, 1.4; $P = .002$
Cookson et al,[59] 2005	Omeprazole, $n = 50$ ARS, $n = 50$	1	Cost-analysis: ARS broke even toward end of year 8, with cost differential between ARS and PPI therapy of ≈$1300 at year 5
Spechler et al,[51] 2001	PPI, $n = 91$ ARS, $n = 38$	10	GRACI score: PPI, 83; ARS, 79; $P = .07$

Abbreviations: ARS, Antireflux surgery; GI, gastrointestinal; GRACI, gastroesophageal reflux disease activity index.
   Data from Refs.[51–53,57]

dose-escalation was completed; however, surgical intervention remained superior. Patients treated with fundoplication experienced more obstructive and gas-bloat symptoms (eg, dysphagia, flatulence, inability to belch) compared with the medically treated cohort. At the 12-year follow-up, the durability of these results remained: Patients who underwent fundoplication had fewer treatment failures compared with patients treated with medical therapy (47% vs 55%, $P = .022$).[53]

Over the past 25 years, surgeon experience with LARS has increased dramatically. With increased experience, the durability of symptom improvement has increased and perioperative complications have decreased. This finding is especially true in high-volume centers. In one single-institution study that followed 100 patients for 10 years after LARS, 90% of patients remained free of GERD symptoms.[54] The authors recently published their experience in a cohort of 288 patients undergoing LARS. With a median follow-up of greater than 5 years, symptom improvement for heartburn was 90% and regurgitation was 92%.[55] These results confirm that LARS can provide excellent durable relief of GERD when patients are appropriately selected and excellent technique is used.

FAILED ANTIREFLUX SURGERY

Antireflux surgery fails because of anatomic problems with the fundoplication or the hiatus. These problems include persistent or recurrent hiatal hernia, slipped fundoplication, and incorrectly constructed fundoplication. The most common symptoms of failed LARS are typical symptoms of GERD (ie, heartburn, regurgitation, and water brash sensation) and dysphagia. One large retrospective review of more than 1700 patients that underwent antireflux surgery found that 5.6% of patients ultimately required a reoperation for symptoms of recurrent GERD or dysphagia.[56]

All patients who present with recurrent or persistent symptoms of GERD should be evaluated with esophageal manometry and ambulatory pH study. If the pH study demonstrates elevated distal esophageal acid exposure, then an esophagram and upper endoscopy should be performed. Once the diagnosis of persistent or recurrent GERD is made, treatment with PPI therapy should be instituted. Most of these patients experience resolution of their symptoms with resumption of PPI therapy. If the patients' symptoms are not effectively managed by medical therapy, then reoperation should be performed to create an effective antireflux valve.

The late development of dysphagia following LARS suggests esophageal obstruction. In this setting, esophageal obstruction most frequently results from a recurrent hiatal hernia or a slipped fundoplication. A UGI and EGD should be the initial study obtained in these patients. If a clear anatomic abnormality is visualized (**Fig. 12**), reoperation can be performed without further investigation. If concurrent GERD symptoms are present, ambulatory pH testing should be performed. To achieve resolution of symptoms, reoperation is almost always necessary in these patients.

Some patients experience no improvement, or even worsened symptoms, following LARS. In these patients, poor operative technique is generally the culprit. An incorrectly constructed fundoplication (generally created out of the body of the stomach and not the fundus) fails to treat GER and can cause new-onset gastroesophageal obstructive symptoms. Failure to completely excise the sac of a hiatal or PEH frequently leads to an early recurrence of hiatal hernia. In the authors' experience, patients who present with persistent symptoms or early recurrence of symptoms following LARS typically require operative management. Following appropriate evaluation with pH testing, manometry, UGI, and EGD, patients should undergo operative

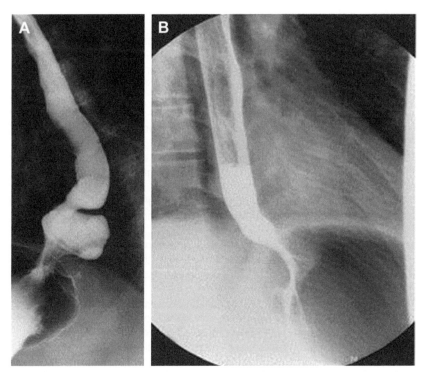

Fig. 12. Esophagram provides excellent assessment of anatomic abnormalities that can cause postoperative dysphagia. (*A*) Patient with dysphagia secondary to postoperative hiatal hernia. (*B*) Normal anatomic appearance of 360° fundoplication. (*From* Oelschlager BK, Eubanks TR, Pellegrini CA. Hiatal hernis and gastroesophageal reflux disease. In: Townsend CM, Beauchamp RD, Evers MB, et al, editors. Sabiston Textbook of Surgery. 19th edition. Philadelphia: Elsevier; 2012; with permission.)

correction of the anatomic problem with creation of an appropriately constructed fundoplication.

It is important to understand that reoperative antireflux surgery comes with higher stakes than first-time antireflux surgery. Tissues are less pliable, making it more challenging for surgeons to construct an effective antireflux valve. In addition, adhesions and less visible tissue planes contribute to increased rates of intraoperative injury of the stomach and esophagus. Consequently, we have a higher threshold to perform reoperative antireflux surgery. With the exceptions described earlier, the authors reserve reoperation for patients with significant symptoms despite maximal nonoperative management.

SUMMARY

Operative treatment of GERD has become more common since the introduction of LARS. Careful patient selection based on symptoms, response to medical therapy, and preoperative testing will optimize the chances for effective and durable postoperative control of symptoms. Complications of the LARS are rare and generally can be managed without reoperation. When reoperation is necessary for failed antireflux surgery, it should be performed by high-volume gastroesophageal surgeons.

REFERENCES

1. Galmiche JP, Janssens J. The pathophysiology of gastro-oesophageal reflux disease: an overview. Scand J Gastroenterol Suppl 1995;211:7–18.
2. Moore JM, Vaezi MF. Extraesophageal manifestations of gastroesophageal reflux disease: real or imagined? Curr Opin Gastroenterol 2010;26(4):389–94.
3. Chang AB, Lasserson TJ, Kiljander TO, et al. Systematic review and meta-analysis of randomised controlled trials of gastro-oesophageal reflux interventions for chronic cough associated with gastro-oesophageal reflux. BMJ 2006; 332(7532):11–7.
4. Vaezi MF, Richter JE. Twenty-four-hour ambulatory esophageal pH monitoring in the diagnosis of acid reflux-related chronic cough. South Med J 1997;90(3): 305–11.
5. Waring JP, Lacayo L, Hunter J, et al. Chronic cough and hoarseness in patients with severe gastroesophageal reflux disease. Diagnosis and response to therapy. Dig Dis Sci 1995;40(5):1093–7.
6. Mainie I, Tutuian R, Shay S, et al. Acid and non-acid reflux in patients with persistent symptoms despite acid suppressive therapy: a multicentre study using combined ambulatory impedance-pH monitoring. Gut 2006;55(10): 1398–402.
7. Vela MF. Non-acid reflux: detection by multichannel intraluminal impedance and pH, clinical significance and management. Am J Gastroenterol 2009;104(2):277–80.
8. Wassenaar E, Johnston N, Merati A, et al. Pepsin detection in patients with laryngopharyngeal reflux before and after fundoplication. Surg Endosc 2011; 25(12):3870–6.
9. Worrell SG, DeMeester SR, Greene CL, et al. Pharyngeal pH monitoring better predicts a successful outcome for extraesophageal reflux symptoms after antireflux surgery. Surg Endosc 2013;27(11):4113–8.
10. Ducoloné A, Vandevenne A, Jouin H, et al. Gastroesophageal reflux in patients with asthma and chronic bronchitis. Am Rev Respir Dis 1987;135(2):327–32.
11. Davis MV. Relationship between pulmonary disease, hiatal hernia, and gastroesophageal reflux. N Y State J Med 1972;72(8):935–8.
12. Bowrey DJ, Peters JH, DeMeester TR. Gastroesophageal reflux disease in asthma: effects of medical and surgical antireflux therapy on asthma control. Ann Surg 2000;231(2):161–72.
13. Bandeira CD, Rubin AS, Cardoso PF, et al. Prevalence of gastroesophageal reflux disease in patients with idiopathic pulmonary fibrosis. J Bras Pneumol 2009; 35(12):1182–9.
14. Raghu G, Freudenberger TD, Yang S, et al. High prevalence of abnormal acid gastro-oesophageal reflux in idiopathic pulmonary fibrosis. Eur Respir J 2006; 27(1):136–42.
15. Salvioli B, Belmonte G, Stanghellini V, et al. Gastro-oesophageal reflux and interstitial lung disease. Dig Liver Dis 2006;38(12):879–84.
16. Tobin RW, Pope CE, Pellegrini CA, et al. Increased prevalence of gastroesophageal reflux in patients with idiopathic pulmonary fibrosis. Am J Respir Crit Care Med 1998;158(6):1804–8.
17. Allaix ME, Fisichella PM, Noth I, et al. Idiopathic pulmonary fibrosis and gastroesophageal reflux. Implications for treatment. J Gastrointest Surg 2014;18(1): 100–4 [discussion: 104–5].
18. Fahim A, Crooks M, Hart SP. Gastroesophageal reflux and idiopathic pulmonary fibrosis: a review. Pulm Med 2010;2011:e634613.

19. Sweet MP, Patti MG, Leard LE, et al. Gastroesophageal reflux in patients with idiopathic pulmonary fibrosis referred for lung transplantation. J Thorac Cardiovasc Surg 2007;133(4):1078–84.
20. Hershcovici T, Jha LK, Johnson T, et al. Systematic review: the relationship between interstitial lung diseases and gastro-oesophageal reflux disease. Aliment Pharmacol Ther 2011;34(11–12):1295–305.
21. Lee JS, Ryu JH, Elicker BM, et al. Gastroesophageal reflux therapy is associated with longer survival in patients with idiopathic pulmonary fibrosis. Am J Respir Crit Care Med 2011;184(12):1390–4.
22. Kilduff CE, Counter MJ, Thomas GA, et al. Effect of acid suppression therapy on gastroesophageal reflux and cough in idiopathic pulmonary fibrosis: an intervention study. Cough 2014;10:4.
23. Raghu G, Yang ST, Spada C, et al. Sole treatment of acid gastroesophageal reflux in idiopathic pulmonary fibrosis: a case series. Chest 2006;129(3):794–800.
24. Linden PA, Gilbert RJ, Yeap BY, et al. Laparoscopic fundoplication in patients with end-stage lung disease awaiting transplantation. J Thorac Cardiovasc Surg 2006;131(2):438–46.
25. D'Ovidio F, Keshavjee S. Gastroesophageal reflux and lung transplantation. Dis Esophagus 2006;19(5):315–20.
26. Kilic A, Shah AS, Merlo CA, et al. Early outcomes of antireflux surgery for United States lung transplant recipients. Surg Endosc 2013;27(5):1754–60.
27. O'Halloran EK, Reynolds JD, Lau CL, et al. Laparoscopic Nissen fundoplication for treating reflux in lung transplant recipients. J Gastrointest Surg 2004;8(1):132–7.
28. Hoppo T, Jarido V, Pennathur A, et al. Antireflux surgery preserves lung function in patients with gastroesophageal reflux disease and end-stage lung disease before and after lung transplantation. Arch Surg 2011;146(9):1041–7.
29. Wong RK, Hanson DG, Waring PJ, et al. ENT manifestations of gastroesophageal reflux. Am J Gastroenterol 2000;95(Suppl 8):S15–22.
30. Luketina RR, Koch OO, Köhler G, et al. Obesity does not affect the outcome of laparoscopic antireflux surgery. Surg Endosc 2014. [Epub ahead of print].
31. Mion F, Dargent J. Gastro-oesophageal reflux disease and obesity: pathogenesis and response to treatment. Best Pract Res Clin Gastroenterol 2014;28(4):611–22.
32. Perez AR, Moncure AC, Rattner DW. Obesity adversely affects the outcome of antireflux operations. Surg Endosc 2001;15(9):986–9.
33. Tekin K, Toydemir T, Yerdel MA. Is laparoscopic antireflux surgery safe and effective in obese patients? Surg Endosc 2012;26(1):86–95.
34. Booth MI, Stratford J, Jones L, et al. Randomized clinical trial of laparoscopic total (Nissen) versus posterior partial (Toupet) fundoplication for gastro-oesophageal reflux disease based on preoperative oesophageal manometry. Br J Surg 2008;95(1):57–63.
35. Oleynikov D, Eubanks TR, Oelschlager BK, et al. Total fundoplication is the operation of choice for patients with gastroesophageal reflux and defective peristalsis. Surg Endosc 2002;16(6):909–13.
36. Fein M, Seyfried F. Is there a role for anything other than a Nissen's operation? J Gastrointest Surg 2010;14(Suppl 1):S67–74.
37. Shan CX, Zhang W, Zheng XM, et al. Evidence-based appraisal in laparoscopic Nissen and Toupet fundoplications for gastroesophageal reflux disease. World J Gastroenterol 2010;16(24):3063–71.
38. Oelschlager BK, Yamamoto K, Woltman T, et al. Vagotomy during hiatal hernia repair: a benign esophageal lengthening procedure. J Gastrointest Surg 2008; 12(7):1155–62.

39. Markar SR, Karthikesalingam AP, Hagen ME, et al. Robotic vs laparoscopic Nissen fundoplication for gastro-oesophageal reflux disease: systematic review and meta-analysis. Int J Med Robot 2010;6(2):125–31.
40. Stefanidis D, Hope WW, Kohn GP, et al. Guidelines for surgical treatment of gastroesophageal reflux disease. Surg Endosc 2010;24(11):2647–69.
41. Wang YR, Dempsey DT, Richter JE. Trends and perioperative outcomes of inpatient antireflux surgery in the United States, 1993-2006. Dis Esophagus 2011; 24(4):215–23.
42. Richter JE. Gastroesophageal reflux disease treatment: side effects and complications of fundoplication. Clin Gastroenterol Hepatol 2013;11(5):465–71 [quiz: e39].
43. Cadiere GB, Himpens J, Rajan A, et al. Laparoscopic Nissen fundoplication: laparoscopic dissection technique and results. Hepatogastroenterology 1997; 44(13):4–10.
44. Bizekis C, Kent M, Luketich J. Complications after surgery for gastroesophageal reflux disease. Thorac Surg Clin 2006;16(1):99–108.
45. Collet D, Cadière GB. Conversions and complications of laparoscopic treatment of gastroesophageal reflux disease. Formation for the Development of Laparoscopic Surgery for Gastroesophageal Reflux Disease Group. Am J Surg 1995; 169(6):622–6.
46. Hunter JG, Smith CD, Branum GD, et al. Laparoscopic fundoplication failures: patterns of failure and response to fundoplication revision. Ann Surg 1999; 230(4):595–604 [discussion: 604–6].
47. Watson DI, de Beaux AC. Complications of laparoscopic antireflux surgery. Surg Endosc 2001;15(4):344–52.
48. Odabasi M, Abuoglu HH, Arslan C, et al. Asymptomatic partial splenic infarction in laparoscopic floppy Nissen fundoplication and brief literature review. Int Surg 2014;99(3):291–4.
49. Bredenoord AJ, Draaisma WA, Weusten BL, et al. Mechanisms of acid, weakly acidic and gas reflux after anti-reflux surgery. Gut 2008;57(2):161–6.
50. Kessing BF, Broeders JAJL, Vinke N, et al. Gas-related symptoms after antireflux surgery. Surg Endosc 2013;27(10):3739–47.
51. Spechler SJ, Lee E, Ahnen D, et al. Long-term outcome of medical and surgical therapies for gastroesophageal reflux disease: follow-up of a randomized controlled trial. JAMA 2001;285(18):2331–8.
52. Lundell L, Miettinen P, Myrvold HE, et al. Seven-year follow-up of a randomized clinical trial comparing proton-pump inhibition with surgical therapy for reflux oesophagitis. Br J Surg 2007;94(2):198–203.
53. Lundell L, Miettinen P, Myrvold HE, et al. Comparison of outcomes twelve years after antireflux surgery or omeprazole maintenance therapy for reflux esophagitis. Clin Gastroenterol Hepatol 2009;7(12):1292–8.
54. Dallemagne B, Weerts J, Markiewicz S, et al. Clinical results of laparoscopic fundoplication at ten years after surgery. Surg Endosc 2006;20(1):159–65.
55. Oelschlager BK, Eubanks TR, Oleynikov D, et al. Symptomatic and physiologic outcomes after operative treatment for extraesophageal reflux. Surg Endosc 2002;16(7):1032–6.
56. Lamb PJ, Myers JC, Jamieson GG, et al. Long-term outcomes of revisional surgery following laparoscopic fundoplication. Br J Surg 2009;96(4):391–7.
57. Grant AM, Wileman SM, Ramsay CR, et al. Minimal access surgery compared with medical management for chronic gastro-oesophageal reflux disease: UK collaborative randomised trial. BMJ 2008;337:a2664.

58. Mahon D, Rhodes M, Decadt B, et al. Randomized clinical trial of laparoscopic Nissen fundoplication compared with proton-pump inhibitors for treatment of chronic gastro-oesophageal reflux. Br J Surg 2005;92(6):695–9.
59. Cookson R, Flood C, Koo B, et al. Short-term cost effectiveness and long-term cost analysis comparing laparoscopic Nissen fundoplication with proton-pump inhibitor maintenance for gastro-oesophageal reflux disease. Br J Surg 2005; 92(6):700–6.

Paraesophageal Hernia

Dmitry Oleynikov, MD[a],*, Jennifer M. Jolley, MD[b]

KEYWORDS

- Hiatal • Paraesophageal • Nissen fundoplication • Hernia • Laparoscopic

KEY POINTS

- A paraesophageal hernia is a common diagnosis with surgery as the mainstay of treatment.
- Accurate arrangement of ports for triangulation of the working space is important.
- The key steps in paraesophageal hernia repair are reduction of the hernia sac, complete dissection of both crura and the gastroesophageal junction, reapproximation of the hiatus, and esophageal lengthening to achieve at least 3 cm of intra-abdominal esophagus.
- On-lay mesh with tension-free reapproximation of the hiatus.
- Anti-reflux procedure is appropriate to restore lower esophageal sphincter (LES) competency.

INTRODUCTION

Hiatal hernias were first described by Henry Ingersoll Bowditch in Boston in 1853 and then further classified into 3 types by the Swedish radiologist, Ake Akerlund, in 1926.[1,2] In general, a hiatal hernia is characterized by enlargement of the space between the diaphragmatic crura, allowing the stomach and other abdominal viscera to protrude into the mediastinum. The cause of hiatal defects is related to increased intra-abdominal pressure causing a transdiaphragmatic pressure gradient between the thoracic and abdominal cavities at the gastroesophageal junction (GEJ).[3] This pressure gradient results in weakening of the phrenoesophageal membrane and widening of the diaphragmatic hiatus aperture. Conditions that are associated with increased intra-abdominal pressure are those linked with all abdominal wall hernias, including obesity, pregnancy, chronic constipation, and chronic obstructive pulmonary disease with chronic cough. There has even been a potential genetic component discovered in the development of hiatal hernias. Specific familial clusters across generations have been identified, indicating a possible autosomal dominant mode of

[a] Center for Advanced Surgical Technology, University of Nebraska Medical Center, 986245 Nebraska Medical Center, Omaha, NE 68198-6245, USA; [b] Department of Surgery, University of Nebraska Medical Center, 986245 Nebraska Medical Center, Omaha, NE 68198-6245, USA
* Corresponding author.
E-mail address: doleynik@unmc.edu

Surg Clin N Am 95 (2015) 555–565
http://dx.doi.org/10.1016/j.suc.2015.02.008
0039-6109/15/$ – see front matter © 2015 Elsevier Inc. All rights reserved.
surgical.theclinics.com

Abbreviations	
EGD	Esophagogastroduodenoscopy
GEJ	Gastroesophageal junction
GERD	Gastroesophageal reflux disease
GI	Gastrointestinal
LES	Lower esophageal sphincter
LUQ	Left upper quadrant
PEH	Paraesophageal hernia

inheritance. Certain evidence has linked a collagen-encoding COL3A1 gene and an altered collagen-remodeling mechanism in the formation of hiatal hernias.[4] This link indicates that there may be both genetic and acquired factors that contribute to the development of hiatal hernias.

Although hiatal hernias were originally only classified into 3 types, the current classification scheme defines 4 types of hiatal or paraesophageal hernias (PEHs).[1] These types are listed next:

Type 1: Sliding hernia, the GEJ migrates into the thorax

Type 2: True PEH or rolling hernia, the herniation of the gastric fundus through a weakness in the phrenoesophageal membrane, the GEJ remains in the normal anatomic location

Type 3: Combination of types 1 and 2, the herniation of the GEJ and stomach into the chest (occasionally they can be larger and are sometimes termed *giant PEHs*)

Type 4: Includes other intra-abdominal viscera, such as colon, small bowel, omentum, or spleen along with the stomach migrating into the chest

Type 1, or sliding hiatal hernias, are the most common type and account for approximately 95% of hiatal hernias. The other 3 types combine to make up the remaining 5% of hiatal hernias.[1] All can be approached with similar preoperative and operative strategies when patients are symptomatic.

CLINICAL PRESENTATION

Although the true prevalence of these hernias is difficult to determine because they are often asymptomatic or poorly defined, more recent epidemiologic studies have shown them to be more common than previously recognized in the Western population.[4] Typical patients are female and elderly, more commonly in or beyond their sixth decade of life. They may present with vague symptoms of intermittent epigastric pain and postprandial fullness. Sliding hiatal hernias are most commonly associated with gastroesophageal reflux disease (GERD). Large hiatal defects tend to present with symptoms of progressive intolerance to solids/liquids with regurgitation, nausea, and vomiting. These defects can also present with symptoms related to the space they occupy, such as chest pain and respiratory problems caused by lung compression or aspiration. These respiratory issues may include shortness of breath, asthma, and bronchitis. Other unpredictable symptoms that may be revealed with a thorough history include hoarseness, cough, laryngitis, and pharyngitis.[4] An unusual cause of gastrointestinal (GI) bleeding and iron deficiency anemia is Cameron lesions related to hiatal hernias. These lesions are linear gastric ulcers or erosions located on the gastric mucosal folds at the diaphragmatic impression of large hiatal hernias.[5] Cameron lesions are prevalent in 5% of patients with a hiatal hernia discovered on upper endoscopy, and the risk of one existing increases with hernia size.[5] More acute complications of PEHs are mechanical problems, such as gastric obstruction, volvulus, incarceration, and strangulation, which require urgent surgical intervention. These problems may be seen in patients who present with obstructive symptoms of new-onset dysphagia, chest pain, and early satiety. There is a well-known triad, Borchardt triad, associated with gastric volvulus that one should look for in patients: epigastric pain, inability to vomit, and failure to pass a nasogastric tube into the stomach.[2] Some long-term effects of hiatal hernias are the development of severe reflux with associated erosive esophagitis, Barrett esophagus, and an increased risk of subsequent esophageal cancer.[4] All symptomatic patients are recommended to undergo PEH repair if deemed to be a good surgical candidate.

PREOPERATIVE EVALUATION

Hiatal hernias may be discovered incidentally on lateral chest radiographs as a retrocardiac bubble or during the work-up of unexplained upper GI symptoms, cardiac, or respiratory symptoms. The evaluation of these patients should follow a standard protocol in all instances including a complete history and physical. The history may reveal symptoms that were not previously apparent. The physical examination of these patients is usually unremarkable unless they are having acute complications related to the hiatal hernia. The best diagnostic study to determine the presence and size of the hernia is an upper GI barium study. It can also demonstrate associated esophageal motility dysfunction or stricture/stenosis related to long-standing GERD.[4] Esophagogastroduodenoscopy (EGD) is essential to evaluating esophageal length and the mucosa of the herniated stomach for any other abnormal pathology, such as ulcers, esophagitis, gastritis, Barrett esophagus, or neoplasms. EGDs should be performed on all patients who are being evaluated for PEH repair in order to better understand the important anatomic landmarks specific to each patient. Esophageal manometry is also essential to assess esophageal motility and lower esophageal sphincter (LES) characteristics (pressure, relaxation, and location), which may alter the operative approach with regard to the choice of fundoplication performed. Although not essential in the preoperative evaluation, an esophageal pH study can help to provide a quantitative analysis of reflux episodes by correlating pH with a patient's subjective complaints of reflux.[3] Often, because these patients are elderly, they have significant comorbidities that require further evaluation, specifically with regard to the assessment of cardiac and respiratory status. With the help of anesthesia, cardiology, and pulmonology preoperative consultations, the necessary additional studies (such as cardiac stress tests or pulmonary function tests) are obtained. All of these examinations help to determine whether or not patients are suitable surgical candidates.

TREATMENT

Most patients who are found to be symptomatic from a hiatal hernia will have experienced little relief for their upper GI symptoms with over-the-counter antacids, histamine receptor antagonists, or proton pump inhibitors. Although it is good to continue these medications to help control symptoms, the definitive management of PEHs is surgery. Historically PEHs were treated with a thoracotomy or laparotomy; but the laparoscopic transabdominal approach has become the gold standard for repair of all hiatal hernias. The first laparoscopic PEH repair was reported in 1991 and continues to evolve with respect to variations in technique, including removal or reduction of the hernia sac, the use of mesh to reinforce the cruroplasty, and whether or not to incorporate an antireflux procedure. Despite these controversies in practice, certain basic tenants exist in laparoscopic hiatal hernia repair: reduction of the hernia sac and its contents, complete dissection of both crura and the GEJ, tension-free reapproximation of the hiatus, and adequate mobilization of the esophagus to achieve at least 3 cm of intra-abdominal esophagus.[3]

LAPAROSCOPIC PARAESOPHAGEAL HERNIA REPAIR PROCEDURE

1. Proper and secure patient placement
   a. Patients are placed in a supine position with both arms tucked and appropriately padded in order to minimize neurologic injury.
   b. Placement of a Foley catheter is important for accurate measurement of urine output, as the procedure may be lengthy.
   c. The author uses a footboard at the base of the bed and a belt strap at the waist for steep reverse Trendelenburg positioning.
   d. The video monitor is located at the head of the bed so that both operators can watch one screen.
   e. An orogastric tube is inserted before beginning the operation for stomach decompression.
   f. Each patient receives preoperative antibiotics and chemical and mechanical venous thromboembolism prophylaxis.
2. Accurate arrangement of ports for triangulation of the working space in the hiatus (**Fig. 1**)
   a. Reminder: The esophageal hiatus is slightly to the patients' left; both it and the mediastinum will be more cephalad after insufflation, so it is necessary to ensure that the trocars are placed high enough and more to the left on the patients' abdominal wall.
   b. The author makes a 2-mm incision in the left upper quadrant (LUQ) and then uses a Veress needle to enter the abdomen.
   c. Once the Veress needle is confirmed to be intra-abdominal via a saline drop test, the author then insufflates to a pressure of 15 mm Hg with carbon dioxide to create pneumoperitoneum.
   d. The author proceeds by placing an 11-mm visualization trocar approximately 10 cm superior and 2 cm lateral to umbilicus (to the patients' left) and then 3 more working ports (11 mm in LUQ, 11 mm more lateral on the left, and a 5 mm in right upper quadrant, which will go through the falciform ligament) and then a Nathanson liver retractor through a 5-mm epigastric incision. This placement is shown in **Fig. 2**.
3. Complete reduction of the hernia sac
   a. Once the ports are in and the liver retractor has been placed, patients are put in steep reverse Trendelenburg and a right-side-down position to optimize the view of the hiatus.
   b. Pull the contents of the hernia sac down below the diaphragm.
   c. Start with a left crus approach using a bipolar energy device to divide the short gastrics beginning approximately at the level of the inferior splenic pole.
   d. Dissect out the left crus at the angle of His and then begin to enter the mediastinal space in the avascular plane directly anterior to the aorta (**Fig. 3**).
   e. Key: Identify the anterior vagus nerve and left pleura as you begin to dissect anteriorly and superiorly in the mediastinal space.
   f. Continue to dissect circumferentially and anterior to the esophagus until you see the medial edge of the right crus (**Fig. 4**).
   g. Switch the dissection to other side and use the bipolar energy device to divide the gastrohepatic ligament.

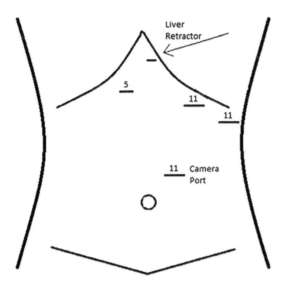

Fig. 1. Port placement.

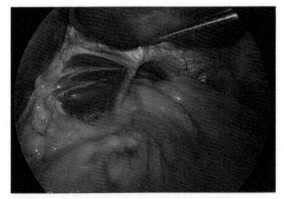

Fig. 2. Large type 3 PEH.

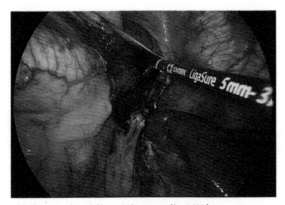

Fig. 3. Dissection of left crus. (Covidien, Minneapolis, MN.)

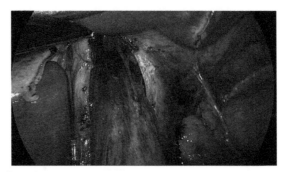

Fig. 4. Anterior dissection.

    h. Continue the dissection just medial to the right crus, starting at the decussation and moving anteriorly, always being aware of the location of the posterior vagus nerve.

    i. A retroesophageal window is created, and a Penrose drain is inserted into this posterior plane in order to have more traction on the esophagus and stomach by the assistant.

4. Extensive mediastinal dissection in order to obtain 3 cm of intra-abdominal esophagus

    a. This step is the important step necessary to achieve adequate esophageal length and avoid having to perform a Collis gastroplasty with its potential associated complications (**Fig. 5**).

    b. This step can be aided with removal of the orogastric tube, which helps in esophageal retraction.

    c. Electrocautery with the hook is advantageous for dissection in this area, as there are often vascular attachments here.

5. Creation of a tension-free posterior cruroplasty with mesh reinforcement

    a. Use a series of interrupted sutures placed posterior to the esophagus every 5 to 8 mm, ensuring adequate bites of tissue on both crura.

    b. For the last 2 sutures, the author decreases the pneumoperitoneum to approximately 8 mm Hg in order to decrease the tension at this point (**Fig. 6**).

    c Secure the absorbable mesh to the right and left crus and posteriorly in a U-shaped, overlay fashion in order to buttress the cruroplasty (**Fig. 7**).

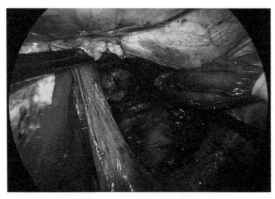

Fig. 5. Complete reduction of hernia sac and esophageal mobilization.

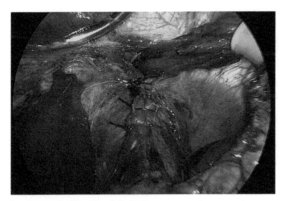

Fig. 6. Plication of crura and closure of defect.

6. Proceed with antireflux procedure
   a. The author chooses between a standard Nissen and Toupet fundoplication based on the results of the preoperative esophageal manometry tests. If there seems to be inadequate esophageal motility, then the author uses a Toupet fundoplication in order to decrease potential postoperative dysphagia.
   b. Start by finding a location on the greater curvature of the stomach that is 3 cm distal and posterior to the GEJ. The author generally marks this spot with a clip.
   c. Then use the standard shoeshine maneuver in order to create a floppy, symmetric fundoplication.
   d. The wrap is secured with interrupted sutures, approximately 2 cm apart, either to the opposing side of the stomach or to the esophagus depending on whether it is a Nissen or Toupet, respectively. (The Penrose is removed after the first suture.)
   e. The fundoplication is then secured to the hiatus via stitches on both crura taking bites of the wrap, esophagus, and diaphragm (**Fig. 8**).
7. Perform routine completion endoscopy
   a. It is used to confirm smooth entry into the stomach at the GEJ and also to visualize a complete, symmetric wrap on retroflexion (**Fig. 9**).
8. Postoperatively
   a. The patients are started on a clear-liquid diet on postoperative day 0 and advanced the next day to a soft mechanical diet.

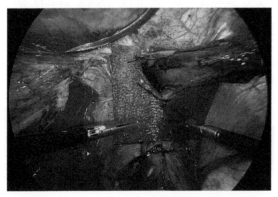

Fig. 7. Mesh insertion and retraction of esophagus with Penrose drain.

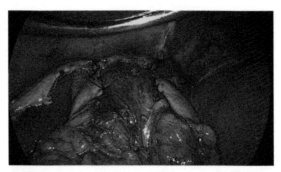

Fig. 8. Toupet fundoplication.

b. An upper GI is not routinely performed postoperatively, and usually patients are discharged home on postoperative day 1.
c. Patients will continue a soft diet for the first 2 weeks until they are seen for their first postoperative follow-up visit in the clinic.
d. All patients are routinely seen again in the clinic at 6 months and 12 months postoperatively.

KEY TECHNICAL POINTS IN LAPAROSCOPIC PARAESOPHAGEAL HERNIA REPAIR

1. Complete reduction of the hernia sac after careful dissection
2. Identification of the GEJ and both crura
3. Obtaining adequate intra-abdominal esophageal length, at least 3 cm
4. Tension-free reapproximation of the crura, using onlay mesh
5. Creation of an antireflux procedure to help restore LES competency and secure the repair
6. Completion endoscopy to ensure proper fundoplication technique

CONTROVERSIES IN TECHNIQUE

Most surgeons now accept that laparoscopic PEH repair, as opposed to open repair, is the standard of care. It provides better visibility during the mediastinal dissection allowing for greater esophageal lengthening and a decreased need to perform a Collis gastroplasty. In addition, patients have shorter hospital stays, faster recovery times, reduced pulmonary complications, and less morbidity compared with open PEH repair. Draaisma and colleagues,[6] in their review of the literature regarding

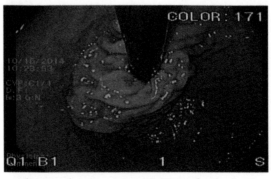

Fig. 9. Completion endoscopy showing symmetric Nissen fundoplication.

laparoscopic versus open PEH repair, found the overall median hospital stay to be 3 days in the laparoscopic group and 10 days for the conventional open patients. The median morbidity rate was 4.3% in the laparoscopically treated patients, which was less than the 16.2% median morbidity rate in the open group. Although not demonstrated in all studies, one area in which the laparoscopic PEH repair has been shown to be less superior than the open repair is in recurrence rates. Thus, modifications have been made to the technical aspects of this surgery in order to lower the recurrence rates, some of which are controversial. These controversial techniques include topics such as complete removal of the hernia sac, the need to perform an antireflux procedure, placement of a gastrostomy tube or gastropexy, or the use of mesh (and which type is best) to reinforce the cruroplasty.

At the University of Nebraska Medical Center, the performance of an antireflux procedure with laparoscopic PEH repair is the standard of care. It not only helps to prevent recurrence but also aids in reestablishing the LES pressure. Most patients with PEHs present with symptoms of reflux that can be improved with a fundoplication. Based on preoperative 24-hour pH studies and manometry, 60% to 100% of these patients will have GERD and/or decreased LES pressure.[2] In addition, during the transhiatal dissection, disruption of the normal anatomy of the LES occurs and, thus, a fundoplication helps to restore this and preemptively treat subsequent postoperative reflux. A prospective study performed in 2011 divided 60 patients into 2 groups based on preoperative evaluation: those who received a fundoplication and those who underwent an Allison-type repair. Their results indicated an increased incidence of new-onset esophagitis in the group with no fundoplication compared with the patients who received a fundoplication, 28% versus 7%, respectively. It also showed an increase in the number of abnormal pH tests postoperatively in the group without a fundoplication, from 29% preoperatively to 44% after surgery.[7] Besides combatting postoperative reflux, the fundoplication may act as an anchor to keep the stomach below the diaphragm and reduce hernia recurrence. The preoperative manometry studies help to determine which fundoplication, either a Nissen or a Toupet, will be best suited for patients. If patients have any esophageal dysmotility, then a Toupet fundoplication is chosen as the more appropriate antireflux procedure.[8] Many studies have published lower dysphagia rates after Toupet fundoplication compared with Nissen with little difference in control of GERD after 1 to 5 years of follow-up.[9] An antireflux procedure, whether a Nissen or a Toupet, is key to restoring the mechanical barrier to reflux and should be part of all laparoscopic PEH repairs.

The use of mesh and what type of mesh are other areas of PEH repair that are debated by surgeons. Certain comparative studies have shown that patients with a prosthetic hiatal closure have a lower rate of postoperative hiatal hernia recurrence in comparison with patients with simple hiatal repair in laparoscopic PEH repair operations.[10] There are concerns, however, with using a prosthetic mesh because of the associated complications, such as adhesion formation, mesh contraction, foreign-body reaction, and tissue erosion that may lead to revision surgery.[11] Another problem associated with mesh hiatoplasty is the increased frequency of patients complaining of late dysphagia with a prevalence of up to 13%.[12] A review of 28 cases of mesh-related complications by Stadlhuber and colleagues[13] demonstrated reoperative findings of intraluminal mesh erosion (n = 17), esophageal stenosis (n = 6), and dense fibrosis (n = 5). There was no relationship in this study to any particular mesh, as these complications occurred in patients who had undergone hiatal hernia repair with polypropylene, polytetrafluoroethylene, biologic, or dual mesh and subsequently presented with symptoms of dysphagia, heartburn, chest pain, fever, epigastric pain, and weight loss. The choice to use absorbable mesh in the place of synthetic meshes is to minimize some of these morbidities. In the literature review by Antoniou and colleagues,[12] porcine dermal collagen mesh was shown by several studies to have decreased adhesion formation and fibrosis and enhanced neovascularization, which demonstrate the advantages of biologic implants over synthetic meshes. Oelschlager and colleagues[14] investigated the use of porcine small intestinal submucosa as a biologic mesh to supplement laparoscopic PEH repair in a multicenter, prospective trial consisting of 108 patients who were randomized to repair with or without this onlay, keyhole-shaped biologic mesh. After 6 months, 90% of the study group underwent upper gastrointestinal series testing; the results indicated a significant reduction in recurrence rates in the mesh patient population versus the nonmesh group (9% compared with 24%, respectively) without any mesh-related complications.[12,14] One study by Schmidt and colleagues[15] compared mesh repair (onlay biologic) versus primary suture repair among 70 patients with small hiatal defects less than 5 cm. At 1 year after surgery, the patients were studied with a barium swallow and/or EGD to assess for recurrence. For the suture cruroplasty group, 5 of 32 patients (16%) demonstrated recurrence, whereas none of the 38 patients that had crural reinforcement with absorbable mesh recurred ($P = .017$). Lee and colleagues[16] studied the results of using human acellular dermal matrix mesh in laparoscopic hiatal hernia repair in 52 patients after 1 year and demonstrated a recurrence rate of only 3.8% and no mesh-related complications. An absorbable mesh cruroplasty helps to decrease the early recurrence rate of PEHs after laparoscopic repair without increasing the complication rate. Further studies are necessary to help determine the long-term recurrence rates and their significance after laparoscopic PEH repair with absorbable mesh.

SUMMARY

The treatment of PEHs is challenging. They tend to occur in patients in their 60s and 70s with multiple medical problems and a variety of associated symptoms. Detailed preoperative evaluation is crucial to determining a safe and effective strategy for repair in the operating room. Laparoscopic PEH repair has shown to be advantageous compared with conventional open repair with regard to hospital stay, recovery time, and decreased complications. Although some results indicate there are higher recurrence rates in laparoscopic PEH repair, the clinical significance of these recurrences has not yet been determined. In order to maximize the efficacy of this procedure, modifications have emerged, such as performing a fundoplication and using an absorbable mesh onlay to reinforce the cruroplasty. Although more prospective, randomized studies are needed to support the superior results of these surgical adjuncts, laparoscopic PEH repair with an antireflux procedure and absorbable mesh should be the current standard of care.

REFERENCES

1. Arafat FO, Teitelbaum EN, Hungness ES. Modern treatment of paraesophageal hernia: preoperative evaluation and technique for laparoscopic repair. Surg Laparosc Endosc Percutan Tech 2012;22(4):297–303.
2. Auyang E, Oelschlager B. Laparoscopic Paraesophageal Hernia Repair. In: Swanstrom L, Soper N, editors. Mastery of Endoscopic and Laparoscopic Surgery, Chapter 23. Philadelphia: Lippincott Williams & Wilkins; 2013. p. 222–30.
3. Oleynikov D, Ranade A, Parcells J, et al. Paraesophageal Hernias and Nissen Fundoplication. In: Oleynikov D, Bills ND, editors. Robotic Surgery for the General Surgeon, Chapter 6. Hauppauge (NY): Nova Science Publishers; 2014. p. 65–74.

4. Tiwari M, Tsang A, Reynoso J, et al. Options for large hiatal defects. In: Murayama KM, Chand B, Kothari S, et al, editors. Evidence-Based Approach to Minimally Invasive Surgery. Woodbury (CT): Cine-Med, Inc; 2011. p. 47–56.

5. Maganty K, Smith RL. Cameron lesions: unusual cause of gastrointestinal bleeding and anemia. Digestion 2008;77(3–4):214–7.

6. Draaisma WA, Gooszen HG, Tournoij E, et al. Controversies in paraesophageal hernia repair: a review of literature. Surg Endosc 2005;19(10):1300–8.

7. DeMeester SR. Laparoscopic paraesophageal hernia repair: critical steps and adjunct techniques to minimize recurrence. Surg Laparosc Endosc Percutan Tech 2013;23(5):429–35.

8. Soper NJ, Teitelbaum EN. Laparoscopic paraesophageal hernia repair: current controversies. Surg Laparosc Endosc Percutan Tech 2013;23(5):442–5.

9. Stefanidis D, Hope WW, Kohn GP, et al. Guidelines for surgical treatment of gastroesophageal reflux disease. Surg Endosc 2010;24(11):2647–69.

10. Granderath FA, Carlson MA, Champion JK, et al. Prosthetic closure of the esophageal hiatus in large hiatal hernia repair and laparoscopic antireflux surgery. Surg Endosc 2006;20(3):367–79.

11. Davis SS Jr. Current controversies in paraesophageal hernia repair. Surg Clin North Am 2008;88(5):959–78, vi.

12. Antoniou SA, Pointner R, Granderath FA. Hiatal hernia repair with the use of biologic meshes: a literature review. Surg Laparosc Endosc Percutan Tech 2011; 21(1):1–9.

13. Stadlhuber RJ, Sherif AE, Mittal SK, et al. Mesh complications after prosthetic reinforcement of hiatal closure: a 28-case series. Surg Endosc 2009;23(6): 1219–26.

14. Oelschlager BK, Barreca M, Chang L, et al. The use of small intestine submucosa in the repair of paraesophageal hernias: initial observations of a new technique. Am J Surg 2003;186(1):4–8.

15. Schmidt E, Shaligram A, Reynoso JF, et al. Hiatal hernia repair with biologic mesh reinforcement reduces recurrence rate in small hiatal hernias. Dis Esophagus 2014;27(1):13–7.

16. Lee YK, James E, Bochkarev V, et al. Long-term outcome of cruroplasty reinforcement with human acellular dermal matrix in large paraesophageal hiatal hernia. J Gastrointest Surg 2008;12(5):811–5.

Endoscopic Dilatation, Heller Myotomy, and Peroral Endoscopic Myotomy
Treatment Modalities for Achalasia

Marco E. Allaix, MD, PhD[a], Marco G. Patti, MD[b],*

KEYWORDS

- Achalasia • Endoscopic botulinum toxin injection • Pneumatic dilatation • Myotomy
- Fundoplication • POEM • Dysphagia • Reflux

KEY POINTS

- Endoscopic botulinum toxin injection (EBTI) should be used only in patients who cannot be treated with pneumatic dilatation (PD) or surgery.
- The short-term results of PD are similar to those of surgery. The available literature, however, suggests that the effect of surgery is for a longer duration.
- Laparoscopic Heller myotomy (LHM) is the approach of choice for achalasia in most centers.
- A partial fundoplication is associated with a lower risk of postoperative reflux compared with myotomy alone.
- A partial fundoplication achieves better functional results than a total fundoplication, with lower rates of postoperative dysphagia.
- There are no significant differences in reflux control after partial anterior or partial posterior fundoplication.
- Peroral endoscopic myotomy (POEM) is a novel promising approach to achalasia with good short-term outcomes.

INTRODUCTION

Esophageal achalasia is a primary esophageal motility disorder characterized by the absence of esophageal peristalsis and failure of the lower esophageal sphincter (LES) to relax in response to swallowing. In about 50% of patients, the LES is

Conflict of Interest: The authors have no conflicts of interest to declare.
[a] Department of Surgical Sciences, University of Torino, Corso A. M. Dogliotti 14, Torino 10126, Italy; [b] Center for Esophageal Diseases, Department of Surgery, University of Chicago Pritzker School of Medicine, 5841 South Maryland Avenue, MC 5095, Room G-207, Chicago, IL 60637, USA
* Corresponding author.
E-mail address: mpatti@surgery.bsd.uchicago.edu

hypertensive. These abnormalities lead to impaired emptying of food from the esophagus into the stomach with consequent food stasis.

This article reviews the most clinically relevant aspects of both diagnosis and management of patients with achalasia, focusing on the several treatment modalities available.

PATHOPHYSIOLOGY

Esophageal achalasia is a rare disease that can occur at any age, even though it is more frequent between 30 and 60 years.[1] The cause is unknown; however, the following 2 theories have been proposed:

1. A degenerative disease of the neurons
2. Infections of the neurons by a virus or another agent, such as *Trypanosoma cruzi.*

In patients with achalasia, the degeneration of the myenteric plexus leads to loss of the postganglionic inhibitory neurons, which mediate LES relaxation by producing nitric oxide and vasoactive intestinal polypeptide. As a consequence, there is unopposed cholinergic stimulation by postganglionic cholinergic neurons, which increases LES resting pressure and decreases LES relaxation. There is no propagation of peristaltic waves in response to swallowing, but rather the presence of simultaneous contractions.[2]

CLINICAL PRESENTATION

- Dysphagia is present in about 95% of patients with achalasia. Often, it occurs for both solids and liquids.
- Regurgitation of retained and undigested food and saliva is the second most frequent symptom, being reported by about 60% of patients. Aspiration of esophageal contents can lead to respiratory symptoms including cough, hoarseness, wheezing, and recurrent episodes of pneumonia.
- Heartburn is present in about 40% of patients, and it is secondary to stasis and fermentation of undigested food in the esophageal lumen.
- Chest pain occurs in about 40% of patients, usually at the time of a meal, and it is probably caused by esophageal distention.

DIAGNOSTIC PROCEDURES

- Upper endoscopy is usually the first test that is performed in patients presenting with dysphagia for ruling out a stricture secondary to gastroesophageal reflux or cancer.
- Barium swallow shows narrowing at the level of the gastroesophageal junction, the presence of an air-fluid level secondary to slow esophageal emptying, and tertiary contractions of the esophageal wall (**Fig. 1**). The barium swallow defines both diameter and axis of the esophagus and reveals the presence of associated pathologic findings, such as an epiphrenic diverticulum.
- Esophageal manometry is the gold standard for the diagnosis of achalasia. Absence of esophageal peristalsis and impaired relaxation of the LES in response to wet swallows are the key criteria for the diagnosis of achalasia. With the adoption of high-resolution manometry (HRM), a new classification of esophageal achalasia has been proposed with 3 distinct manometric patterns: type I, classic, with minimal esophageal pressurization; type II, with panesophageal pressurization; and type III, with spasm, characterized by rapidly propagated esophageal pressurization attributable to spastic contractions (**Fig. 2**).[3]

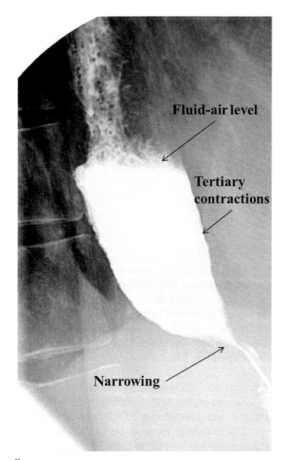

Fig. 1. Barium swallow.

Patients with type II achalasia have the best prognosis, because they are significantly more likely to respond to PD or LHM than patients with type I or type III achalasia.[4] These 3 subtypes may represent 3 distinct pathophysiologic conditions, thus explaining some of the observed variability in treatment response.

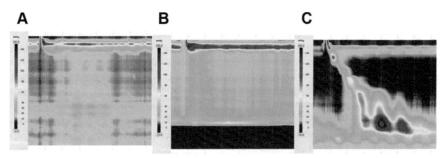

Fig. 2. Achalasia patterns according to the Chicago classification: (A) type I, (B) type II, (C) type III.

- Ambulatory pH monitoring differentiates between gastroesophageal reflux and achalasia when the diagnosis is uncertain in untreated patients who complain of heartburn, and it assesses the presence of pathologic reflux after treatment.

TREATMENT

Because the pathogenesis of achalasia is unknown, treatment aims to improve esophageal emptying and the patient's symptoms by relieving the functional obstruction at the level of the gastroesophageal junction. The following treatment modalities are available:

1. EBTI
2. PD
3. LHM
4. POEM

Endoscopic Botulinum Toxin Injection

EBTI into the LES decreases the LES pressure by preventing acetylcholine release at the level of the cholinergic synapses. This treatment option is safe and achieves immediate symptom relief or improvement in about 80% of patients.[5] Lack of an initial symptomatic response to EBTI and residual LES pressure of 18 mm Hg or greater after EBTI are associated with a poor response. The effect progressively declines over time, with only about 40% patients being symptom free at 12 months.[6] Most patients need repeated EBTIs, with short-lasting clinical benefits, probably secondary to the formation of antibodies.[7-9]

Transmural inflammation and fibrosis frequently occur at the level of the gastroesophageal junction after repeated EBTI, making a subsequent LHM more challenging and the outcome less predictable.[10,11] Horgan and colleagues[12] analyzed the effect of EBTI on the technical aspects and outcome of LHM in 57 patients with achalasia. Of these patients, 15 had received 1 or more EBTIs preoperatively. Dissection of the submucosal plane was difficult in 8 patients (53.3%), and esophageal perforation occurred in 2 cases (13.3%). Among the 42 patients who had not received any EBTI, difficulty in identifying or following the submucosal plane was encountered in 3 patients (7%), and esophageal perforation occurred in 1 patient only (2.4%). All mucosal injuries were repaired laparoscopically, with no clinical sequelae.

Smith and colleagues[11] reported the outcomes in 209 patients with achalasia undergoing HM, with most cases completed laparoscopically (98%). Of these, 154 had undergone EBTI and/or PD preoperatively (100 PD only, 33 EBTI only, and 21 both). Intraoperative complications were more common in the endoscopically treated group, with gastroesophageal perforation being the most common complication (9.7% vs 3.6%). Of note, esophageal perforation was experienced only by patients who had undergone prior endoscopic treatment. Postoperative complications, primarily severe dysphagia, and pulmonary complications were more common after endoscopic treatment (10.4% vs 5.4%). The rate of myotomy failure was higher in the endoscopically treated group (19.5% vs 10.1%).

Compared with PD, ETBI is associated with significantly higher symptom recurrence rates at 12 months. Vaezi and colleagues[13] randomized patients who had symptoms of achalasia to EBTI (22 patients) or PD (20 patients). Symptom scores were assessed at baseline and at 1, 3, 6, 9, and 12 months after treatment. Esophageal manometry was performed before treatment, while a barium esophagram was obtained initially and at 1, 6, and 12 months posttreatment. At 12 months, 14 of 20 (70%) patients who received PD and 7 of 22 (32%) patients who received EBTI showed symptom remission ($P = .017$).

Similarly, EBTI is less effective than LHM at 2-year follow-up. In 2004, Zaninotto and colleagues[14] randomized 40 patients with achalasia to 2 EBTIs 1 month apart (100 units each) and 40 patients with achalasia to LHM. At 2-year follow-up, 34% of patients who received EBTI were asymptomatic compared with 87.5% of those who received LHM.

Based on the evidence currently available, EBTI should be used only in patients who are not candidates for more effective therapeutic options, such as PD and LHM.

Pneumatic Dilatation

PD is currently the most effective nonsurgical treatment of achalasia.[15] This procedure has been standardized with the introduction of Rigiflex balloons (Boston Scientific Corporation, MA, USA). A 30-mm, 35-mm, or 40-mm balloon is inserted fluoroscopically over a guidewire and inflated at the level of the gastroesophageal junction to achieve progressive and controlled tearing of the muscle fibers. Esophageal perforation after PD is the most common complication, with a rate that ranges between 0% and 8%.[5] PD relieves or improves dysphagia in about 85% of patients at 1 month after the procedure, while it has little effect on chest pain.[16] PD success rate steadily declines over time to less than 60% after 3 years. Additional PDs are necessary in about 25% of patients, with poorer results in those with persistent or early recurrent dysphagia after the first PD session. After PD, abnormal gastroesophageal reflux is detected by 24-hour pH monitoring in up to 33% of the patients studied.[17–19]

Eckardt and colleagues[20] reported the late results of a prospective study including 54 patients with achalasia treated with PD and followed up for a median of 13.8 years. A single PD resulted in a 5-year remission rate of 40% and a 10-year remission rate of 36%. Repeated PDs only mildly improved the clinical response. Patients undergoing more than 1 PD had a slightly better outcome after the second dilatation: the 5-year remission rate was 6% after the first and 28% after the second PD. Patients requiring 3 PDs did not have a better long-term response after the second PD compared with after the first PD. After 5 years, only 12% and 6% remained in clinical remission after the first and second PD, respectively. A third PD improved the clinical remission rate to 35% at 5 years but to only 19% at 10 years. Significant predictors of favorable long-term outcome were age greater than 40 years ($P = .0014$) and a post-PD LES pressure of less than 10 mm Hg ($P = .0001$).

Therefore, young patients (<40 years) and those who do not respond to a single PD should be referred for LHM.

The past 3 decades have witnessed a progressive shift from PD to surgery for the treatment of achalasia. In the 1980s and in the 1990s, PD was considered the main treatment modality for the patient with achalasia, while surgery had a secondary role in case of PD failure (perforation or recurrent dysphagia). The beginning of this century has witnessed a progressive greater use of minimally invasive surgery for the treatment of achalasia.[21,22]

Laparoscopic Heller Myotomy

In 1991, the first minimally invasive esophageal myotomy was performed in the United States by a left thoracoscopic approach. Pellegrini and colleagues[23] treated 17 patients with achalasia by a thoracoscopic Heller myotomy (15 patients) or LHM (2 patients). The mean hospital stay was 3 days; no deaths or major complications occurred. With regard to dysphagia, final results were excellent in 12 patients (70%), good in 2 patients (12%), fair in 2 patients (12%), and poor in 1 patient (6%). In 3 patients the myotomy was not carried far enough onto the stomach; in 2 patients dysphagia resolved after a second myotomy was performed laparoscopically. Postoperative esophageal manometry was done in 8 patients, and a mean LES pressure of 10 ± 2 mm Hg was obtained. Ambulatory 24-hour pH monitoring was performed in 4 patients 1 to 13 months after the operation, showing abnormal acid exposure in 2 cases.

The quick introduction and widespread use of the laparoscopic approach to many digestive diseases has raised the debate about the best minimally invasive approach to achalasia: thoracoscopic or laparoscopic? For instance, Patti and colleagues[24] compared 30 patients with achalasia who had undergone thoracoscopic Heller myotomy with 30 patients who had an LHM with a Dor fundoplication. There were no differences between the 2 groups in terms of demographic data, symptoms, and manometric findings. Pathologic gastroesophageal reflux was present at the preoperative pH monitoring in 2 patients who had undergone laparoscopy. The mean hospital stay was shorter after laparoscopic surgery (42 hours vs 84 hours). Similar results were achieved in terms of relief of dysphagia, with excellent (no dysphagia) or good (dysphagia less than once a week) outcomes in 87% of patients in the thoracoscopic group and in 90% of patients in the laparoscopic group. Esophageal manometry and 24-hour pH monitoring were performed 2 to 3 months after surgery in 10 patients in each group. No changes in esophageal body motility were noted in either group of patients. Postoperative 24-hour pH monitoring showed pathologic gastroesophageal reflux in 6 (60%) of 10 patients in the thoracoscopic group and in 1 (10%) of 10 patients in the laparoscopic group. The 2 patients in the laparoscopic group who had preoperative evidence of pathologic reflux had normal reflux scores postoperatively.

LHM with partial fundoplication has several advantages when compared with thoracoscopic Heller myotomy. First, the thoracoscopic approach is more challenging because (1) it requires the use of a double-lumen endotracheal tube and the lateral decubitus position of the patient, (2) the distal extent of the myotomy on the gastric wall is difficult, and (3) intraoperative upper endoscopy is necessary to check the completion of the LES myotomy. Second, the postoperative course after LHM is simpler, with less pain and shorter hospital stay, mainly because a chest tube is not necessary. Third, even though both approaches are similar in relieving dysphagia, the incidence of postoperative pathologic gastroesophageal reflux (by 24-hour pH monitoring) is lower after LHM and partial fundoplication. As patients are often asymptomatic, pH monitoring is recommended to assess the presence of reflux postoperatively.[25] Finally, the fundoplication may correct pathologic reflux when present preoperatively because of a prior PD.

LHM alone is associated with postoperative reflux in about 50% to 60% of patients. Richards and colleagues[26] conducted a prospective randomized clinical trial comparing 21 patients treated by LHM alone and 22 patients undergoing LHM and Dor fundoplication. Patients underwent esophageal manometry and 24-hour pH study at 6 months after surgery. Pathologic gastroesophageal reflux was present in 10 of 21 patients (47.6%) after LHM alone and in 2 of 22 patients (9.1%) after LHM plus Dor ($P = .005$). Postoperative LES pressure and postoperative dysphagia score were similar in the 2 groups.

Therefore, LHM with partial fundoplication is currently the preferred treatment modality for achalasia in most centers in Europe and the United States, with durable relief of dysphagia in most patients at 5 years[27] and beyond.[28,29]

Briefly, the operation consists of the following steps:

- Division of the gastrohepatic ligament.
- Dissection of the right and left pillars of the crus from the anterior wall of the esophagus after division of the phrenoesophageal ligament. No posterior dissection is necessary if a partial anterior fundoplication is planned.
- Division of the short gastric vessels.
- Excision of the fat pad to expose the gastroesophageal junction, after identification of the anterior vagus nerve.
- Myotomy on the right side of the esophagus in the 11-o'clock position; it is extended proximally for about 6 cm above the gastroesophageal junction and distally for 2.5 to 3 cm onto the gastric wall.
- Construction of a partial fundoplication to relieve dysphagia and prevent gastroesophageal reflux.

A partial fundoplication added to the myotomy is associated with lower rates of postoperative dysphagia than a total fundoplication. Rebecchi and colleagues[30] randomized 144 patients with achalasia to LHM and anterior partial fundoplication or to LHM and total fundoplication. With a mean follow-up of 125 months, they found no significant differences in postoperative pathologic reflux, whereas a significantly higher dysphagia rate was observed after total fundoplication (2.8% vs 15%; $P<.001$).

Based on the evidence currently available, both partial anterior and partial posterior fundoplication achieve similar results in terms of control of reflux after LHM. In 2012, Rawlings and colleagues[31] published the results of a multicenter, prospective, randomized controlled trial aiming to compare Dor versus Toupet fundoplication after LHM in patients with achalasia in terms of reflux control at 6 to 12 months. A total of 60 patients (36 Dor and 24 Toupet fundoplications) were available for analysis. The analysis of 24-hour pH monitoring in 43 patients (24 Dor and 19 Toupet) showed similar reflux scores and total acid exposure between the 2 groups.

Some investigators argue that partial posterior fundoplication should be the antireflux procedure of choice because it may be more effective in preventing reflux and keeps the distal edges of the myotomy separated.[32] Others prefer the partial anterior fundoplication because it is simpler to perform and covers the exposed esophageal mucosa (**Fig. 3**).

Increased age and esophageal diameter do not adversely influence the outcome of LHM. For instance, Salvador and colleagues[33] analyzed the influence of age on the surgical outcomes of 571 patients with achalasia treated by LHM and Dor fundoplication. Patients were classified into 3 age groups: group A ($\leq$45 years), group B (45–70 years), and group C ($\geq$70 years). A similar rate of esophageal perforation in the 3 groups of patients and a trend toward a longer postoperative hospital stay for older patients was reported. The treatment failure rate based on the postoperative symptom score did not differ significantly between the 3 groups of patients: 31 failures in group A (10.1%), 19 in group B (8.4%), and 3 in group C (7.5%; $P = .80$).

Sweet and colleagues[34] divided 113 patients with achalasia into 4 groups according to the maximal diameter of the esophageal lumen and the shape of the esophagus: group A, diameter less than 4.0 cm (46 patients); group B, esophageal diameter 4.0 to 6.0 cm (32 patients); group C, diameter greater than 6.0 cm and straight axis (23 patients); and group D, diameter greater than 6.0 cm and sigmoid-shaped esophagus (12 patients). All patients underwent LHM and Dor fundoplication. The median length of follow-up was 45 months (range, 7 months–12.5 years). Excellent or good results were obtained in 89% of group A and 91% of groups B, C, and D. Postoperative

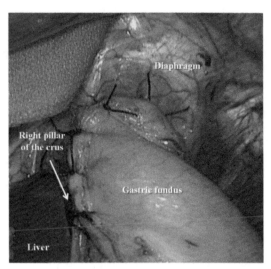

Fig. 3. Partial anterior fundoplication.

PDs were necessary in 23 patients (20%) to treat dysphagia, whereas a second myotomy was performed in 5 patients (4%). No patient required an esophagectomy.

Therefore, LHM can also be performed in elderly patients and in those with a dilated and sigmoid esophagus, whereas esophagectomy should be considered only in case of failure of LHM.

At present, even though there is evidence supporting the long-lasting results of surgery, the role of PD and LHM is under debate. In 2011, a randomized, multicenter European trial[35] aimed to compare the outcomes at 2-year follow-up in 201 patients with untreated esophageal achalasia: 95 underwent PD and 106 underwent LHM and Dor fundoplication. The primary outcome was therapeutic success (defined as a drop in the Eckardt score to ≤3) at the yearly follow-up assessment. The secondary outcomes included the need for re-treatment, LES pressure, esophageal emptying on a timed barium esophagram, quality of life, and the complications rate.

The investigators found no significant difference in the outcome between PD and LHM (at 1 year: PD 90% vs LHM 93%; at 2 years: PD 86% vs LHM 90%). At 2-year follow-up, LES pressure was similar in the 2 groups; no differences were observed in terms of esophageal emptying and quality of life. Esophageal perforation occurred in 4% of the patients who underwent PD and in 12% of the patients who underwent LHM. The study confirmed the superiority of LHM for patients younger than 40 years.

Even though in this study the short-term results of PD and LHM were similar, longer follow-up is needed to support the equivalence of these procedures.

Per Oral Endoscopic Myotomy

Recently, a novel procedure for the treatment of achalasia termed peroral endoscopic myotomy has been proposed. POEM is an endoscopic procedure performed under general anesthesia. Briefly, saline with indigocarmine and epinephrine is injected in the submucosal layer approximately 12 to 13 cm proximal to the gastroesophageal junction at the 2-o'clock position. Then, a 2-cm longitudinal incision is made on the mucosal surface and the submucosal space is entered. A submucosal tunnel is created on the anterior wall of the esophagus extending down onto the first 3 cm of the stomach. After completing the submucosal tunnel, the circular muscular fibers are selectively sectioned beginning 2 to 3 cm distal to the mucosal entry and extending about 3 cm distal to the gastroesophageal junction. Hemostatic clips are used to close the site of the mucosal entry.

The first report of POEM in 17 consecutive patients with achalasia was published by Inoue and colleagues[36] in 2010. Mean length of the myotomy was 8.1 cm (about 6 cm on the esophagus and 2 cm on the proximal stomach). In all cases, the resting LES pressure significantly decreased after POEM (from mean 52.4 mm Hg to 19.9 mm Hg; P = .0001). With a mean follow-up of 5 months, no patient had recurrent dysphagia, while 1 patient developed grade B esophagitis according to Los Angeles classification. No patient underwent further endoscopic or surgical procedures during the follow-up.

In 2012, Swanstrom and colleagues[37] published the outcomes in 18 patients with achalasia treated with POEM. Median length of myotomy was 9 cm. The investigators reported 3 intraoperative complications, including 2 gastric mucosotomies and 1 full-thickness esophagotomy, which were all repaired endoscopically with no postoperative sequelae. Median hospital stay was 1 day. At a mean follow-up of 11.4 months, relief of dysphagia was reported in all patients, with a significant drop of the median Eckardt score from 6 to 0. Postoperative upper endoscopy was performed in 14 patients, showing esophagitis in 4 cases (28%). Postoperative HRM performed in 12 patients showed significant improvements in LES resting pressure (from 45 to 16.8 mm Hg; P = .009). The 24-hour pH monitoring performed in 13 patients objectively diagnosed pathologic gastroesophageal reflux in 46% of cases.

In 2013, von Renteln and colleagues[38] reported the results of a prospective, international, multicenter trial including 70 patients with achalasia undergoing POEM in 5 centers in Europe and North America. The mean length of the myotomy was 13 cm (range, 5–23 cm). The number of patients available for analysis progressively decreased during the follow-up period from 70 at 3 months, to 61 at 6 months, and 51 at 1 year. At 3 months after POEM, esophageal manometry was obtained in 61 patients: mean LES pressure significantly decreased from 28 to 9 mm Hg (P<.001). An upper endoscopy revealed the presence of esophagitis in 42% of patients. The symptom remission rate at 3, 6, and 12 months was 97%, 89%, and 82%, respectively. Symptoms of gastroesophageal reflux were reported by 37% of patients at 12 months after the procedure. However, no objective evaluation of reflux by 24-hour pH monitoring was performed.

Only a few nonrandomized studies comparing POEM and LHM have been published. For instance, Hungness and colleagues[39] reported the short-term outcomes in 18 patients with achalasia undergoing POEM and in 55 patients treated by LHM. Length of the myotomy, complication rate, and length of hospital stay were similar in the 2 groups. At 6 weeks after POEM, normalization of esophagogastric junction pressure and contrast column height were showed by esophageal HRM and timed esophagram, respectively. Postoperative upper endoscopy was obtained in 15 patients at a median follow-up interval of 1.5 (1.5–12) months after POEM, showing esophagitis in 5 (33%) patients. Treatment success, defined as Eckardt score less than or equal to 3 after POEM, was achieved in 16 (89%) patients at median 6-month follow-up.

Recently, a comparative study by Bhayani and colleagues[40] including 64 patients with achalasia undergoing LHM (42% with Toupet and 58% with Dor fundoplication) and 37 undergoing POEM showed significantly longer median operative time (149 vs 120 min, P<.001) and median hospitalization (2.2 vs 1.1 days, P<.0001) among patients undergoing LHM, with no differences in postoperative morbidity. Patients underwent esophageal manometry at a median of 6.8 (range, 5.7–10) months. Significant improvement in LES pressure was observed in both groups of patients postoperatively; however, LES resting pressure was lower after LHM than after POEM (7.1 vs 16 mm Hg, $P = .006$). Abnormal acid exposure documented by 24-hour pH monitoring was observed in 39% of patients after POEM and in 32% of patients after LHM. At 6-month follow-up, 29% of patients who underwent LHM reported dysphagia to solids compared with none of the patients who underwent POEM ($P = .001$).

Based on the limited evidence available, POEM seems to be a promising new procedure. Even though it has been claimed that POEM has the surgical efficacy of an LHM with the recovery profile of an endoscopy,[41] there are some concerns about this new technique:

1. Superior endoscopic skills are required to perform this demanding procedure.
2. Even though significant reduction in post-POEM LES pressure has been reported, it is greater than 10 mm Hg, a value that predicts long-term failure.
3. Pathologic gastroesophageal reflux is common after POEM.
4. The formation of adhesions between the submucosal and the longitudinal muscular layer after POEM might make the dissection at this level challenging in case a surgical revision is needed to treat recurrent or persistent dysphagia after POEM.

Therefore, the authors believe that longer follow-up and large randomized clinical trials are needed before validating the use of POEM in the routine clinical practice for the treatment of esophageal achalasia.

SUMMARY

At present, LHM with partial fundoplication is considered the gold standard for the treatment of patients with esophageal achalasia. Endoscopic procedures such as EBTI and PD should be considered as primary treatment modalities only in frail patients. POEM is a new approach with promising short-term results.

REFERENCES

1. Mayberry JF. Epidemiology and demographics of achalasia. Gastrointest Endosc Clin N Am 2001;11:235–48.
2. Park W, Vaezi MF. Etiology and pathogenesis of achalasia: the current understanding. Am J Gastroenterol 2005;100:1404–14.
3. Pandolfino JE, Ghosh SK, Rice J, et al. Classifying esophageal motility by pressure topography characteristics: a study of 400 patients and 75 controls. Am J Gastroenterol 2008;103:27–37.
4. Pandolfino JE, Kwiatek MA, Nealis T, et al. Achalasia: a new clinically relevant classification by high- resolution manometry. Gastroenterology 2008;135:1526–33.
5. Campos GM, Vittinghoff E, Rabl C, et al. Endoscopic and surgical treatments for achalasia: a systematic review and meta-analysis. Ann Surg 2009;249:45–57.
6. Allescher HD, Storr M, Seige M, et al. Treatment of achalasia: botulinum toxin injection vs. pneumatic balloon dilation. A prospective study with long-term follow-Up. Endoscopy 2001;33:1007–17.
7. Pasricha PJ, Rai R, Ravich WJ, et al. Botulinum toxin for achalasia: long-term outcome and predictors of response. Gastroenterology 1996;110:1410–5.
8. Fishman VM, Parkman HP, Schiano TD, et al. Symptomatic improvement in achalasia after botulinum toxin injection of the lower esophageal sphincter. Am J Gastroenterol 1996;91:1724–30.

9. Annese V, Basciani M, Perri F, et al. Controlled trial of botulinum toxin injection versus placebo and pneumatic dilation in achalasia. Gastroenterology 1996;111: 1418–24.
10. Patti MG, Feo CV, Arcerito M, et al. Effects of previous treatment on results of laparoscopic Heller myotomy for achalasia. Dig Dis Sci 1999;44(11):2270–6.
11. Smith CD, Stival A, Howell DL, et al. Endoscopic therapy for achalasia before Heller myotomy results in worse outcomes than Heller myotomy alone. Ann Surg 2006;243:579–86.
12. Horgan S, Hudda K, Eubanks T, et al. Does botulinum toxin injection make esophagomyotomy a more difficult operation? Surg Endosc 1999;13:576–9.
13. Vaezi MF, Richter JE, Wilcox CM, et al. Botulinum toxin versus pneumatic dilatation in the treatment of achalasia: a randomised trial. Gut 1999;44:231–9.
14. Zaninotto G, Annese V, Costantini M, et al. Randomized controlled trial of botulinum toxin versus laparoscopic Heller myotomy for esophageal achalasia. Ann Surg 2004;239:364–70.
15. Stefanidis D, Richardson W, Farrell TM, et al. Society of American Gastrointestinal and Endoscopic Surgeons. SAGES guidelines for the surgical treatment of esophageal achalasia. Surg Endosc 2012;26:296–311.
16. Katz PO, Gilbert J, Castell DO. Pneumatic dilatation is effective long-term treatment for achalasia. Dig Dis Sci 1998;43:1973–7.
17. Wehrmann T, Jacobi V, Jung M, et al. Pneumatic dilation in achalasia with a low-compliance balloon: results of a 5-year prospective evaluation. Gastrointest Endosc 1995;42:31–6.
18. Aguilar-Paiz LA, Valdovinos-Diaz MA, Flores-Soto C, et al. Prospective evaluation of gastroesophageal reflux in patients with achalasia treated with pneumatic dilatation, thoracic or abdominal myotomy. Rev Invest Clin 1999;51:345–50.
19. Karamanolis G, Sgouros S, Karatzias G, et al. Long-term outcome of pneumatic dilation in the treatment of achalasia. Am J Gastroenterol 2005;100:270–4.
20. Eckardt VF, Gockel I, Bernhard G. Pneumatic dilation for achalasia: late results of a prospective follow-up investigation. Gut 2004;53:629–33.
21. Patti MG, Fisichella PM, Perretta S, et al. Impact of minimally invasive surgery on the treatment of esophageal achalasia: a decade of change. J Am Coll Surg 2003;196:698–705.
22. Wang YR, Dempsey DT, Friedenberg FK, et al. Trends of Heller myotomy hospitalizations for achalasia in the United States, 1993–2005: effect of surgery volume on perioperative outcomes. Am J Gastroenterol 2008;103:2454–64.
23. Pellegrini CA, Wetter LA, Patti MG, et al. Thoracoscopic esophagomyotomy. Initial experience with a new approach for the treatment of achalasia. Ann Surg 1992; 216:291–6.
24. Patti MG, Arcerito M, De Pinto M, et al. Comparison of thoracoscopic and laparoscopic Heller myotomy for achalasia. J Gastrointest Surg 1998;2:561–6.
25. Patti MG, Arcerito M, Tong J, et al. Importance of preoperative and postoperative pH monitoring in patients with esophageal achalasia. J Gastrointest Surg 1997;1:505–10.
26. Richards WO, Torquati A, Holzman MD, et al. Heller myotomy versus Heller myotomy with Dor fundoplication. A prospective randomized double-blind clinical trial. Ann Surg 2004;240:405–15.
27. Wright AS, Williams CW, Pellegrini CA, et al. Long-term outcomes confirm the superior efficacy of extended Heller myotomy with Toupet fundoplication for achalasia. Surg Endosc 2007;21:713–8.
28. Patti MG, Pellegrini CA, Horgan S, et al. Minimally invasive surgery for achalasia. An 8-year experience with 168 patients. Ann Surg 1999;230:587–93.

29. Cowgill SM, Villadolid D, Boyle R, et al. Laparoscopic Heller myotomy for achalasia: results after 10 years. Surg Endosc 2009;23:2644–9.
30. Rebecchi F, Giaccone C, Farinella E, et al. Randomized controlled trial of laparoscopic Heller myotomy plus Dor fundoplication versus Nissen fundoplication for achalasia. Ann Surg 2008;248:1023–30.
31. Rawlings A, Soper NJ, Oelschlager B, et al. Laparoscopic Dor versus Toupet fundoplication following Heller myotomy for achalasia: results of a multicenter, prospective, randomized-controlled trial. Surg Endosc 2012;26:18–26.
32. Hunter JG, Trus TL, Branum GD, et al. laparoscopic Heller myotomy and fundoplication for achalasia. Ann Surg 1997;225:655–65.
33. Salvador R, Costantini M, Cavallin F, et al. Laparoscopic Heller myotomy can be used as primary therapy for esophageal achalasia regardless of age. J Gastrointest Surg 2014;18:106–11.
34. Sweet MP, Nipomnick I, Gasper WJ, et al. The outcome of laparoscopic Heller myotomy for achalasia is not influenced by the degree of esophageal dilatation. J Gastrointest Surg 2008;12:159–65.
35. Boeckxstaens GE, Annese V, des Varannes SB, et al. European Achalasia Trial Investigators. Pneumatic dilation versus laparoscopic Heller's myotomy for idiopathic achalasia. N Engl J Med 2011;364:1807–16.
36. Inoue H, Minami H, Kobayashi Y, et al. Peroral endoscopic myotomy (POEM) for esophageal achalasia. Endoscopy 2010;42:265–71.
37. Swanstrom LL, Kurian A, Dunst CM, et al. Long-term outcomes of an endoscopic myotomy for achalasia: the POEM procedure. Ann Surg 2012;256:659–67.
38. Von Renteln D, Fuchs KH, Fockens P, et al. Peroral endoscopic myotomy for the treatment of achalasia: an international prospective multicenter study. Gastroenterology 2013;145:309–11.e1–3.
39. Hungness ES, Teitelbaum EN, Santos BF, et al. Comparison of perioperative outcomes between peroral esophageal myotomy (POEM) and laparoscopic Heller myotomy. J Gastrointest Surg 2013;17:228–35.
40. Bhayani NH, Kurian AA, Dunst CM, et al. A comparative study on comprehensive, objective outcomes of laparoscopic Heller myotomy with per-oral endoscopic myotomy (POEM) for achalasia. Ann Surg 2014;259:1098–103.
41. Swanstrom LL. Poetry is in the air: first multi-institutional results of the per-oral endoscopic myotomy procedure for achalasia. Gastroenterology 2013;145: 272–3.

Gastroesophageal Reflux Disease After Bariatric Procedures

Maria S. Altieri, MD, MS, Aurora D. Pryor, MD*

KEYWORDS

- GERD • Roux-en-Y gastric bypass • Sleeve gastrectomy

KEY POINTS

- There is a clear relationship between gastroesophageal reflux disease (GERD) and obesity.
- Roux-en-Y gastric bypass (RYGB) is associated with decreased incidence of GERD and is the procedure of choice for obese patients with GERD seeking a bariatric procedure.
- The information regarding GERD after adjustable gastric banding (AGB) and sleeve gastrectomy (SG) is contradictory, thus surgeons should avoid these procedures for patients with GERD seeking weight loss surgery.
- In case of de novo GERD after AGB or SG, in severe cases, conversion to RYGB is safe and effective.

INTRODUCTION

Obesity has reached epidemic proportions in the United States and around the world. Recent reports show that up to 35% of adults in the United States are considered obese.[1] With the number of obese individuals increasing, there is an exponential increase in the number of weight loss surgeries being performed. As we are gaining knowledge about the different comorbidities and complications after weight loss surgery, gastroesophageal reflux disease (GERD) remains an important and controversial topic among bariatric surgeons. This article reviews the current knowledge of GERD after bariatric surgery.

GASTROESOPHAGEAL REFLUX DISEASE

GERD refers to symptoms or pathologic findings produced by stomach contents flowing backward into the esophagus or beyond.[2] It is one of the most commonly encountered gastrointestinal diagnoses for gastroenterologists and primary care doctors. A systematic review cited a prevalence of GERD between 10% and 20% of the

Division of Bariatric, Foregut and Advanced Gastrointestinal Surgery, Department of Surgery, Stony Brook University Medical Center, 101 Nicolls Road, Stony Brook, NY 11794, USA
* Corresponding author. 100 Nichols Road, HSC T18-040, Stony Brook, NY 11794.
E-mail address: aurora.pryor@stonybrookmedicine.edu

surgical.theclinics.com

Abbreviations	
AGB	Adjustable gastric banding
GERD	Gastroesophageal reflux disease
LAGB	Laparoscopic adjustable gastric banding
LES	Lower esophageal sphincter
LSG	Laparoscopic sleeve gastrectomy
RYGB	Roux-en-Y gastric bypass
SG	Sleeve gastrectomy

Western population to have weekly symptoms of GERD,[3] and others have cited between 60 and 70 million Americans as being affected annually.[4] It has significant impact on quality of life and health care costs.[5,6] The pathogenic pathway commonly described is owing to lower esophageal sphincter (LES) dysfunction, which prevents the LES from contracting and allows reflux of gastric contents into the esophagus.

GASTROESOPHAGEAL REFLUX DISEASE AND OBESITY

More than one-third of the adult population in the United States is now considered obese.[7] The association between GERD and obesity has generated great interest, because obesity has been indicated as a potential risk factor for reflux disease.[8] A directly dependent relationship has been reported because an increase in body mass index has mirrored an increase in the risk of GERD.[9] The incidence of reflux in the obese population has been cited as high as 61%.[10] The pathophysiologic mechanism underlying the link between obesity and GERD has not been fully elucidated and seems to be multifaceted. As the number of obese patients is increasing, so is the volume and variety of bariatric procedures. The effect of bariatric surgery on preexisting GERD or newly developed GERD differs by procedure.

GASTROESOPHAGEAL REFLUX DISEASE AFTER ROUX-EN-Y GASTRIC BYPASS

Roux-en-Y gastric bypass (RYGB) has been used as a standalone reflux procedure. Mechanisms of the antireflux effect of RYGB include diverting bile from the Roux limb, promoting weight loss, lowering acid production in the gastric pouch, rapid pouch emptying, and decreasing abdominal pressure over the LES. Several studies have examined the relationship between GERD and RYGB.[11] Studies have also analyzed symptomatic relief by using questionnaires before and after the procedure.[12–15] These studies have shown improvement in symptoms after surgery. Others have also shown symptomatic improvement when using 24-hour pH-metry[15,16] and manometric studies.[16] One study has examined further the incidence of esophagitis postoperatively on endoscopy.[16] Merrouche and colleagues[16] showed a 6% incidence of esophagitis on endoscopy after RYGB; however, the preoperative incidence was not mentioned.

Pallati and colleagues[17] also examined the GERD symptoms after several bariatric procedures by using the Bariatric Outcomes Longitudinal Database. GERD score improvement was highest in the RYGB group; 56.5% of patients showed improvement of symptoms. The study concluded that RYGB was superior to all other procedures in improving GERD. The proposed but unproven mechanisms included a greater weight loss and a decrease in the amount of gastric juice in the proximal pouch.[17] The study, however, did not show any objective measures of GERD improvement.

Another study by Frezza and colleagues[18] showed a significant decrease in GERD-related symptoms over the 3-year study after laparoscopic RYGB, with decrease in reported heartburn from 87% to 22% ($P<.001$). The authors proposed that, in addition to volume reduction and rapid egress, the mechanism of how this procedure affects symptoms of GERD is through weight loss and elimination of acid production in the gastric pouch. The gastric pouch lacks parietal cells; thus, there is minimal to no acid production and also, owing to its small size, it minimizes any reservoir capacity to promote regurgitation.

Varban and colleagues[19] examined the utilization of acid-reducing medications (proton pump inhibitor and H2-blockers) at 1 year after various bariatric procedures. The groups reported that at 1 year after RYGB, 56.2% of patients would discontinue an acid-reducing medication that they had been using at baseline. Interestingly, the group also showed that 19.2% of patients would also start a new acid-reducing medication after RYGB.

Given the number of studies that have reported improvement in GERD symptoms after RYGB, this procedure is now widely accepted as the procedure of choice for treatment of GERD in the morbidly obese patient.[18,20] Although no increased risk is conferred to patients with a body mass index of 35 kg/m^2 or higher who undergo fundoplication for GERD,[21,22] the recommendation and practice of many surgeons is to perform a laparoscopic gastric bypass in lieu of fundoplication owing to its favorable effect on other comorbid conditions. In addition, advocates of the RYGB are promoting a conversion to an RYGB instead of a redo fundoplication.[22–24] In a recent study, Stefanidis and colleagues[25] followed 25 patients who had previous failed fundoplication, which was taken down and converted to an RYGB. Patients were followed with the Gastrointestinal Quality of Life Index and the Gastrointestinal Symptoms Rating Sale. The revision surgery led to resolution of GERD symptoms for a majority of the patients. The authors concluded that an RYGB after a failed fundoplication has excellent symptomatic control of symptoms and excellent quality of life.[25] However, owing to the technical challenges of the procedure and the potential for high morbidity, it should only be performed by experienced surgeons.

GASTROESOPHAGEAL REFLUX DISEASE AFTER ADJUSTABLE GASTRIC BAND

The adjustable gastric band became a popular procedure owing to its simplicity and perceived safety profile. The association between the band and GERD is conflicting. The majority of studies show that symptoms and pH improve after gastric band placement, although some suggest an increase in GERD after placement.

A recent review by Ardila-Hani and Soffer[26] reviewed the effect of the 3 common bariatric procedures on gastrointestinal motility. The authors reported that the LAGB was associated with esophageal motor dysfunction and esophageal dilation. Several mechanisms may play a role, such as esophageal outflow obstruction or dysmotility from higher pressure. Animal studies have showed that placement of a nonobstructive band around the esophagogastric junction results in dilation proximal to the band[27] and an increase in resting LES pressure and frequency of aperistalsis.[28] O'Rourke and colleagues[28] further showed that, when the band is placed at the esophagogastric junction, symptoms developed sooner compared with when placed around the proximal stomach. However, both placements resulted in esophageal motility disorder or abnormal peristaltic sequences. Tolonen and colleagues[29] showed that reflux episodes significantly decreased postoperatively in patients analyzed with 24-hour pH monitor. The group concluded that a gastric band that is correctly placed and adjusted leads to relief of GERD symptoms.

Other studies have showed esophageal dilation on radiographic studies after band placement, which is explained by the band causing an outflow obstruction.[30–34]

Although this finding is significant, it may not translate into symptomatic findings.[32] In addition, dilation can be reversed after emptying of band.[30,33] Thus, an overly tightened band can induce reflux. Even if asymptomatic, patients with ABG will need follow-up for appropriate band adjustments.

Studies have examined symptomatic relief and decreased use of medication after LAGB.[17,19,30,35–39] Most of these studies have shown a decrease in symptoms and use of medication; however, 1 study has shown an increase in heartburn.[36] A systematic review cited newly developed symptoms after LAGB between 6% and 50%.[40] Although relief of symptoms can be explained by weight loss in the first year,[19,35,37] some studies have shown relief shortly after a band placement or within 6 months, citing these outcomes on the direct mechanical effect of the band, which could function as an antireflux barrier.[30,35,37] Overtightening of the band has been implicated as the reason for development of symptoms after a longer period of time.[28,35,39]

Owing to the conflicting results of studies evaluating laparoscopic adjustable gastric banding and GERD, many surgeons would not recommend this procedure if the patient has symptoms of GERD preoperatively.

GASTROESOPHAGEAL REFLUX DISEASE AFTER SLEEVE GASTRECTOMY

Sleeve gastrectomy (SG), which was originally described as a first stage of the biliopancreatic diversion, is a relatively new treatment alternative for morbid obesity. It has become popular owing to its technical simplicity and its proven weight loss outcomes.[41] Although it has many positive effects on obesity and obesity-related comorbidities, the association between GERD and SG remains controversial.

Although some studies have reported improvement in GERD symptoms after SG, the majority of studies have reported an increase in GERD symptoms.[42–47] The International Sleeve Gastrectomy Expert Panel reported a postoperative rate of GERD symptoms after SG in up to 31%[48]; however, others cited increased GERD prevalence after surgery between 2.1% and 34.9%.[49]

Studies Showing an Increase in Gastroesophageal Reflux Disease After Sleeve Gastrectomy

Several studies have shown an increase of GERD after SG at various time points. The comparison between different studies is difficult owing to variations in the definition of GERD. Although some have utilized the use of proton pump inhibitors as a diagnostic tool,[43] others have used the definition of typical heartburn and/or acid regurgitation occurring at least once per week.[42] Few studies used objective data to define reflux. Tai and colleagues[42] examined symptoms of GERD and erosive esophagitis at 1 year after laparoscopic sleeve gastrectomy (LSG). The groups concluded that there was a significant increase in the prevalence of GERD symptoms and erosive esophagitis (P<.001), in addition to a significant increase in the prevalence of hiatal hernias (P<.001), which was higher in patients who presented with erosive esophagitis after LSG. Others have shown a similar increase of GERD at 1 year.[43,44] Himpens and colleagues[46] compared adjustable gastric banding (AGB) and SG at 1 and 3 years after procedures. GERD seemed de novo after 1 year in 8.8% and 21.8% of patients with AGB and SG, respectively. At 3 years, however, rates changed to 20.5% and 3.1% in the ABG and SG groups. Another study followed patients for more than 6 years and reported 23% to 26% of patients reporting frequent episodes of GERD.

Various mechanisms have been postulated to cause symptoms of GERD after LSG (Table 1). As SG alters the gastroesophageal anatomy, it has been hypothesized that the anatomic abnormalities created contribute to the development of GERD in

Table 1
Proposed mechanisms leading to gastroesophageal reflux disease after SG

Anatomy	
Tubular sleeve with inferior pouch	50
Concomitant presence of a hiatal hernia	45,55,60–62
Decrease in lower esophageal sphincter resting pressure	42,44,53,60,62–64
Increased intragastric pressure	53,62–64
Esophageal motility disorders	45,53
Increase in anatomic abnormalities	42,43,45,50,53,65–67
Incompetent pylorus	55
Intrathoracic sleeve migration	55
Fundal dilatation with distal narrowing	46,63,65
Reduced gastric compliance and reduces gastric volume	43,64
Altered gastric emptying	43,45,50,65,66
Technique	
Disrupt the integrity of sling fibers of Helvetius at esophagogastric junction	52
Stapling close to the angle of His	68
Narrowing incisura angularis leading to dilation of fundus	55,61
Dissection of phrenoesophageal ligament	55
Narrowing sleeve gastrectomy	67

Data from Refs.[42–45,50,53,55,60–67]

patients. Lazoura and colleagues[50] showed that the final shape of the sleeve can influence the development of GERD. The group showed that patients with tubular pattern and inferior pouch (preservation of the antrum) did better in terms of regurgitation and vomiting compared with a tubular sleeve with a superior pouch. Others have also suggested the importance of antral preservation to avoid GERD development.[51] An increase in acid production capacity can cause reflux in the case of an overly dilated sleeve, whereas impaired esophageal acid clearance can lead to reflux in a smaller sleeve.[52,53] Formation of a neofundus can in an effort to avoid fistulas may also lead to development of GERD.[46]

Daes and colleagues[54] further concentrated on describing and standardizing the procedure to reduce GERD symptoms. The authors identified 4 technical errors that led to development of GERD after the procedure: relative narrowing at the junction of the vertical and horizontal parts of the sleeve, dilation of the fundus, twisting of the sleeve, and persistence of hiatal hernia or a patulous cardia. By ensuring careful attention to surgical technique and performing a concomitant hiatal hernia repair in all patients, they reduced the rate of postoperative GERD to only 1.5%. The group concluded that hiatal hernia is the most important predisposing factor.[54]

Studies Showing Reduction of Gastroesophageal Reflux Disease After Sleeve Gastrectomy

Several studies have reported either decreased or no association between GERD and LSG. Interestingly, in some of these studies, GERD improvement has been reported as a secondary outcome. Rawlins and colleagues[55] reported an improvement of symptoms in 53% of patients, but de novo GERD in 16% of patients. A multicenter prospective database review examined GERD in all 3 major bariatric procedures and reported improvement in all. The authors used medication use to define GERD. A small portion of patients reported worsening GERD, which was highest in the SG group.[17] Sharma and colleagues[56] also reported an improvement of GERD as assessed by symptom questionnaires, as well as improvement in grade of esophagitis on endoscopy.

The possible mechanisms for improvement of GERD postoperatively are faster gastric emptying, reduction in gastric reservoir function, gastrointestinal hormonal modifications, decrease in acid secretions, and decrease in weight. Daes and colleagues[54] reported a decrease in incidence of GERD by using a standardized operative technique and concomitant repair of hiatal hernia. Other techniques used to minimize reflux after SG are listed in **Table 2**.

Summary

Owing to conflicting reports about the association between GERD and LSG, this procedure is controversial in patients with preexisting GERD. If LSG is considered in this population, hiatal hernia repair and meticulous technique are essential. We would like to emphasize the importance of preoperative testing to define the anatomy and evaluate preexisting GERD, esophagitis, Barrett's esophagus, or the presence of hiatal hernia. Based on these findings, we council patients to the best procedure choice for them.

PRESENTATION OF POSTPROCEDURE REFLUX DISEASE

GERD is treated initially by clinical diagnosis on the basis of history and physical evaluation. Symptoms include heartburn, chest pain, regurgitation, nausea, and coughing. In postbariatric patients, symptoms of GERD can mask other postoperative complications. Previous undiagnosed motility disorders can worsen after bariatric surgery. In addition, surgery-specific postoperative complications can present as newly developed reflux symptoms. For example, in the case of the LABG, newly developed symptoms can be owing to malpositioned or an overtight band, band slippage, or

Table 2	
Proposed mechanisms to minimize gastroesophageal reflux disease after sleeve gastrectomy	
Study	Recommendations
Daes et al,[54] 2014	Avoid twisting of the sleeve Avoid narrowing at the junction of the vertical and horizontal parts of the sleeve Avoid dilation of the fundus Repair of a hiatal hernia
Del Genio et al,[52] 2014	Preserve integrity of the sling fibers of Helvetius Avoid small bougie size (<40 Fr) Straight lumen Avoid leaving an excessive posterior gastric fundus
Dupree et al,[53] 2014	Avoid narrowing the gastric body or pylorus Repair concomitant hiatal hernias Attention to crural repair Attention to sleeve size and volume
Keidar et al,[65] 2010	Avoid creation of a narrow sleeve Do not place an excessive tension to the stomach Do not oversuture with overly big bites

Data from Refs.[52–54,65]

herniation. In the case of the RYGB, development of GERD can be owing to stenosis of the gastrojejunal anastomosis. Sleeve patients can also experience reflux with herniation, stricture, kinking, or dysmotility.

DIAGNOSIS

Initial treatment of GERD in the postbariatric patient is medical therapy similar to that used in the general population. If symptoms continue or worsen despite pharmacologic therapy, further evaluation is needed. In case the bariatric procedure is performed at another institution, information about previous studies is helpful.[57] Several tests can aid the diagnosis of GERD, such as the 24-hour pH study, an upper gastrointestinal endoscopy and manometry. Of these studies, the 24-hour pH study is the gold standard for detection of GERD. Specifically, impedance studies can differentiate acid and nonacid reflux as well. Barium esophogram may also be helpful for detection of hiatal hernia or to help identify an outlet problem. An endoscopy can evaluate for Barrett's esophagus, esophagitis, or presence of a hiatal hernia. When

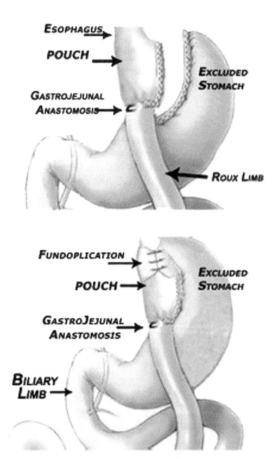

Fig. 1. Fundoplication over bypassed stomach. (*From* Kawahara NT, Alster C, Fauze MF, et al. Modified Nissen fundoplication: laparoscopic anti-reflux surgery after Roux-en-Y gastric bypass for obesity. Clinics (Sao Paulo) 2012;67(5):532.)

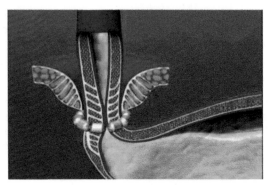

Fig. 2. Linx procedure. (*Courtesy of* Torax Medical, Inc, Shoreview, MN; with permission.)

performing an endoscopy, the gastroenterologist or surgeon should be aware of the exact bariatric procedure performed and the resulting anatomy, specifically gastric pouch or sleeve size, anastomotic characteristics, and potential fistulae.

TREATMENT

As described, initial treatment is similar to that in the general population. Proton pump inhibitors are first-line medications. Promotility agents can also be used. When symptoms persist and further evaluation cannot find a specific cause for the symptoms, revision surgery can be considered.

AVAILABLE PROCEDURES

Inadequate weight loss and uncontrollable reflux are the most common indications for revisional bariatric surgery. Depending on procedure, there are several possibilities. In case of the AGB and SG, conversion to RYGB has been shown to be safe and successful. Langer and colleagues[58] demonstrated a successful conversion of SG to RYGB for 3 patients. After surgery, improved reflux in all 3 patients was reported and patients were able to discontinue acid-suppressive medications.[58]

Patients with newly developed GERD symptoms after RYGB may have several possibilities. A revision of the bypass is a possibility to lengthen the Roux limb and/or downsize the gastric pouch. A case of conversion to a Belsey Mark IV fundoplication has also been described in the literature, although that is not standard.[59] Other surgeons have proposed fundoplication using the bypassed stomach (**Fig. 1**).

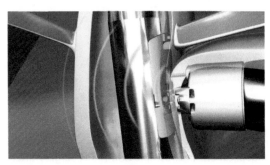

Fig. 3. The MUSE system. (*Courtesy of* Medigus LTD, Omer, Israel; with permission.)

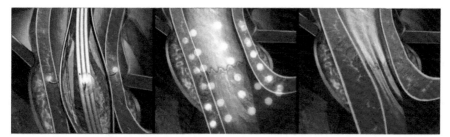

Fig. 4. Stretta procedure. (*Courtesy of* Mederi Therapeutics Inc, Norwalk, CT; with permission. © 2015 Mederi Therapeutics Inc.)

As new techniques continue to develop, such as the Linx device (**Fig. 2**), the MUSE system (**Fig. 3**), Stretta Procedure (**Fig. 4**), and EsophyX (**Fig. 5**), among other endoluminal therapies, new choices emerge. These procedures may be performed either postoperatively in patients with newly developed reflux or concurrently in patients

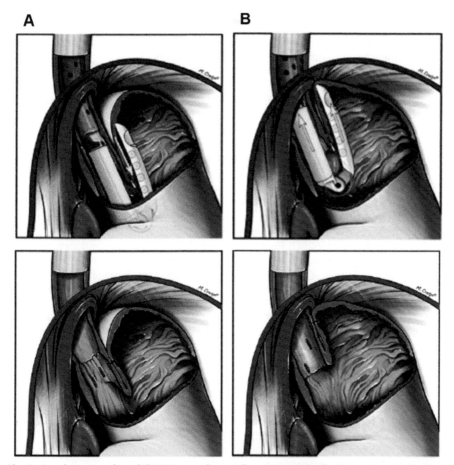

Fig. 5. Esophyx procedure. (*A*) TIF 1 procedure with gastrogastric plications placed at the level of the Z-line. (*B*) TIF 2 creates an esophagogastric fundoplication proximal to the Z-line. (*From* Bell RC, Cadiere GB. Transoral rotational esophagogastric fundoplication: technical, anatomical, and safety considerations. Surg Endosc 2011;25(7):2387–99.)

desiring procedures such as a Sleeve; however, no data are available currently for these approaches.

SUMMARY

GERD is a significant comorbidity in bariatric patients preoperatively and postoperatively. Surgeons should be aware of appropriate evaluation, procedures choices, and management options. Revision surgery for reflux symptoms is common and appropriate anatomy and outcomes should be considered when offering these interventions to our patients. Patient selection is important to ensure avoiding postoperative development or worsening of GERD.

REFERENCES

1. Ogden CL, Carroll MD, Kit BK, et al. Prevalence of obesity in the United States, 2009-2010. NCHS Data Brief 2012;82:1–8.
2. Katz PO, Gerson LB, Vela MF. Guidelines for the diagnosis and management of gastroesophageal reflux disease. Am J Gastroenterol 2013;108:308–28.
3. Dent J, El-Serag HB, Wallander MA, et al. Epidemiology of gastro-oesophageal reflux disease: a systematic review. Gut 2005;54:710–7.
4. Peery AF, Dellon ES, Lund J, et al. Burden of gastrointestinal disease in the United States: 2012 update. Gastroenterology 2012;143:1179–87.
5. Camilleri M, Dubois D, Coulie B, et al. Prevalence and socioeconomic impact of upper gastrointestinal disorders in the United States: results of the US Gastrointestinal Study. Clin Gastroenterol Hepatol 2005;3:543–52.
6. Locke GR, Talley NG, Fett SL, et al. Prevalence and clinical spectrum of gastroesophageal reflux: a population-based study in Olmsted Country, Minnesota. Gastroenterology 1997;112:1448–56.
7. Ogden CL, Carroll MD, Kit BK, et al. Prevalence of childhood and adult obesity in the United States, 2011-2012. JAMA 2014;311(8):806–14.
8. Corley DA, Kubo A. Body mass index and gastroesophageal reflux disease: a systematic review and meta-analysis. Am J Gastroenterol 2006;101:2619–28.
9. Jacobson BC, Somers SC, Fuchs CS, et al. Body-mass index and symptoms of gastroesophageal reflux in women. N Engl J Med 2006;354:2340–8.
10. Iovino P, Angrisani L, Galloro G, et al. Proximal stomach function in obesity with normal and abnormal oesophageal acid exposure. Neurogastroenterol Motil 2006;18:425–32.
11. Kawahara NT, Alster C, Maluf-Filho F, et al. Modified Nissen fundoplication: laparoscopic antireflux surgery after Roux-en-Y gastric bypass for obesity. Clinics (Sao Paulo) 2012;67(5):531–3.
12. Nelson LG, Gonzalez R, Haines K, et al. Amelioration of gastroesophageal reflux symptoms following Roux-en-Y-gastric bypass for clinically significant obesity. Ann Surg 2005;71:950–4.
13. Clements RH, Gonzalez QH, Foster A, et al. Gastrointestinal symptoms are more intense in morbidly obese patients and are improved with laparoscopic Roux-en Y gastric bypass. Obes Surg 2003;13:610–4.
14. Foster A, Laws HL, Gonzales QH, et al. Gastrointestinal outcome after laparoscopic Roux-en-Y gastric bypass. J Gastrointest Surg 2003;7:750–3.
15. Mejia-Rivas M, Herrera-Lopez A, Hernandez-Calleros J, et al. Gastroesophageal reflux disease in morbid obesity: the effect of roux-en-y gastric bypass. Obes Surg 2008;18:1217–24.

16. Merrouche M, Sebate JM, Jouet P, et al. Gastro-esophageal reflux and esophageal motility disorders in morbidly obese patients before and after bariatric surgery. Obes Surg 2007;17:894–900.
17. Pallati PK, Shaligram A, Shostrom VK, et al. Improvement in gastroesophageal reflux disease symptoms after various bariatric procedures: review of the bariatric outcomes longitudinal database. Surg Obes Relat Dis 2014;10:502–7.
18. Frezza EE, Ikramuddin S, Gourash W, et al. Symptomatic improvement in gastroesophageal reflux disease (GERD) following laparoscopic Roux-en-Y gastric bypass. Surg Endosc 2002;16:1027–31.
19. Varban OA, Hawasli AA, Carlin AN, et al. Variation in utilization of acid-reducing medications at 1 year following bariatric surgery: results from the Michigan Bariatric Surgery Collaborative. Surg Obes Relat Dis 2015;11(1):222–8.
20. Raftopoulos I, Awais O, Courcoulas AP, et al. Laparoscopic gastric bypass after antireflux surgery for the treatment of gastroesophageal reflux in morbidly obese patients: initial experience. Obes Surg 2004;14:1373–80.
21. Telem DA, Altieri M, Gracia G, et al. Perioperative outcome of esophageal fundoplication for gastroesophageal reflux disease in obese and morbidly obese patients. Am J Surg 2014;208(2):163–8.
22. Varela JE, Hinojosa MW, Nguyen NT. Laparoscopic fundoplication compared with laparoscopic gastric bypass in morbidly obese patients with gastroesophageal reflux disease. Surg Obes Relat Dis 2009;5:139–43.
23. Nguyen SQ, Grams J, Tong W, et al. Laparoscopic Roux-en-Y gastric bypass after previous Nissen fundoplication. Surg Obes Relat Dis 2009;5:280–2.
24. Ibele A, Garren J, Gould J. The impact of previous fundoplication on laparoscopic gastric bypass outcomes: a case control evaluation. Surg Endosc 2012;26:177–81.
25. Stefanidis D, Navarro F, Augenstein VA, et al. Laparoscopic fundoplication takedown with conversion to Roux-en-Y gastric bypass leads to excellent reflux control and quality of life after fundoplication failure. Surg Endosc 2012;26:3521–7.
26. Ardila-Hani A, Soffer EE. Review article: the impact of bariatric surgery on gastrointestinal motility. Aliment Pharmacol Ther 2011;34:825–31.
27. Tung H, Schulze-Delrieu K, Shirazi S, et al. Hypertrophic smooth muscle in the partially obstructed opossum esophagus. The model: histological and ultrastructural observations. Gastroenterology 1991;100:853–64.
28. O'Rourke R, Seltman AK, Chang E, et al. A model for gastric banding in the treatment of morbid obesity. The effect of chronic partial gastric outlet obstruction on esophageal physiology. Ann Surg 2006;244:723–33.
29. Tolonen P, Victorzon M, Niemi R, et al. Does gastric banding for morbid obesity reduce or increase gastroesophageal reflux? Obes Surg 2006;16(11):1469–74.
30. Weiss HG, Nehoda H, Labeck B, et al. Treatment of morbid obesity with laparoscopic adjustable gastric banding affects esophageal motility. Am J Surg 2000; 180:479–82.
31. Weiss H, Nehoda H, Labeck B, et al. Adjustable gastric and esophagogastric banding: a randomized clinical trial. Obes Surg 2002;12:573–8.
32. Milone L, Daud A, Durak E, et al. Esophageal dilation after laparoscopic adjustable gastric banding. Surg Endosc 2008;22:1482–6.
33. de Jong JR, Tiethof C, van Ramshorst B, et al. Esophageal dilation after laparoscopic adjustable gastric banding: a more systematic approach is needed. Surg Endosc 2009;23(12):2802–8.
34. Naef M, Mouton WG, Naef U, et al. Esophageal dysmotility disorders after laparoscopic gastric banding-an underestimated complication. Ann Surg 2011;253: 285–90.

35. De Jong JR, Van Ramshorst B, Timmer R, et al. The influence of laparoscopic adjustable gastric banding on gastroesophageal reflux. Obes Surg 2004;14: 399–406.

36. Gutschow CA, Collet P, Prenzel K, et al. Long-term results and gastroesophageal reflux in a series of laparoscopic adjustable gastric banding. J Gastrointest Surg 2005;9:941–8.

37. Dixon JB, O'Brien PE. Gastroesophageal reflux in obesity: the effect of Lap-Band placement. Obes Surg 1999;9:527–31.

38. Spivak H, Hewitt MF, Onn A, et al. Weight loss and improvement of obesity-related illness in 500 U.S. patients following laparoscopic adjustable gastric banding procedure. Am J Surg 2005;189:27–32.

39. Suter M, Dorta G, Giusti V, et al. Gastric banding interferes with esophageal motility and gastroesophageal reflux. Arch Surg 2005;140:639–43.

40. de Jong JR, Besselink MG, van Ramshorst B, et al. Effects of adjustable gastric banding on gastroesophageal reflux and esophageal motility: a systematic review. Obes Surg 2010;11(4):297–305.

41. Hutter MM, Schimer DB, Jones DB, et al. First report from the American College of Surgeons Bariatric Surgery Center Network: laparoscopic sleeve gastrectomy has morbidity and effectiveness positioned between the band and the bypass. Ann Surg 2011;254(3):410–20.

42. Tai CM, Huang CK, Lee YC, et al. Increase in gastroesophageal reflux disease symptoms and erosive esophagitis 1 year after laparoscopic sleeve gastrectomy among obese adults. Surg Endosc 2013;27:1260–6.

43. Himpens J, Dapri G, Cadiere GB. A prospective randomized study between laparoscopic gastric banding and laparoscopic isolated sleeve gastrectomy: results after 1 and 3 years. Obes Surg 2006;16:1450–6.

44. Braghetto I, Csendes A, Korn O, et al. Gastroesophageal reflux disease after sleeve gastrectomy. Surg Laparosc Endosc Percutan Tech 2010;20:148–53.

45. Carter PR, Leblank KA, Hausmann MG, et al. Association between gastroesophageal reflux disease and laparoscopic sleeve gastrectomy. Surg Obes Relat Dis 2011;7:569–72.

46. Himpens J, Dobbeleir J, Peeters G. Long-term results of laparoscopic sleeve gastrectomy for obesity. Ann Surg 2010;252(2):319–24.

47. Menenakos E, Stamou KM, Albanopoulos K, et al. Laparoscopic sleeve gastrectomy performed with intent to treat morbid obesity: a prospective single-center study of 261 patients with a median follow-up of 1 year. Obes Surg 2010;20(3):276–82.

48. Rosenthal RJ. International sleeve gastrectomy expert panel. International sleeve gastrectomy expert panel consensus statement: best practice guidelines based on experience of >12,000 cases. Surg Obes Relat Dis 2012;132(1):8–19.

49. Laffin M, Chau J, Gill RS, et al. Sleeve gastrectomy and gastroesophageal reflux disease. J Obes 2013;2013:741097.

50. Lazoura O, Zacharoulis D, Triantafyllidis G, et al. Symptoms of gastroesophageal reflux following laparoscopic sleeve gastrectomy are related to the final shape of the sleeve as depicted by radiology. Obes Surg 2011;21:295–9.

51. Nocca D, Krawczykowsky D, Bomans B, et al. A prospective multicenter study of 163 sleeve gastrectomies: results at 1 and 2 years. Obes Surg 2008;18(5):560–5.

52. Del Genio G, Tolone S, Limongelli P, et al. Sleeve gastrectomy and development of "de novo" gastroesophageal reflux. Obes Surg 2014;24(1):71–7.

53. Dupree CE, Blair K, Steele SR, et al. Laparoscopic sleeve gastrectomy in patients with preexisting gastroesophageal reflux disease: a national analysis. JAMA 2014;149(4):328–34.

54. Daes J, Jimenez M, Said N, et al. Improvement of gastroesophageal reflux symptoms after standardized laparoscopic sleeve gastrectomy. Obes Surg 2014;24: 536–40.

55. Rawlins L, Rawlins MP, Brown CC, et al. Sleeve gastrectomy: 5 year-outcomes of a single institution. Surg Obes Relat Dis 2013;9(1):21–5.

56. Sharma A, Aggarwal S, Ahuja V, et al. Evaluation of gastroesophageal reflux before and after sleeve gastrectomy using symptom scoring, scintigraphy, and endoscopy. Surg Obes Relat Dis 2014;10(4):600–5.

57. ASGE Standards of Practice Committee. Role of endoscopy in the bariatric surgery patient. Gastrointest Endosc 2008;68(1):1–10.

58. Langer FB, Bohdjalian A, Shakeri-Leidenmuhler S, et al. Conversion from sleeve gastrectomy to Roux-en-Y gastric bypass- indications and outcome. Obes Surg 2010;20:835–40.

59. Chen RH, Lautz D, Gilbert RJ, et al. Antireflux operation for gastroesophageal reflux after Roux-en-Y gastric bypass for obesity. Ann Thorac Surg 2005;80: 1938–40.

60. Burgehart JS, Schotborgh CA, Schoon EJ, et al. Effect of sleeve gastrectomy on gastroesophageal reflux. Obes Surg 2007;17:57–62.

61. Zhang N, Maffei A, Cerabona T, et al. Reduction in obesity-related comorbidities: is gastric bypass better than sleeve gastrectomy? Surg Endosc 2013;27: 1273–80.

62. Soricelli E, Iossa A, Casella G, et al. Sleeve gastrectomy and crural repair in obese patients with gastroesophageal reflux disease and/or hiatal hernia. Surg Obes Relat Dis 2013;9(3):356–61.

63. Chopra A, Chao E, Etkin Y, et al. Laparoscopic sleeve gastrectomy for obesity: can it be considered a definitive procedure? Surg Endosc 2012;26(3):831–7.

64. Howard DD, Caban AM, Cendan JC, et al. Gastroesophageal reflux after sleeve gastrectomy in morbidly obese patients. Surg Obes Relat Dis 2011;7(6):544–8.

65. Keidar A, Appelbaum L, Schweiger C, et al. Dilated upper sleeve can be associated with severe postoperative gastroesophageal dysmotility and reflux. Obes Surg 2010;20(2):140–7.

66. Lakdawala MA, Bhasker A, Mulchandani D, et al. Comparison between the results of laparoscopic sleeve gastrectomy and laparoscopic Roux-en-Y gastric bypass in the Indian population: a retrospective 1 year study. Obes Surg 2010; 20(1):1–6.

67. Abd Ellatif ME, Abdallah E, Askar W, et al. Long term predictors of success after laparoscopic sleeve gastrectomy. Int J Surg 2014;12(5):504–8.

68. Kleidi E, Theodorou D, Albanopoulos K, et al. The effect of laparoscopic sleeve gastrectomy on the antireflux mechanism: can it be minimized? Surg Endosc 2013;27:4625–30.

Barrett Esophagus

Mark Splittgerber, MD, Vic Velanovich, MD*

KEYWORDS

- Barrett esophagus • Gastroesophageal reflux • Barrett prevention
- Esophageal adenocarcinoma prevention • Endoscopic ablation • Esophagectomy

KEY POINTS

- Barrett esophagus has a prevalence of 1.6% of the general population and an incidence of 9.9/1000 patients/year. Gastroesophageal reflux, male gender, Caucasian race, and obesity are the primary risk factors.
- Duodenogastroesophageal reflux is the primary causative agent.
- Screening should be considered for high-risk populations.
- Endoscopic radiofrequency ablation is the preferred treatment modality for high-grade dysplasia and should be considered for low-grade dysplasia.
- Esophagectomy should only be considered for persistent high-grade dysplasia or high suspicion of invasive carcinoma.

INTRODUCTION

Barrett esophagus is a change in the normal squamous epithelium of the esophagus to specialized columnar-lined epithelium. Barrett esophagus is of interest to surgeons in that it is associated with gastroesophageal reflux disease (GERD) and is a risk factor for esophageal adenocarcinoma. Beyond that, nearly every other aspect of Barrett esophagus has been an area of controversy among surgeons, gastroenterologists, pathologists, and epidemiologists. The purpose of this article is to review the disease Barrett esophagus with emphasis on current clinical management.

EPIDEMIOLOGY AND RISK FACTORS
Prevalence

It is difficult to know the true prevalence of Barrett esophagus because many individuals are asymptomatic and, therefore, will never be evaluated. Prevalence may also vary from location to location based on variable population risk factors. However, the best estimate of the population prevalence of Barrett esophagus is 1.6% of the general population.[1] Although probably related to GERD, the prevalence of Barrett esophagus has increased, paralleling the increase in esophageal

Division of General Surgery, University of South Florida, Tampa, FL, USA
* Corresponding author. Division of General Surgery, One Tampa General Circle, F145, Tampa, FL 33606.
E-mail address: vvelanov@health.usf.edu

Surg Clin N Am 95 (2015) 593–604
http://dx.doi.org/10.1016/j.suc.2015.02.011
0039-6109/15/$ – see front matter © 2015 Elsevier Inc. All rights reserved.
surgical.theclinics.com

Abbreviations	
AGA	American Gastroenterological Association
EMR	Endoscopic mucosal resection
GERD	Gastroesophageal reflux disease
HGD	High-grade dysplasia
LGD	Low-grade dysplasia
OR	Odds ratio
PDT	Photodynamic therapy
PPI	Proton pump inhibitor
RFA	Radiofrequency ablation

adenocarcinoma; the true cause is unknown.[2] In a study conducted in Sweden, symptomatic subjects had a prevalence of Barrett esophagus of 2.3%, compared with 1.4% in asymptomatic individuals.[3] Paradoxically, patients with short-segment Barrett esophagus seem to have more frequent and intense symptoms than did those with long-segment Barrett esophagus.[4]

Incidence

The incidence of Barrett esophagus is even more difficult to estimate than its prevalence. Most studies have relied on follow-up of patients who have manifestations of GERD or calculations based on estimates. The Kalixanda study[5] of a general Swedish population initially found endoscopic or histologic diagnosis of GERD and nonerosive reflux disease, of these patients 9.7% of patients with nonerosive reflux disease progressed to erosive esophagitis, and 1.8% to Barrett esophagus. In patients initially with erosive esophagitis, 13.3% progress to a more severe grade and 8.9% to Barrett esophagus.[6] The overall incidence of Barrett esophagus was 9.9 per 1000 person-years.[6]

The incidence of Barrett esophagus seems to be increasing. A study from Northern Ireland by Coleman, and colleagues[7] found that the annual incidence from 2002 to 2005 was 62.0 per 100,000 persons per year, showing an increase 159% compared with 1993 through 1997. This incidence increased most markedly in patients younger than 60 years, especially in men younger than 40 years. Two studies from The Netherlands also documented a similar increased incidence.[6,8]

Risk Factors

Risk factors for the development of Barrett esophagus include GERD, obesity, male gender, Caucasian ethnicity, and increasing age (**Box 1**). Smoking might increase the risk of Barrett esophagus, whereas *Helicobacter pylori* infection, and specific "healthy" dietary factors may lower the risk.[9] Nelsen and colleagues[10] compared 50 Barrett esophagus patients to matched controls with CT to determine gastroesophageal junction fat area, visceral fat area, and abdominal circumference. Visceral and gastroesophageal junction fat were significantly greater among patients with Barrett esophagus (odds ratio [OR], 6.0; 95%, CI 1.3–27.7) independent of body mass index.

Tobacco smoking increases the risk of Barrett esophagus. Subjects with Barrett esophagus were significantly more likely to have ever smoked cigarettes than the population-based controls (OR, 1.67; 95% CI, 1.04–2.67) or GERD controls (OR, 1.61; 95% CI, 1.33–1.96).[11] Increasing pack-year history of smoking increased the risk of Barrett esophagus. There was synergy of smoking with GERD with the attributable proportion of disease among individuals who ever smoked and had heartburn or regurgitation was 0.39 (95% CI, 0.25–0.52).[11]

| Box 1 |
| Risk factors for GERD |

- GERD
- Male gender
- Caucasian race
- Obesity
- Smoking
- Diet

Abbreviation: GERD, gastroesophageal reflux disease.

Diets high in fiber and "good" fats reduce the risk of Barrett esophagus. Greater intake of omega-3 fatty acids (OR, 0.46; 95% CI, 0.22–0.97), polyunsaturated fat, total fiber (OR, 0.34; 95% CI, 0.15–0.76), and fiber from fruits and vegetables (OR, 0.47; 95% CI, 0.25–0.88) were associated with a lower risk. Higher meat intakes were associated with a lower risk of "long-segment" Barrett esophagus (OR, 0.25; 95% CI, 0.09–0.72). Conversely, higher trans-fat intakes were associated with increased risk of Barrett esophagus (OR, 1.11; 95% CI, 1.03–1.21). Total fat intake, barbecued foods, and fiber intake from sources other than fruits and vegetables were not associated with Barrett esophagus.[12]

Some social issues may be associated with Barrett esophagus. German patients with Barrett esophagus and adenocarcinoma tend to have higher incomes.[13] Barrett esophagus seems to be less prevalent among persons of Asian, Caribbean, African, Middle Eastern, and South American origin.[14] African Americans with Barrett esophagus are less likely than whites to have long-segment disease (12% vs 26%) and dysplasia (0% vs 7%).[15]

Progression to Adenocarcinoma

Progression of Barrett esophagus is primarily dependent on histologic grade (**Box 2**). Nondysplastic epithelium progresses at a rate of 3.86 per 1000 persons per year,[16] low-grade dysplasia (LGD) at 7.66 per 1000 persons per year,[16] and high-grade dysplasia (HGD) at 146 per 1000 persons per year.[17] The progression rate of HGD seems to be lower than the occult carcinoma rate discovered in esophagectomy specimens of HGD of 30%.[18] Age, male gender, and Barrett metaplasia length only modestly increase the risk of progression to carcinoma.[19,20] Current smoking, former smoking, and more than 40 years of smoking increased the risk of progression to HGD and esophageal adenocarcinoma; current alcohol use did not, but former alcohol use did.[19,21]

Multiplex familial kindreds, defined as families with 3 or more members with Barrett esophagus or esophageal adenocarcinoma,[21] have a younger median age at diagnosis of esophageal adenocarcinoma (57 vs 62 years old) and a lower body mass

| Box 2 |
| Progression to esophageal adenocarcinoma related to histologic grade of Barrett esophagus |

- Nondysplastic Barrett esophagus: 3.86 per 1000 persons per year
- Low-grade dysplasia: 7.66 per 1000 persons per year
- High-grade dysplasia: 146 per 1000 persons per year

index.[22] It is estimated that 6.2% of patients with Barrett esophagus, 9.5% of patients with esophageal adenocarcinoma, and 9.5% of patients with gastroesophageal junction adenocarcinoma have a first- or second-degree relative with familial Barrett esophagus.[23]

Acid and Bile Esophageal Reflux

Development of Barrett esophagus is related to abnormal acid and bile exposure. Specifically, duodenogastroesophageal reflux seems to be an important driver of Barrett esophagus.[24] Esophageal exposure to both acid and duodenogastroesophageal reflux 100% in patients with complicated Barrett esophagus, 89% with uncomplicated Barrett esophagus, 79% with esophagitis, and 50% without esophagitis. There was a correlation between acid exposure and bilirubin absorbance.[25] Nevertheless, the exact mechanism by which bile acids produce mucosal damage is not certain.

DIAGNOSIS

The definition of Barrett esophagus remains controversial. The proximal displacement of the squamocolumnar junction is essential for the diagnosis, but there are different methodologies used to identify the gastroesophageal junction.[26] Identification of the "palisade" of vessels in the lower esophagus with identification of the top of the gastric folds and the diaphragmatic pinch, constitute the essential endoscopic landmarks. Endoscopically, Barrett esophagus appears as a salmon-colored epithelium extending proximal from the gastroesophageal junction (**Fig. 1**A). In cases where the border between the abnormal Barrett epithelium and normal squamous epithelium is difficult to distinguish, narrow band imaging can bring out the distinction (see **Fig. 1**B). Barrett esophagus length should be classified using the Prague system based on circumferential and total length of metaplasia. For example, if 2 cm of esophagus is involved circumferentially with Barrett metaplasia and there is an additional 2 cm tongue of Barrett metaplasia extending from this, this would be classified as C2M4.

In Europe, the histologic diagnosis is based on detection of any type of glandular mucosa with goblet cells,[27] whereas in the United States, intestinal metaplasia with periodic acid-Schiff–positive staining goblet cells is the most widely used histologic criteria. The key basis for this recommendation is the increased incidence of

A   **B**

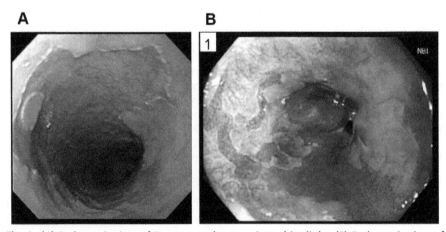

Fig. 1. (*A*) Endoscopic view of Barrett esophagus using white light. (*B*) Endoscopic view of Barrett esophagus using narrow band imaging.

esophageal adenocarcinoma among patients with endoscopic Barrett esophagus with intestinal metaplasia compared with patients who have endoscopic Barrett esophagus without intestinal metaplasia.[28]

Grading of dysplasia is a pathologic determination. There are several possible interpretations from the pathologist[29]:

1. Negative for dysplasia;
2. Positive for dysplasia, either LGD or HGD; or
3. Indefinite for dysplasia.

However, the interobserver variability is substantial. Comparing histologic samples of HGD, intramucosal carcinoma, or submucosal invasive adenocarcinoma, there was consensus among gastrointestinal pathologists (4 out of 7) in 85.9% of the cases, with overall agreement for all 4 diagnostic categories 0.30 kappa score.[30] Therefore, expert review or a review by a panel of experts is essential to ensure the most accurate diagnosis.

MANAGEMENT OF BARRETT ESOPHAGUS
Prevention

There are 2 types of prevention associated with Barrett esophagus: primary prevention of Barrett esophagus and prevention of progression of Barrett esophagus to esophageal adenocarcinoma. Chemoprevention is related to either prevention of esophageal acid exposure or modulation of proinflammatory mechanisms. Chemoprevention with proton pump inhibitors (PPIs), statins, and aspirin or nonsteroidal antiinflammatory drugs is based on epidemiologic evidence.[9] Patients who consume aspirin had a reduced prevalence of Barrett esophagus (OR, 0.56; 95% CI, 0.39–0.80).[31] Regular use of statins was associated with a significantly lower incidence of esophageal cancer in patients with Barrett esophagus (OR, 0.45; 95% CI, 0.24–0.84). The combination of statins with aspirin further reduced the risk (OR, 0.31; 95% CI, 0.04–0.69).[32] During a median follow-up period of 4.5 years, nonsteroidal antiinflammatory drug and statin use were each associated with a reduced risk of neoplastic progression (hazard ratio, 0.47 and 0.48, respectively) and the combination increased the protective effect (hazard ratio, 0.22).[33]

Screening

For the general population, the American Gastroenterological Association (AGA) does not recommend endoscopic screening for Barrett esophagus. However, in patients with multiple risk factors associated with esophageal adenocarcinoma (age >50 years, male sex, white race, chronic GERD, hiatal hernia, increased body mass index, and intraabdominal distribution of fat), the AGA suggests screening for Barrett esophagus may be appropriate.[34]

Treatment

Acid suppression without surveillance is based on the premise that screening has not been shown to improve mortality from adenocarcinoma or to be cost effective.[35] Barbiere and Lyratzapoulos[36] have questioned a variety of assumptions made for these recommendations. Therefore, the recommendation for acid suppression without surveillance should be made with caution and thorough patient counseling.

Acid suppression with surveillance identifies early stage esophageal adenocarcinoma. Because there are no reliable data on the duration of PPI treatment, most practitioners keep patients on PPI therapy indefinitely. Wong and colleagues[37] showed that 80% of esophageal adenocarcinomas found in patients undergoing surveillance were stage I cancers, compared with only 6.5% in patients who were not in the surveillance program ($P<.001$). These data imply that cancers are indeed found earlier when patients are undergoing surveillance. Although the optimal frequency of surveillance has not been determined, most authorities recommend surveillance at intervals of 3 to 5 years for patients with nondysplastic metaplasia, 6 to 12 months for LGD, and every 3 months for HGD in patients not receiving invasive therapy.[1]

Antireflux surgery in experienced hands usually in the form of some type of fundoplication, eliminates acid, and bile reflux in more than 90% of patients with Barrett esophagus.[38] Factors to consider in the choice between medical and surgical management include reflux-related symptoms, comorbidities, patient choice, adverse effects of medications, and individual surgeon skill. Biertho and colleagues[39] showed that, in patients with Barrett esophagus who underwent laparoscopic Nissen fundoplication, 33% had complete regression, 21% had a decrease in the degree of metaplasia or dysplasia, and 7% showed progression. No patients developed HGD or adenocarcinoma. A metaanalysis of antireflux surgery compared with medical treatment in GERD patients with Barrett esophagus demonstrated a pooled estimate of 15.4% of patients who have undergone antireflux surgery will have regression of Barrett esophagus compared with 1.9% of medically managed patients.[40] Nevertheless, the evidence that antireflux surgery lowers the risk for progression to adenocarcinoma is mixed.[41–43] Therefore, although antireflux surgery can successfully treat reflux-related symptoms in patients with Barrett esophagus, caution should be used when discussing its role in Barrett regression or protection against progression to adenocarcinoma. **Box 3** states the various treatment options for Barrett esophagus.

Although different types of endoscopic ablative therapies are available, the AGA,[34] the National Institute for Health and Clinical Excellence in the United Kingdom,[44] and the Society of American Gastrointestinal and Endoscopic Surgeons[45] have recommended ablation only with radiofrequency ablation (RFA), photodynamic therapy (PDT), or endoscopic mucosal resection (EMR) for patients with Barrett esophagus with HGD.

PDT consists of injecting a light-sensitizing drug into the patient, then exposing the portion of the esophagus to light of a specific wavelength, which then leads to metaplasia and dysplasia cell death.[46] However, eradication of both nondysplastic

---

Box 3
Treatment options for Barrett esophagus

- Acid suppression without surveillance
- Acid suppression with surveillance
- Antireflux surgery
- Endoscopic ablation
  - Photodynamic therapy
  - Radiofrequency ablation
  - Cryoablation
- Endoscopic mucosal resection
- Ablation with antireflux surgery
- Esophagectomy

metaplasia and HGD and prevention of adenocarcinoma has been variable,[47,48] with issues involving "buried glands." In addition, especially with long segments of Barrett esophagus, stricture formation was up to 40%,[49] with these strictures being difficult to dilate. For these reasons, PDT, although still considered an acceptable treatment, has lost favor.

RFA applies bipolar electrical energy to the mucosal surfaces at energy levels of 10 J for 1 second. With this technique, the mucosa is ablated to the submucosal level.[50,51] Generally, within several weeks to a few months after ablation, the exposed submucosal esophageal surface resurfaces with a "neosquamous" epithelium (**Fig. 2**). Endoscopic RFA is an effective means of eliminating Barrett metaplasia.[47] Using standardized follow-up protocols, complete ablation can be achieved in more than 90% of patients.[52,53] A metaanalysis and systematic review of the incidence of adenocarcinoma in patients with Barrett esophagus treated with ablative therapies compared with historical controls showed a reduction in carcinoma progression in nondysplastic metaplasia, in LGD, and especially in HGD.[54] A landmark randomized trial has demonstrated superiority of endoscopic RFA compared with sham procedure in reducing the progression to adenocarcinoma of HGD.[55] RFA has been shown to be durable,

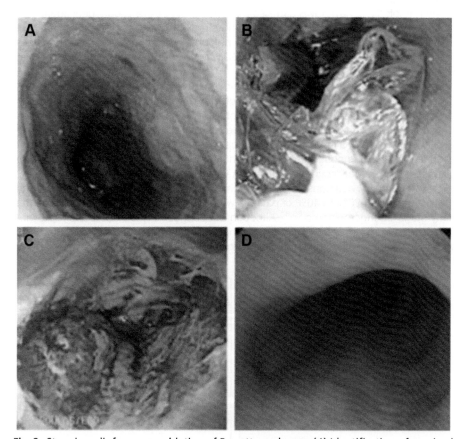

Fig. 2. Steps in radiofrequency ablation of Barrett esophagus. (*A*) Identification of proximal extent of Barrett metaplasia. (*B*) Deflated ablation balloon after ablation completed. (*C*) Immediate ulcer caused by ablation. (*D*) Normal squamous epithelium after completion of healing.

complete eradication of intestinal metaplasia 91%, 96% for HGD, and 100% for LGD, with no disease progression occurring in 1 per 73 patient-years of follow-up and progression to adenocarcinoma occurring in 1 per 181 patient-years.[56] However, ablation of longer segments of Barrett esophagus is associated with a higher rate of both persistent and recurrent metaplasia compared with segments shorter than 3 cm in length.[52] A recent randomized, controlled trial comparing surveillance to RFA in patients with LGD demonstrated at 3 years of follow-up a reduction in the progression to adenocarcinoma from 8.8% in the surveillance group to 1.5% in the RFA-treated group.[57]

Cryoablation involves endoscopically directed spray of liquid nitrogen at −196°C directly onto the Barrett epithelium.[58] Complete eradication of Barrett HGD has been reported in 68% to 97% of patients,[59,60] of intestinal metaplasia occurs in 57%,[60] and intramucosal adenocarcinoma in 80%.[59] Nevertheless, cryoablation is not as well-studied as RFA and is yet to be determined if it is an alternative or complementary treatment.

EMR is a valuable technique to remove nodular Barrett esophagus with HGD. The technique is most useful when either a visible nodule is present or only a short segment of Barrett epithelium is seen. A particular advantage of EMR is that it provides tissue pathologic review. EMR can also be used for Tis or T1a esophageal adenocarcinoma. However, an endoscopic ultrasound examination is essential to ensure that the submucosa is not involved.[47] EMR can be combined with RFA to allow for resection of the nodular component of Barrett HGD with ablation of the remaining field of flat Barrett metaplasia.[61]

Endoscopic RFA has been used in conjunction with antireflux operations. First, RFA in patient with preexisting antireflux operation was associated with no change in reflux symptoms after ablation.[62] Second, combining endoscopic ablation with an antireflux operation reduces the overall number of procedures that a patient must undergo.[63] Last, the presence of a fundoplication reduces the recurrence or persistence of Barrett esophagus.[64] This is consistent with the findings of Krishnan and colleagues,[65] who also have shown that recurrence after RFA was related to uncontrolled reflux.

Esophagectomy was considered a reasonable approach to patients with HGD. The rationale was that 20% to 40% of patients with HGD on biopsy will actually harbor an early stage adenocarcinoma.[66,67] Although esophagectomy can be performed with very low mortality, morbidity remains high. Even if the operation is accomplished without morbidity, the detrimental effects on quality of life are significant.[68] Therefore,

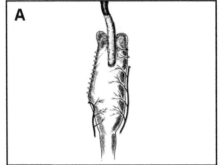 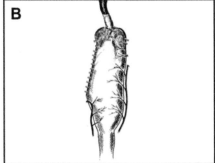

Fig. 3. (*A*) Creation of 2 gastric flaps at the apex of the gastric remnant to be used in the fundoplication. (*B*) The gastric flaps are brought around the anastomosis and sutured together to create the fundoplication.

esophagectomy should be reserved only for patients for whom ablation has not led to durable eradication of HGD or if suspicion for carcinoma is high. When esophagectomy is performed for Barrett esophagus, vagus-preserving esophagectomy should be considered.[69] The addition of a fundoplication after an esophagectomy has been shown to decrease the incidence of recurrent Barrett esophagus in the remnant esophagus from 18% to 6%.[70] The type of fundoplication used involves created gastric flaps from the apex of the gastric remnant, then creating the esophagogastrostomy inferior to the flaps, then bringing the flaps around to create the fundoplication (**Fig. 3**).

SUMMARY

Although there are many unanswered questions with Barrett esophagus, we can safely say that the incidence is increasing, chemoprevention strategies for the prevention of Barrett metaplasia and its progression to adenocarcinoma may be in the offing, surveillance should be considered for all patients who are discovered to have Barrett esophagus, RFA is the treatment of choice for those with HGD and strongly considered in those with LGD, EMR should be the treatment of choice for patients with nodular high-grade Barrett esophagus, and, finally, vagal-sparing esophagectomy reserved for patients with persistent HGD or a strong suspicion of carcinoma, with consideration of a concomitant fundoplication.

REFERENCES

1. Wang KK, Sampliner RE, Practice Parameters Committee of the American College of Gastroenterology. Updated guidelines 2008 for the diagnosis, surveillance and therapy of Barrett's esophagus. Am J Gastroenterol 2008;103:788–97.
2. Spechler SJ. Clinical practice. Barrett's esophagus. N Engl J Med 2002;346: 836–42.
3. Ronkainen J, Aro P, Storskrubb T, et al. Prevalence of Barrett's esophagus in the general population: an endoscopic study. Gastroenterology 2005;129:1825–31.
4. Dickman R, Kim JL, Camargo L, et al. Correlation of gastroesophageal reflux disease symptom characteristics with long-segment Barrett's esophagus. Dis Esophagus 2006;19:360–5.
5. Ronkainen J, Talley NJ, Storskrubb T, et al. Erosive esophagitis is a risk factor for Barrett's esophagus: a community-based endoscopic follow-up study. Am J Gastroenterol 2011;106:1946–52.
6. Post PN, Siersma PD, Van Dekken H. Rising incidence of clinically evident Barrett's esophagus in the Netherlands: a nation-wide registry of pathology reports. Scand J Gastroenterol 2007;42:17–22.
7. Coleman HG, Bhat S, Murray LJ, et al. Increasing incidence of Barrett's oesophagus: a population-based study. Eur J Epidemiol 2011;26:739–45.
8. Van Soest EM, Dieleman JP, Siersema PD, et al. Increasing incidence of Barrett's esophagus in the general population. Gut 2005;54:1062–6.
9. Winberg H, Lindblad M, Lagergren J, et al. Risk factors and chemoprevention in Barrett's esophagus—an update. Scand J Gastroenterol 2012;47:397–406.
10. Nelsen EM, Kirihara Y, Takahashi N, et al. Distribution of body fat and its influence on esophageal inflammation and dysplasia in patients with Barrett's esophagus. Clin Gastroenterol Hepatol 2012;10:728–34.
11. Cook MB, Shaheen NJ, Anderson LA, et al. Cigarette smoking increases the risk of Barrett's esophagus: an analysis of the Barrett's and Esophageal Adenocarcinoma Consortium. Gastroenterology 2012;142:744–53.

12. Kubo A, Block G, Queensberry CP Jr, et al. Effects of dietary fiber, fats, and meat intakes on the risk of Barrett's esophagus. Nutr Cancer 2009;61:607–16.

13. Gao L, Weck MN, Rothenbacher D, et al. Body mass index, chronic atrophic gastritis and heartburn: a population-based study among 8936 older adults from Germany. Aliment Pharmacol Ther 2010;32:296–302.

14. Falk GW, Jacobson BC, Riddell RH, et al. Barrett's esophagus: prevalence-incidence and etiology-origins. Ann N Y Acad Sci 2011;1232:1–17.

15. Khoury JE, Chisholm S, Jamal MM, et al. African Americans with Barrett's esophagus are less likely to have dysplasia at biopsy. Dig Dis Sci 2012;57:419–23.

16. Sharma P, Falk GW, Weston AP, et al. Dysplasia and cancer in a large multicenter cohort of patients with Barrett's esophagus. Clin Gastroenterol Hepatol 2006;4:566–72.

17. Verbeek RE, van Oijen MG, ten Kate FJ, et al. Surveillance and follow-up strategies in patients with high-grade dysplasia in Barrett's esophagus: a Dutch population-based study. Am J Gastroenterol 2012;107:534–42.

18. Buttar NS, Wang KK, Sebo TJ, et al. Extent of high-grade dysplasia in Barrett's esophagus correlates with risk of adenocarcinoma. Gastroenterology 2001;120:1630–9.

19. Prasad GA, Bansal A, Sharma P, et al. Predictors of progression in Barrett's esophagus: current knowledge and future directions. Am J Gastroenterol 2010; 105:1490–502.

20. Coleman HG, Bhat S, Johnston BT, et al. Tobacco smoking increases the risk of high-grade dysplasia and cancer among patients with Barrett's esophagus. Gastroenterology 2012;142:233–40.

21. de Jorge PJ, Steyerberg EW, Kuipers EJ, et al. Risk factors for the development of esophageal adenocarcinoma in Barrett's esophagus. Am J Gastroenterol 2006; 101:1421–9.

22. Chak A, Chen Y, Vengoechea J, et al. Variation in age at cancer diagnosis in familial versus nonfamlial Barrett's esophagus. Cancer Epidemiol Biomarkers Prev 2012;21:376–83.

23. Chak A, Ochs-Balon A, Falk G, et al. Familiality in Barrett's esophagus adenocarcinoma of the esophagus and adenocarcinoma of the gastroesophageal junction. Cancer Epidemiol Biomarkers Prev 2006;15:1668–73.

24. Richter JE. What is the role of duodenogastroesophageal reflux in the development of BE. Ann N Y Acad Sci 2011;1232:10–1.

25. Vaezi MF, Richter JE. Role of acid and duodenogastroesophageal reflux in gastroesophageal reflux disease. Gastroenterology 1996;111:1192–9.

26. Boyce HW. Endoscopic definitions of esophagogastric junction regional anatomy. Gastrointest Endosc 2000;51:586–92.

27. Spechlar SJ, Sharma P, Souza RF, et al. American Gastroenterological Association technical review on the management of Barrett's esophagus. Gastroenterology 2011;140:e18–52.

28. Murray L, Watson P, Johnston B, et al. Risk of adenocarcinoma in Barrett's oesophagus: population based study. BMJ 2003;327:534–5.

29. Goldblum JR. Controversies in the diagnosis of Barrett esophagus and Barrett-related dysplasia: one pathologist's perspective. Arch Pathol Lab Med 2010;134:1479–84.

30. Downs-Kelly E, Mendelin JE, Bennett AE, et al. Poor interobserver agreement in the distribution of high-grade dysplasia and adenocarcinoma in pretreatment Barrett's esophagus biopsies. Am J Gastroenterol 2008;103:2333–40.

31. Omer ZB, Ananthakrishnan AN, Nattinger KJ, et al. Aspirin protects against Barrett's esophagus in a multivariate logistic regression analysis. Clin Gastroenterol Hepatol 2012;10:722–7.

32. Beales IL, Vardi I, Dearman L. Regular statin and aspirin use in patients with Barrett's oesophagus is associated with a reduced incidence of oesophageal adenocarcinoma. Eur J Gastroenterol Hepatol 2012;24(8):917–23.

33. Kastelein F, Spaander MC, Beirmann K, et al. Nonsteroidal anti-inflammatory drugs and statins have chemopreventative effects in patients with Barrett's esophagus. Gastroenterology 2011;141:2000–8.

34. AGA Institute Medical Position Panel. American Gastroenterological Association medical position statement on the management of Barrett's esophagus. Gastroenterology 2011;140:1084–91.

35. Garside R, Pitt M, Somerville M, et al. Surveillance of Barrett's oesophagus: exploring the uncertainty through systematic review, expert workshop and economic modeling. Health Technol Assess 2006;10:1–142.

36. Barbiere JM, Lyratzopoulos G. Cost-effectiveness of endoscopic screening followed by surveillance for Barrett's esophagus: a review. Gastroenterology 2009;137:1869–76.

37. Wong T, Tian J, Nager AB. Barrett's surveillance identifies patients with early esophageal adenocarcinoma. Am J Med 2010;123:462–7.

38. Oelschlager BK, Barreca M, Chang L, et al. Clinical and pathologic response of Barrett's esophagus to laparoscopic antireflux surgery. Ann Surg 2003;238:458–64.

39. Biertho L, Dallemagne B, Dewandre JM, et al. Laparoscopic treatment of Barrett's esophagus: long-term results. Surg Endosc 2007;21:11–5.

40. Chang EY, Morris CD, Seltman AK, et al. The effect of antireflux surgery on esophageal carcinogenesis in patients with Barrett's esophagus: a systematic review. Ann Surg 2007;246:11–21.

41. Gurski RR, Peters JH, Hagen JA, et al. Barrett's esophagus can and does regress after antireflux surgery: a study of prevalence and predictive features. J Am Coll Surg 2003;196:706–12.

42. Bowers SP, Mattar SG, Smith CD, et al. Clinical and histologic follow-up after antireflux surgery for Barrett's esophagus. J Gastrointest Surg 2002;6:532–8.

43. Lagergren J, Ye W, Lagergren P, et al. The risk of esophageal adenocarcinoma after antireflux surgery. Gastroenterology 2010;138:1297–301.

44. National Institute for Health and Clinical Excellence. CG 106 Barrett's oesophagus—ablative therapy: NICE guideline. Available at: http://guidance.nice.org.uk/CG106S. Accessed October 14, 2012.

45. Stefandis D, Hope WW, Kohn GP, et al. Guidelines for surgical treatment of gastroesophageal reflux disease. Surg Endosc 2010;24:2647–69.

46. Wang KK, Song LM, Buttar N, et al. Barrett's esophagus after photodynamic therapy: risk of cancer development during long-term follow-up. Gastroenterology 2004;126(Suppl 2):A50.

47. Menon D, Stafinski T, Wu H, et al. Endoscopic treatments for Barrett's esophagus: a systematic review of safety and effectiveness compared to esophagectomy. BMC Gastroenterol 2010;10:111.

48. Overholt BF, Wang KK, Burdick JS, et al. Five-year efficacy and safety of photodynamic therapy with Photofrin in Barrett's high-grade dysplasia. Gastrointest Endosc 2007;66:460–8.

49. Prasad GA, Wang KK, Buttar NS, et al. Predictors of stricture formation after photodynamic therapy for high grade dysplasia in Barrett's esophagus. Gastrointest Endosc 2007;65:60–6.

50. Dunkin BJ, Martinez J, Bejarano PA, et al. Thin-layer ablation of human esophageal epithelium using a bipolar radiofrequency balloon device (BARRx). Surg Endosc 2006;20:125–30.

51. Smith CD, Bejarano PA, Melvin WS, et al. Endoscopic ablation of intestinal meta-plasia containing high-grade dysplasia in esophagectomy patients using a balloon-based ablation system. Surg Endosc 2007;21:560–9.

52. Velanovich V. Endoscopic endoluminal radiofrequency ablation of Barrett's esophagus: initial results and lessons learned. Surg Endosc 2009;23:2175–80.

53. Wani S, Puli SR, Shaheen NJ, et al. Esophageal adenocarcinoma in Barrett's esophagus after endoscopic ablative therapy: a meta-analysis and systematic review. Am J Gastroenterol 2009;104:502–13.

54. Li YM, Li L, Yu CH, et al. A systematic review and meta-analysis of the treatment for Barrett's esophagus. Dig Dis Sci 2008;53:2837–46.

55. Shaheen NJ, Sharma P, Overholt BF, et al. Radiofrequency ablation in Barrett's esophagus with dysplasia. N Engl J Med 2009;360:2277–88.

56. Shaheen NJ, Overholt BF, Sampliner RE, et al. Durability of radiofrequency abla-tion in Barrett's esophagus with dysplasia. Gastroenterology 2011;141:460–8.

57. Phoa KN, van Vilsteren FG, Weusten BL, et al. Radiofrequency ablation vs. endo-scopic surveillance for patients with Barrett esophagus and low-grade dysplasia: a randomized clinical trial. JAMA 2014;311:1209–17.

58. Johnston MH, Eastone JA, Horwhat JD, et al. Cryoablation of Barrett's esoph-agus: a pilot study. Gastrointest Endosc 2005;62:842–8.

59. Dumot JA, Vargo JJ II, Falk GW, et al. An open-label prospective trial of cryospray ablation for Barrett's esophagus high-grade dysplasia and early esophageal can-cer in high-risk patients. Gastrointest Endosc 2009;70:635–44.

60. Shaheen NJ, Greenwald BD, Peery AF, et al. Safety and efficacy of endoscopic spray cryotherapy for Barrett's esophagus with high-grade dysplasia. Gastroint-est Endosc 2010;71:680–5.

61. Bisschops R. Optimal endoluminal treatment of Barrett's esophagus: integrating novel strategies into clinical practice. Expert Rev Gastroenterol Hepatol 2011;4: 319–33.

62. Hubbard N, Velanovich V. Endoscopic endoluminal radiofrequency ablation of Barrett's esophagus in patients with fundoplications. Surg Endosc 2007;21:625–8.

63. Goers TA, Leao P, Cassera MA, et al. Ablation and laparoscopic reflux operative results in more effective and efficient treatment of Barrett's esophagus. J Am Coll Surg 2011;213:486–92.

64. O'Connell K, Velanovich V. Effects of Nissen fundoplication on endoscopic endo-luminal radiofrequency ablation of Barrett's esophagus. Surg Endosc 2011;25: 830–4.

65. Krishnan K, Pandolfino JE, Kahrilas PJ, et al. Increased risk for persistent intes-tinal metaplasia in patients with Barrett's esophagus and uncontrolled reflux exposure before radiofrequency ablation. Gastroenterology 2012;143:576–81.

66. Rice TW, Sontag SJ. Debate: esophagectomy is the treatment of choice for high grade dysplasia in Barrett's esophagus. Am J Gastroenterol 2006;101:2177–84.

67. Williams VA, Watson TJ, Herbella FA, et al. Esophagectomy for high-grade dysplasia is safe, curative and results in good alimentary outcome. J Gastrointest Surg 2007;11:1589–97.

68. Djarv T, Lagegren J, Blazeby JM, et al. Long-term health-related quality of life following surgery for oesophageal cancer. Br J Surg 2008;95:1121–6.

69. DeMeester SR. Vagal-sparing esophagectomy: is it a useful addition? Ann Thorac Surg 2010;89:S2156–8.

70. Tsiouris A, Hammoud Z, Velanovich V. Barrett's esophagus after resection of the gastroesophageal junction: effects of concomitant fundoplication. World J Surg 2011;35:1867–72.

Minimally Invasive Esophagectomy for Benign Disease

Blair A. Jobe, MD

KEYWORDS

- Minimally invasive esophagectomy • Open esophagectomy • Benign conditions
- Complications

KEY POINTS

- Minimally invasive esophagectomy (MIE) can provide patients with reduced morbidity and a rapid recovery in the treatment of benign conditions.
- There are few data examining the long-term outcomes of MIE, specifically in the context of benign disease.
- At present, MIE should be performed in centers with experience in advanced minimally invasive esophageal surgery, and it requires a team approach.
- Multicenter, prospective randomized controlled trials will be required to determine the superiority of MIE compared with open esophagectomy.

INTRODUCTION

With the introduction of laparoscopic cholecystectomy in 1989, the practice of general surgery was transformed. Laparoscopic cholecystectomy provided the platform for widespread innovation and the ultimate adoption of complex minimal access procedures.[1] This transformation in surgery has been coupled with the development of advanced surgical instrumentation and applied for more complicated disease processes. Since Dallemange described the first laparoscopic fundoplication in 1991,[2] esophageal surgeons have uniformly incorporated laparoscopic approaches into practice. Clinical series have demonstrated that minimally invasive surgery for the treatment of gastroesophageal reflux disease[3–5] and achalasia[6,7] shows efficacy, with decreased recovery times compared with open approaches.

Esophagectomy is often performed in elderly patients who have many coexisting comorbidities, including pulmonary and cardiovascular disease. Open esophagectomy is associated with significant morbidity and mortality even in experienced centers.[8,9] For example, patients who develop pneumonia after esophagectomy have

Esophageal and Lung Institute, Allegheny Health Network, 320 E. North Avenue, Pittsburgh, PA 15212, USA
E-mail address: Bjobe1@wpahs.org

Surg Clin N Am 95 (2015) 605–614
http://dx.doi.org/10.1016/j.suc.2015.02.012
0039-6109/15/$ – see front matter © 2015 Elsevier Inc. All rights reserved.
surgical.theclinics.com

up to a 20% risk of death.[10] The avoidance of laparotomy and thoracotomy may have an impact on the incidence of postoperative complications, particularly respiratory failure, by reducing postoperative pain and convalescence. Based on this, there has been a great interest in minimally invasive esophagectomy (MIE), which has the theoretic advantages of being less traumatic, with a shortened postoperative recovery and fewer cardiopulmonary complications. In addition, enhanced visualization afforded by high-definition imaging and magnification may facilitate a safer approach, with a resultant reduction in blood loss and complications.

MIE has been adopted in many centers. This article describes the history of MIE in the context of benign disease, the surgical technique, and the outcomes of minimally invasive approaches compared with those of the open approach.

HISTORY OF MINIMALLY INVASIVE ESOPHAGECTOMY

MIE was developed based on the experience obtained with benign minimal access surgeries such as Nissen fundoplication, Heller myotomy, and repair of giant paraesophageal hernia. Nascent efforts consisted of hybrid operations that blended traditional open surgery with the minimally invasive approach. In 1993, Collard and colleagues[11] published the first report of MIE, and included 12 patients who underwent thoracoscopic esophageal mobilization followed by laparotomy. Several subsequent reports established the feasibility of this approach, thereby providing the foundation for development expansion. Despite these efforts, the definitive benefit of MIE over the open approach remained dubious.[12,13]

In 1995, DePaula and colleagues[14] reported a series of laparoscopic transhiatal esophagectomy. Twelve patients underwent laparoscopic transhiatal esophagectomy for end-stage achalasia. One patient required conversion to laparotomy, and no procedure-related mortality occurred. In 1997, Swanstrom and Hansen[15] reported the first experience with laparoscopic esophagectomy in the United States. Nine patients were selected based on the presence of cancer, benign strictures, and Barrett's esophagus. Eight patients underwent a transhiatal MIE with cervical anastomosis. One patient in this series underwent video-assisted thoracoscopic surgery with intrathoracic anastomosis. In 1998, Luketich and colleagues[16] reported 8 cases of minimally invasive approach to esophagectomy including a single case of combined thoracoscopic and laparoscopic esophagectomy with cervical anastomosis. Subsequently, Watson and colleagues[17] reported a minimally invasive Ivor Lewis approach in 1999, which described 2 cases of hand-assisted laparoscopic construction of the gastric conduit followed by thoracoscopic mobilization with a hand-sewn intrathoracic anastomosis. In single-institution case series, minimally invasive Ivor Lewis technique was shown to be associated with shortened postoperative hospital stay and recovery.

Indication for Minimally Invasive Esophagectomy in Benign Disease

Unlike MIE in the treatment of esophageal cancer, patients who undergo this procedure for benign disease tend to have a superior functional status and few comorbidities. In addition, the debilitation and malnutrition associated with induction therapy are typically absent. As a result, the outcomes of MIE tend to be improved in patients with benign disease compared with those undergoing resection for malignancy. The potential indications for MIE in the face of benign disease include

End-stage achalasia—patients present with anatomic obstruction and aspiration secondary to esophageal redundancy and dilation in the face of a prior complete myotomy

Severe gastroesophageal reflux disease with associated esophageal motility disorder—patients suffer from volume regurgitation, dysphagia. and chest pain with poor esophageal clearance

Failed antireflux surgery—most patients have undergone 2 to 3 prior antireflux surgeries and are not candidates for roux en y esophagojejunostomy because of functional obstruction proximal to the esophagogastric junction (ie, peristaltic failure)

Severe esophageal motility disorder unresponsive to prior medical and surgical therapy

1. These patients typically have a spastic motility disorder and present with severe dysphagia and regurgitation secondary to functional obstruction and bolus escape with retrograde bolus propagation.

2. Most of these patients have had a prior long myotomy with continued chest pain and dysphagia.

Refractory peptic stricture (rare in the era of proton pump inhibitor therapy)—it is important to screen these patients for gastrinoma and pill-induced injury

Idiopathic inflammatory disorders of the esophagus

Large benign tumors of the esophagus such as leiomyoma—the need for MIE in these patients is rare

Caustic injury to esophagus with refractory stricture

The selection of MIE approach (ie, transhiatal, inversion, Ivor Lewis) should be guided by the type and location of benign disease. For example, a patient with a transmural inflammatory process would not be a good candidate for a minimally invasive inversion esophagectomy, because the periesophageal fibrosis and thickening would preclude a safe stripping technique and increase the chances of hemorrhage and injury to vital structures.

Current Approaches to Minimally Invasive Esophagectomy

The laparoscopic transhiatal (inversion) esophagectomy (LIE) is a modification based on the open inversion technique with vagal preservation described by Akiyama and colleagues[18] in 1994. The LIE is an entirely laparoscopic approach, whereby a vein stripper is attached to the distal esophagus through a cervical esophagotomy, and distal-to-proximal inversion (outside in) of the esophagus is performed by drawing back on the vein stripper, thereby facilitating the transhiatal dissection from below. Attaching to the proximal esophagus, delivering the vein stripper through a laparoscopic port, and drawing from below also can be used to facilitate proximal-to-distal inversion. The esophagus is then placed into a specimen bed and delivered through a 12 mm port site.

This approach provides enhanced mediastinal working space and visualization with the countertraction between the esophagus and its surrounding mediastinal attachments and directed dissection as the esophagus is inverted. Advantages of this approach include the elimination of the need for single-lung ventilation or patient repositioning during the procedure. Perry and colleagues[19] reported a series of 40 consecutive patients who underwent LIE. Four patients (10%) required laparotomy because of adhesions (2 patients), severe kyphosis (1 patient), and a tracheal tear occurred during the mediastinal dissection (1 patient). Median intensive care unit (ICU) and hospital stays were 2 days and 9 days, respectively. There was no operative mortality. The rates of recurrent nerve injury and anastomotic leak were 10% and 27.5%, respectively. The LIE may be particularly useful for patients with end-stage benign esophageal diseases such as achalasia and complicated gastroesophageal reflux disease.

For patients with inflammatory esophageal diseases, long-segment strictures, and benign tumors, the exposure, need for mediastinal dissection, and pliability of the esophageal body may preclude a safe operation.

The thoracoscopic and laparoscopic approaches were initially performed using the McKeown approach, with thoracoscopic esophageal mobilization performed initially, followed by laparoscopy for gastric conduit preparation and feeding jejunostomy placement, and finally the esophagogastrostomy was then performed in the neck. Outstanding thoracoscopic visualization of intrathoracic structures facilitates the safe mobilization of a thoracic esophagus and the radical dissection of lymphatic tissue when performed for malignancy. In 2003, Luketich and colleagues[20] reported the results of 222 consecutive patients who underwent this approach. The operation was successfully completed in 93% of patients. There were no emergent conversions to laparotomy for hemorrhage. The rates of hospital mortality and anastomotic dehiscence were 1.4% and 11.7%, respectively. Median ICU time and hospital stay were 1 day and 7 days, respectively. Using the gastroesophageal reflux disease health-related quality of life (GERD-HRQL), the quality of life was preserved based on pre and postoperative scores on relatively short-term follow-up. However, the potential pitfall with this approach is related to the cervical dissection and risk for recurrent nerve injury, pharyngeal dysfunction, and a higher anastomotic dehiscence rate. Because of this, an alternative method is to use a completely thoracoscopic–laparoscopic Ivor Lewis approach with a proximal intrathoracic anastomosis (TLE), in which laparoscopic gastric conduit creation followed by thoracoscopic mobilization and removal of thoracic esophagus, gastric pull-up, and construction of an esophagogastric anastomosis are performed. In 2006, Bizekis and colleagues[21] reported a series of TLE in 50 patients for cancer. Twenty-five patients (50%) received preoperative chemotherapy or chemoradiation. There was 1 nonemergent conversion to laparotomy. The rates of operative mortality and anastomotic dehiscence were both 6%. Four patients (8%) developed pneumonia postoperatively. There were no recurrent nerve injuries. It is important to emphasize that most data are obtained in populations with malignancy, and to date, there have been no large series examining the long-term outcomes of MIE as a treatment for benign disease.

Preoperative Preparation

Optimal outcomes depend on obtaining a complete preoperative risk assessment with the mitigation of modifiable risks (eg, coronary artery stenosis, active tobacco use, uncontrolled diabetes, cardiac dysrhythmia, celiac artery stenosis). The possibility of conversion to thoracotomy or laparotomy should be discussed preoperatively. Cardiac clearance and pulmonary function testing should be obtained to assess the risk for cardiopulmonary complications such as myocardial infarction and pneumonia. Smoking cessation is critically important, and assistance with quitting should be provided. All patients should meet with the dietician before and after surgery to discuss caloric optimization and postoperative diet. Prophylactic anticoagulation in conjunction with sequential compression devices is routinely employed. For thoracoscopic procedures, a double-lumen endotracheal tube is placed, and proper location is confirmed with bronchoscopy after patient positioning into the left lateral decubitus position.

SURGICAL TECHNIQUE

The technical details of LIE[22] and TLE[23] have been described previously. The characteristics and indications for each procedure are summarized in **Table 1**. Both procedures are complicated and ideally require 2 experienced surgeons to deliver a

Table 1
Characteristics of minimally invasive laparoscopic transhiatal (inversion) esophagectomy and Ivor Lewis esophagectomy

	Laparoscopic Transhiatal (Inversion) Esophagectomy	Thoracoscopic–Laparoscopic Ivor Lewis Esophagectomy
Approach	Laparoscopic	Thoracoscopic and laparoscopic
Single-lung ventilation	No	Yes
Patient position	Supine	Supine to left lateral decubitus
Laparoscopic ports	6-port technique	5-port technique
Thoracoscopic ports	N/A	5-port technique
Anastomosis	Neck	High chest
Advantage	No need for patient repositioning/single-lung ventilation/thoracoscopy	Rare recurrent laryngeal nerve injury, low anastomotic leak/stricture rates, less gastric conduit required, good intrathoracic visualization
Disadvantage	Limited mediastinal working space, higher anastomotic leak/stricture, pharyngeal dysfunction, requires longer gastric conduit length	Need for single-lung ventilation, potentially fatal intrathoracic anastomotic leak

successful outcome in an appropriate time frame. Important technical tips that need to be emphasized include

- Attention should be paid to preserve the right gastroepiploic arcade while mobilizing the stomach during division of the gastrocolic ligament and elevation of antrum away from the pancreatic bed. Every effort should be made to dissect all lymphatic tissue en bloc with surgical specimen throughout the procedure. the authors include the common hepatic lymph nodes along with the celiac nodes when performing MIE for malignancy.
- For benign diseases, the left gastric artery can be preserved in continuity with the right gastric artery. This maneuver may enhance arterial inflow to the neoesophagus. The pyloroantral area must be mobilized (including Kocher maneuver) until the pylorus can be elevated to the right crus in a tension-free manner.
- Circumferential mediastinal dissection should be performed as far proximally as can be safely visualized through the hiatus. This action facilitates the dissection of diaphragmatic hiatus from the chest, and the retrieval of the surgical specimen with neoesophagus pull-up into the chest.
- The authors favor a narrow (5 cm wide) neoesophagus because of its superior long-term functional benefits such as improved emptying and less reflux. During the creation of gastric conduit, the first assistant grasps the tip of the fundus along the greater curvature and stretches it toward the spleen, while a second grasper is placed on the antral area and a slight downward retraction is applied. This maneuver facilitates a straight application stapler, thus preventing spiraling and subsequent ischemia of the conduit.
- A key initial step in the chest part of TLE is to place a retracting suture through the central tendon of the diaphragm, which is brought out through the anterior chest wall via a 1 mm incision. This suture retracts the diaphragm inferiorly and anteriorly, and allows excellent visualization of the crural diaphragm and esophagogastric junction.

- The dissection of proximal esophagus above the azygos vein arch should be maintained on the esophageal wall to prevent injury of the recurrent laryngeal nerve.
- All aortoesophageal vessels and any lymphatic branches arising from the thoracic duct should be meticulously clipped prior to division to prevent unexpected bleeding and chylothorax.
- With the TLE approach, the esophagus is divided proximal to the level of the azygos arch.
- The proximal esophagus is divided at the level of the azygos arch, ensuring that the site of division is proximal to squamocolumnar junction in patients with long-segment Barrett esophagus.
- The gastric conduit needs to be positioned without redundancy or tension. With the TLE approach, the authors use a 28 or 25 mm circular stapler for the esophagogastrostomy. First, a gastrotomy is created parallel to the staple line at the most proximal aspect of the neoesophagus; the stapler is introduced into the chest through a 5 cm minithoracotomy made at the surgeon right hand port. The stapler is then introduced into the lumen of the neoesophagus, and the pin is deployed along the greater curvature after assessing for tension. After esophagogastrostomy, the opening in the gastrotomy is closed with an endoscopic stapler.
- After the stapler is removed at the completion of anastomosis, it is important to verify that the stapler contains 2 complete tissue rings, as this indicates that a complete circumferential anastomosis has been established.
- With the Ivor Lewis approach, the neoesophagus should be sutured to the right crus from the thoracic side to prevent small bowel herniation from the abdominal cavity.

POSTOPERATIVE MANAGEMENT

All patients who undergo MIE are placed in the intensive care unit (ICU), and every effort is made to extubate the patient immediately following surgery. Prior to extubation, therapeutic bronchoscopy is performed to clear the airway as much as possible to minimize atelectasis and mucous plugging. A nasogastric tube is place intraoperatively, and the patient should be maintained in a 45° head-up position to prevent aspiration and improve functional residual capacity. Prophylactic anticoagulation with heparin in conjunction with sequential compression devices is critical to prevent deep vein thrombosis (DVT) and pulmonary embolism. Aggressive pulmonary toileting and early ambulation should be implemented to maximize pulmonary function and prevent DVT. Electrolytes should be monitored and corrected to prevent postoperative arrhythmia. On postoperative day 2, continuous tube feeding is started at 10 mL/h, and the rate of tube feeding is advanced to goal over the following day. Prior to discharge, tube feeding is changed to cyclic (3 PM–9 AM), thereby enabling patients to maintain daily activities without a connection to tube feeding. On day 5, a water-soluble contrast examination should be obtained to inspect the anastomosis for leak, anatomic features, and emptying. Patients are then initiated on 30 to 60 mL of clear fluids by mouth every 1 to 2 hours. The patients are discharged with sips of liquid, cyclic tube feeding at goal rate, and a Jackson-Pratt (JP) drain (placed at the level of the anastomosis); they should be seen in the clinic after 2 weeks with a chest radiograph and blood work.

Prevention of Anastomotic Leak

Anastomotic dehiscence remains a potentially life-threatening complication associated with MIE. A prospective, randomized study by Bhat and colleagues[24] demonstrated that a pedicled omental transposition to reinforce the esophagogastrostomy significantly reduced the incidence of dehiscence, thus decreasing the morbidity and mortality of the procedure.

Several methods to improve the microcirculation of the neoesophagus have been investigated. Akiyama and colleagues[25] performed preoperative angiographic embolization of the left gastric, right gastric, and splenic arteries in a group of patients, followed 2 days later by esophagogastrectomy with gastric tubularization and esophagogastrostomy. In the control group, esophagectomy was performed without preoperative embolization. There was improved circulation in the embolization group compared with the control group (33% vs 67%, respectively) as measured by laser flowmetry. Anastomotic dehiscence rates were higher in the control group. Supercharging of the neoesophagus by vascular anastomoses has been investigated as another approach. Nagawa and colleagues[26] performed intraoperative anastomoses between the left gastroepiploic and transverse cervical arteries, resulting in no anastomotic dehiscence compared with the 10% to 25% dehiscence rate previously experienced by the group using unaugmented techniques. The drawback to this procedure is that it required multiple surgical teams with experience in microvascular anastomoses. In their practice, the authors have used preoperative gastric ischemic conditioning by laparoscopic ligation of left gastric vessels 2 weeks prior to esophagectomy, potentially decreasing the rate of dehiscence and stricture[27–29] in high-risk patients. Combining a minimally invasive approach with these methods for prevention of anastomotic leak, the outcomes of MIE would improve further.

Is Minimally Invasive Esophagectomy Superior to Open Esophagectomy?

No randomized controlled trials comparing MIE with open esophagectomy have been conducted. Several retrospective studies have shown MIE to be equivalent or improved compared with the open approach.[20,30,31] In a case–control study comparing LIE (n = 21) with open transhiatal esophagectomy (n = 21),[30] LIE was associated with less blood loss and shorter hospital stay without increasing the operative time, morbidity, or mortality related to esophagectomy. In the report of 222 consecutive patients who underwent combined thoracoscopic–laparoscopic esophagectomy, Luketich and colleagues[20] demonstrated a low mortality rate (1.4%) and short hospital stay (7 days) compared with most open series published.[9,32] Pham and colleagues[31] reported the results of a retrospective study comparing TLE (n = 44) with open Ivor Lewis esophagectomy (n = 46). TLE was associated with less blood loss and wound problems. However, TLE required longer operative times, and there was no significant difference in hospital stay, 30-day mortality, or cardiopulmonary complications.

A meta-analysis by Biere and colleagues[33] demonstrated no significant difference for major morbidity or pulmonary complications between the groups, although there was a trend toward mortality rate reduction in the MIE group. A meta-analysis by Nagpal and colleagues[34] showed that MIE was associated with less blood loss, shorter operative time and length of hospital stay, and lower respiratory complications compared with open esophagectomy. As such, a quicker recovery and a reduction in morbidity can be achieved with MIE, but outcomes of MIE remain variable. For example, in a recent report of 1033 MIEs using the combined laparoscopic and thoracoscopic approach,[35] Luketich and colleagues demonstrated an overall mortality rate of 1.7% and a median length of stay of 8 days. Patients spent a median of 2 days in the ICU. However, the mortality rate after 30 days was not reported. Multicenter, prospective randomized trials comparing MIE with open esophagectomy will be required to determine if MIE is superior to open esophagectomy. Esophagectomy remains one of the most complicated and technically demanding procedures performed in the field of surgery, and the outcomes are tightly linked to case volume and experience of surgeons and hospitals.[36]

SUMMARY

MIE can provide patients with reduced morbidity and a rapid recovery in the treatment of benign conditions. There is few data examining the long-term outcomes of MIE specifically in the context of benign disease. At present, MIE should be performed in centers with experience in advanced minimally invasive esophageal surgery, and it requires a team approach. Multicenter, prospective randomized controlled trials will be required to determine the superiority of MIE compared with open esophagectomy. Further investigation will be required to determine the effect of MIE on quality of life and long-term outcomes in the treatment of benign conditions.

REFERENCE

1. Vierra M. Minimally invasive surgery. Annu Rev Med 1995;46:147–58.
2. Dallemagne B, Weerts JM, Jehaes C, et al. Laparoscopic Nissen fundoplication: preliminary report. Surg Laparosc Endosc 1991;1(3):138–43.
3. Ackroyd R, Watson DI, Majeed AW, et al. Randomized clinical trial of laparoscopic versus open fundoplication for gastro-oesophageal reflux disease. Br J Surg 2004;91(8):975–82.
4. DeMeester TR, Bonavina L, Albertucci M. Nissen fundoplication for gastroesophageal reflux disease. Evaluation of primary repair in 100 consecutive patients. Ann Surg 1986;204(1):9–20.
5. Hunter JG, Trus TL, Branum GD, et al. A physiologic approach to laparoscopic fundoplication for gastroesophageal reflux disease. Ann Surg 1996;223(6): 673–85 [discussion: 685–7].
6. Khajanchee YS, Kanneganti S, Leatherwood AE, et al. Laparoscopic Heller myotomy with Toupet fundoplication: outcomes predictors in 121 consecutive patients. Arch Surg 2005;140(9):827–33 [discussion: 833–4].
7. Patti MG, Pellegrini CA, Horgan S, et al. Minimally invasive surgery for achalasia: an 8-year experience with 168 patients. Ann Surg 1999;230(4):587–93 [discussion: 593–4].
8. Millikan KW, Silverstein J, Hart V, et al. A 15-year review of esophagectomy for carcinoma of the esophagus and cardia. Arch Surg 1995;130(6):617–24.
9. Orringer MB, Marshall B, Iannettoni MD. Transhiatal esophagectomy: clinical experience and refinements. Ann Surg 1999;230(3):392–400 [discussion: 400–3].
10. Atkins BZ, Shah AS, Hutcheson KA, et al. Reducing hospital morbidity and mortality following esophagectomy. Ann Thorac Surg 2004;78(4):1170–6 [discussion: 1170–6].
11. Collard JM, Lengele B, Otte JB, et al. En bloc and standard esophagectomies by thoracoscopy. Ann Thorac Surg 1993;56(3):675–9.
12. Akaishi T, Kaneda I, Higuchi N, et al. Thoracoscopic en bloc total esophagectomy with radical mediastinal lymphadenectomy. J Thorac Cardiovasc Surg 1996; 112(6):1533–40 [discussion: 1540–1].
13. Robertson GS, Lloyd DM, Wicks AC, et al. No obvious advantages for thoracoscopic two-stage oesophagectomy. Br J Surg 1996;83(5):675–8.
14. DePaula AL, Hashiba K, Ferreira EA, et al. Laparoscopic transhiatal esophagectomy with esophagogastroplasty. Surg Laparosc Endosc 1995;5(1):1–5.
15. Swanstrom LL, Hansen P. Laparoscopic total esophagectomy. Arch Surg 1997; 132(9):943–7 [discussion: 947–9].

16. Luketich JD, Nguyen NT, Weigel T, et al. Minimally invasive approach to esophagectomy. JSLS 1998;2(3):243–7.
17. Watson DI, Davies N, Jamieson GG. Totally endoscopic Ivor Lewis esophagectomy. Surg Endosc 1999;13(3):293–7.
18. Akiyama H, Tsurumaru M, Ono Y, et al. Esophagectomy without thoracotomy with vagal preservation. J Am Coll Surg 1994;178(1):83–5.
19. Perry KA, Enestvedt CK, Diggs BS, et al. Perioperative outcomes of laparoscopic transhiatal inversion esophagectomy compare favorably with those of combined thoracoscopic-laparoscopic esophagectomy. Surg Endosc 2009;23(9):2147–54.
20. Luketich JD, Alvelo-Rivera M, Buenaventura PO, et al. Minimally invasive esophagectomy: outcomes in 222 patients. Ann Surg 2003;238(4):486–94 [discussion: 494–5].
21. Bizekis C, Kent MS, Luketich JD, et al. Initial experience with minimally invasive Ivor Lewis esophagectomy. Ann Thorac Surg 2006;82(2):402–6 [discussion: 406–7].
22. Jobe BA, Kim CY, Minjarez RC, et al. Simplifying minimally invasive transhiatal esophagectomy with the inversion approach: lessons learned from the first 20 cases. Arch Surg 2006;141(9):857–65 [discussion: 865–6].
23. Kent MS, Schuchert M, Fernando H, et al. Minimally invasive esophagectomy: state of the art. Dis Esophagus 2006;19(3):137–45.
24. Bhat MA, Dar MA, Lone GN, et al. Use of pedicled omentum in esophagogastric anastomosis for prevention of anastomotic leak. Ann Thorac Surg 2006;82(5): 1857–62.
25. Akiyama S, Kodera Y, Sekiguchi H, et al. Preoperative embolization therapy for esophageal operation. J Surg Oncol 1998;69(4):219–23.
26. Nagawa H, Seto Y, Nakatsuka T, et al. Microvascular anastomosis for additional blood flow in reconstruction after intrathoracic esophageal carcinoma surgery. Am J Surg 1997;173(2):131–3.
27. Holscher AH, Schneider PM, Gutschow C, et al. Laparoscopic ischemic conditioning of the stomach for esophageal replacement. Ann Surg 2007;245(2): 241–6.
28. Varela E, Reavis KM, Hinojosa MW, et al. Laparoscopic gastric ischemic conditioning prior to esophagogastrectomy: technique and review. Surg Innov 2008; 15(2):132–5.
29. Enestvedt CK, Hosack L, Winn SR, et al. VEGF gene therapy augments localized angiogenesis and promotes anastomotic wound healing: a pilot study in a clinically relevant animal model. J Gastrointest Surg 2008;12(10):1762–70 [discussion: 1771–2].
30. Perry KA, Enestvedt CK, Pham T, et al. Comparison of laparoscopic inversion esophagectomy and open transhiatal esophagectomy for high-grade dysplasia and stage I esophageal adenocarcinoma. Arch Surg 2009;144(7):679–84.
31. Pham TH, Perry KA, Dolan JP, et al. Comparison of perioperative outcomes after combined thoracoscopic-laparoscopic esophagectomy and open Ivor-Lewis esophagectomy. Am J Surg 2010;199(5):594–8.
32. Bailey SH, Bull DA, Harpole DH, et al. Outcomes after esophagectomy: a ten-year prospective cohort. Ann Thorac Surg 2003;75(1):217–22 [discussion: 222].
33. Biere SS, Cuesta MA, van der Peet DL. Minimally invasive versus open esophagectomy for cancer: a systematic review and meta-analysis. Minerva Chir 2009; 64(2):121–33.
34. Nagpal K, Ahmed K, Vats A, et al. Is minimally invasive surgery beneficial in the management of esophageal cancer? A meta-analysis. Surg Endosc 2010;24(7): 1621–9.

35. Luketich JD, Pennathur A, Levy RM, et al. Outcomes after minimally invasive esophagectomy: review of over 1000 patients. Ann Surg 2012;256:95–103.
36. Hulscher JB, van Sandick JW, de Boer AG, et al. Extended transthoracic resection compared with limited transhiatal resection for adenocarcinoma of the esophagus. N Engl J Med 2002;347(21):1662–9.

Preoperative Evaluation of Gastroesophageal Reflux Disease

 CrossMark

Vikas Singhal, MBBS[a], Leena Khaitan, MD, MPA[b],*

KEYWORDS

- GERD evaluation • Preoperative assessment • Diagnostic evaluation

KEY POINTS

- Gastroesophageal reflux disease (GERD) causes troublesome symptoms, mucosal injury in the esophagus, or both of these.
- The objective diagnosis of GERD should be made with an ambulatory acid or nonacid reflux study before proceeding with surgical intervention to get the best outcome.
- The preoperative evaluation of GERD should not only confirm the diagnosis of GERD but also help to determine the true cause of the GERD to help guide treatment.
- Symptom correlation is a key aspect when diagnosing GERD to help predict outcome of a procedure and set patient expectation.
- GERD can be caused by poor gastric emptying and this should be evaluated as part of the work-up either symptomatically or with objective evaluation.
- GERD can be caused by some dysfunction of the LES, such as hiatal hernia, hypotensive LES, or transient inappropriate LES relaxations that result from gastric distention.
- Once the cause of GERD is elucidated, the surgeon can determine whether medications, surgical intervention with Nissen fundoplication, partial fundoplication, Linx placement, hiatal hernia repair, or an endoscopic treatment will have the desired outcome for the patient.
- Esophageal motility disorders should be assessed before any surgery with manometry and esophagram.

INTRODUCTION: NATURE OF THE PROBLEM

Gastroesophageal reflux disease (GERD) has been defined per the Montreal definition as "Reflux that causes troublesome symptoms, mucosal injury in the esophagus, or both of these."[1] The prevalence of GERD has been noted to be extremely high in Western countries. In 2004, approximately 20% of the US population reported reflux symptoms that occurred at least weekly.[2] According to data from the Gallup organization (1988) approximately 44% of Americans experience heartburn at least

[a] Department of GI and Bariatric Surgery, Jaypee Hospital, Wishtown Sector 128, Noida, UP 201304, India; [b] Department of Surgery, University Hospitals Case Medical Center, 11100 Euclid Avenue, Cleveland, OH 44106, USA
* Corresponding author.
E-mail address: Leena.khaitan@uhhospitals.org

Surg Clin N Am 95 (2015) 615–627
http://dx.doi.org/10.1016/j.suc.2015.02.013
0039-6109/15/$ – see front matter © 2015 Elsevier Inc. All rights reserved.
surgical.theclinics.com

Abbreviations	
GERD	Gastroesophageal reflux disease
HRQL	Health-related quality of life
LES	Lower esophageal sphincter
MII	Multichannel intraluminal impedance
PPI	Proton pump inhibitor
SAP	Symptom Associated Probability
SI	Symptom Index
TLESR	Transient inappropriate relaxations of the LES

once per month. Almost 18% of Americans take nonprescription drugs for reflux-related symptoms.[3] It is remarkable that this disease is so prevalent and yet the treatment options are significantly underused. Despite the availability of multiple treatments on the market, medications remain the primary treatment modality offered to patients.

Adaptations to equipment and technique have resulted in newer laparoscopic and endoscopic procedures being approved for GERD. If patients decide to proceed with a procedure for their reflux, there are several options available. Apart from the gold standard Nissen fundoplication, newer laparoscopic procedures, such as lower esophageal sphincter (LES) augmentation with the LINX reflux (Torax Medical, Shoreview, MN) management system, are now in the armamentarium of surgeon and patient. Endoscopic procedures, such as radiofrequency ablation (Stretta procedure) and transoral incisionless fundoplication, are also becoming popular because patients are desiring less invasive procedures for reflux disease. In addition, multiple new interventional treatments for GERD are on the horizon. Each of these treatments addresses a different mechanism of GERD. As a result the preoperative assessment for treatment of GERD now includes not only confirmation of the diagnosis of GERD but also the determination of the cause of GERD to tailor the appropriate treatment option to the patient.

RELEVANT ANATOMY AND PATHOPHYSIOLOGY
Etiology of Gastroesophageal Reflux Disease

Stein and DeMeester[4] provided the concept of the plumbing circuit where the esophagus functions as an antegrade pump, the LES as a valve, and stomach as a reservoir. Problems with any component of the circuit (either poor esophageal motility, a dysfunctional LES, or delayed gastric emptying) can lead to GERD. From a medical or surgical standpoint, it is extremely important to identify which of these components is defective so that effective therapy can be applied.

The LES is defined by manometry as a zone of elevated intraluminal pressure at the esophagogastric junction. It is a 3- to 5-cm segment of contracted circular smooth muscle at the distal end of the esophagus, the resting tone of which varies from 10 to 35 mm Hg when measured at end expiration. Hypotensive pressure within the sphincter is often a cause of severe reflux. At least 2 cm of the sphincter should be intra-abdominal.

Another cause of reflux is transient inappropriate LES relaxations (relaxation in the absence of swallowing). These transient LES relaxations (TLESRs) are vagally mediated reflexes triggered by gastric distention and serve to vent the stomach. Prolonged or more frequent TLESRs have been investigated as a cause of reflux disease and it is agreed that TLESRs are a common mechanism of reflux.[5] Patients with reflux have a low gastric yield pressure such that these relaxations can be stimulated by minimal gastric distention and volume intake.

Apart from the LES itself there are two other anatomic structures that contribute to preventing reflux at the esophagogastric junction: the diaphragmatic crura, and the phrenoesophageal ligament, which help form the angle of His. For proper LES function, this junction must be located in the abdomen so that the diaphragmatic crura can assist the action of the LES, thus functioning as an extrinsic sphincter. If this mechanism is defective, GERD is exacerbated. A hiatal hernia may contribute to reflux because proximal migration of the LES may result in loss of its abdominal high-pressure zone, or the length of the high-pressure zone may decrease. Also the crural mechanisms are not effective in preventing reflux. Hence reduction of hiatal hernia with re-establishing the intra-abdominal length of the esophagus, with proper crural closure, apart from a fundic wrap are key components to surgical correction of GERD.

A chronically increased intragastric pressure and increased frequency of TLESRs are thought to play the major role in obesity-related GERD and reflux disease in pregnancy. Another mechanism of GERD to be considered is poor gastric emptying. If the stomach empties poorly, there is a backup in the plumbing circuit that then leads to reflux of gastric contents into the esophagus.

A newer line of investigation is the realization that not all reflux is acid. Other components of the reflux fluid, such as bile acids, pepsin, and gas, apart from hypersensitivity to the volume of reflux itself have all been thought to contribute to reflux disease, especially reflux with atypical symptoms and those symptoms that do not respond to proton pump inhibitors (PPIs). This makes sense with the various mechanisms outlined previously.

CLINICAL PRESENTATION AND EXAMINATION

A thorough assessment of symptoms preoperatively is important as an initial screening for the causes of the patient's reflux. Symptoms related to reflux disease can be extensive and varied (**Table 1**). The most typical symptoms of GERD are heartburn and regurgitation, belching, and sometimes epigastric discomfort. Atypical symptoms of GERD are many including bloating; dysphagia; and oropharyngeal symptoms, such as hoarseness, globus, and chronic cough. Patients can also present with chest symptoms or etiologies, such as chest pain, pneumonia, chronic aspiration, and asthma. It is key in such patients to exclude cardiac causes of pain before labeling it as noncardiac chest pain. Other manifestations include dental erosions, sinusitis, otitis media, and sleep apnea. Finally, patients can have complications of GERD that include stricture, ulceration, and Barrett esophagus. The timing of the reflux, relationship to meals, exacerbation of symptoms with upright or supine position, and

Table 1
Various manifestations of GERD

Typical Symptoms	Atypical Symptoms	Complications
Heartburn	Chronic cough	Stricture
Regurgitation[a]	Hoarseness	Esophagitis
Epigastric pain	Globus	Ulceration
Belching	Dysphagia	Barrett esophagus
	Chest pain	Adenocarcinoma
	Chronic aspiration	
	Bronchitis	
	Sinusitis	

[a] Regurgitation is one of the most important symptoms that can be impacted by a surgical intervention for GERD.

difficulty swallowing should be noted. Elicitation of this history can help the surgeon to set patient expectation for success of a procedure once the work-up is completed. Symptoms alone can never be the only tool used for the diagnosis of reflux. It is well established that symptoms alone have limited positive predictive value for success with intervention.[6,7]

Patients should also be assessed for their surgical candidacy. Patients should be able to withstand surgery and should also be mentally prepared for surgery. There are studies that suggest patients with psychiatric diagnoses may do poorly with antireflux surgery.

Patients who present with typical symptoms usually respond the most to treatment either medical or surgical. To objectively stratify GERD symptoms, such questionnaires as GERD-Q and GERD-HRQL (health-related quality of life) have been developed. These may be used to screen patients with GERD and assess response to intervention by comparing preintervention with postintervention surveys. The GERD-HRQL has been validated by Velanovich[8] for this purpose. Through these questionnaires it has become clear that GERD can affect quality of life as severely as other chronic diseases, such as diabetes, arthritis, and heart failure.[9]

Physical examination is usually not very contributory in the assessment of GERD.

DIAGNOSTIC PROCEDURES
Presumptive Treatment As a Diagnostic Measure

GERD is unusual in that one of the initial modes of diagnosis is by initiating therapy. Patients with reflux symptoms are frequently started on antiacid medications as a diagnostic and therapeutic maneuver. This has been the standard for several years. These medications are extremely effective at blocking acid and are thought to have few side effects. The recent American College of Gastroenterology guidelines recommend that in patients with symptoms and history consistent with uncomplicated GERD, the diagnosis of GERD may be assumed and empirical therapy begun. Patients who show signs of GERD complications or other illness or who do not respond to therapy should be considered for further diagnostic testing.[10] However, these recommendations are now being challenged because there is growing evidence that an endoscopy at baseline can be very helpful in determining further management of the patient's GERD and can evaluate for a complication of reflux, such as inflammation, strictures, or Barrett-type changes. In addition, the long-term use of medications, such as PPIs, is now being shown to have serious potential side effects (**Box 1**). These side effects may drive more patients to think about a procedure for treatment of their GERD rather than remain on medications.

Upper Gastrointestinal Tract Endoscopy

Upper endoscopy is often the first diagnostic test in a GERD evaluation. Endoscopy itself has a low sensitivity to diagnose reflux disease. However, it is useful in the diagnosis of complications of GERD, such as inflammation, strictures, and Barrett esophagus. It is also essential to rule out cancer. Biopsies can be taken of erosive disease to identify reflux-related changes in the esophagus. If erosive disease is found there is a school of thought that no further testing is necessary before doing an antireflux procedure. However, studies have shown that even with erosive disease, a 24-hour pH test maybe negative. These patients often have poor outcomes with surgical intervention.[11] However, patients may have reflux and no evidence of erosive disease or mucosal changes in the esophagus. The authors recommend doing ambulatory pH monitoring before making a final diagnosis of GERD.

Box 1
Side effects of PPIs

Possible increase *Clostridium difficile* overgrowth caused by increased gastric pH.

Histamine agonists and PPIs have been implicated in community- and hospital-acquired pneumonias.

Higher risk of bone fractures (wrist, hip, and spine) caused by decreased calcium absorption from lower gastric pH.

Interactions of some PPIs with clopidogrel leading to less effectiveness of the medication.

Acid suppression may affect iron absorption in those with low baseline stores.

Long-term PPI use linked to chronic atrophic gastritis, hypergastrinemia, and fundic gland polyps.

Long-term PPI use is associated with hypomagnesemia caused by reduced intestinal absorption.

Adapted from Ament PW, Dicola DB, James ME. Reducing adverse effects of proton pump inhibitors. Am Fam Physician 2012;86(1):68.

With endoscopy, a retroflexed view at the cardia can help to identify hiatal hernias and visualize the flap at the LES. The endoscopist can make a subjective assessment of the LES as to its "looseness" and function. Furthermore, a poor man's assessment can be made of gastric yield pressure in that in patients with low gastric yield pressure, it is difficult to fully insufflate the stomach when retroflexing at the cardia. Endoscopy can also be therapeutic to dilate strictures and take biopsies at the time of the study. The endoscopy can be performed by gastroenterology or by the surgeon who is considering a procedure for the patient. Because of the increasing incidence of Barrett esophagus, many physicians now advocate that any patient requiring long-term PPIs should have at least one endoscopy to look for any anatomic abnormalities. Of note, if the patient complains of dysphagia, an esophagram should be done first to alert the endoscopist to strictures or diverticula that may complicate the endoscopy.

Esophagram

An esophagram is a useful test in assessing function of the proximal gastrointestinal tract. It is a noninvasive way to look for structural abnormalities, such as stricture, paraesophageal hernia, hiatal hernia (sliding or fixed), and diverticula. Extrinsic compression of the esophagus and mucosal abnormalities can be seen in addition to a real-time view of the anatomy and function of the gastroesophageal junction (**Figs. 1** and **2**). The physician performing the procedure can give a subjective assessment of reflux; however, this should not be a substitute for ambulatory pH. Barium swallow has a sensitivity of only 34% and cannot be definitively diagnostic for GERD.[12]

Many patients with GERD may have no significant findings on radiographic study. Additionally, this radiologic study can elucidate other motility disorders that may mimic reflux, such as achalasia.

Ambulatory pH Testing

If further evaluation is warranted or a procedure for reflux is being considered then an ambulatory pH study needs to be done to objectively measure the patient's reflux. Ambulatory pH monitoring is considered the gold standard confirmatory test. The testing is done with patients off PPIs for a minimum of 7 days and H_2 receptor blockers

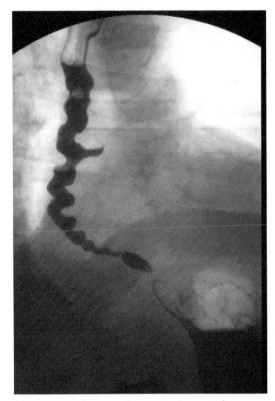

Fig. 1. An abnormal barium esophagram demonstrating a corkscrew pattern.

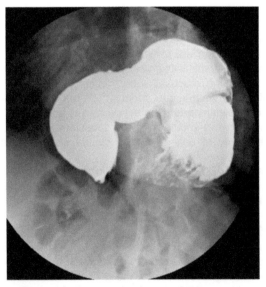

Fig. 2. Hiatal hernia with upside down stomach.

for 3 days. The gold standard is a catheter-based study first described by DeMeester and colleagues.[13] The endoscope is placed and the gastroesophageal junction is measured. Then 5 cm above the gastroesophageal junction the pH probe is placed with the aid of a suction device that helps it to hook on the mucosa. The total time with pH less than 4 is considered acid reflux and is transduced and recorded. A drop of pH below 4 for more than 4% of the time in a 24-hour period is considered an abnormal study.

Scoring systems have been developed and used to derive results from the pH testing study. Several parameters are considered and a composite score is calculated. One of the most commonly used scores initially designed by Johnson and DeMeester and later modified by Jameison and DeMeester comprises six variables.[13] The components of the DeMeester score are (normal <14.72) as follows:

1. Total esophageal acid exposure time
2. Upright acid exposure time
3. Supine acid exposure time
4. Number of episodes of reflux
5. Number of reflux episodes lasting more than 5 minutes
6. The duration of the longest reflux episode

A total acid reflux time greater than 4.2% is considered a positive study for pathologic acid reflux disease. A DeMeester score greater than 14.72 is considered positive for pathologic acid reflux disease.[13] In addition to these two parameters, the most important piece of information gleaned from this study is the symptom correlation.

The patients chart their symptoms during the period of testing and the symptoms are then correlated with periods of acid reflux on pH testing. The Symptom Index (SI),[14] Symptom Sensitivity Index, and Symptom-Associated Probability (SAP)[15] scores are then derived. SI is the percentage of symptom episodes that were associated with reflux during the study period. For example, if the patients noted 10 symptom episodes and five of them were associated with positive reflux on pH testing, then the SI would be 50% or 0.5. An SI value greater than 0.5 is generally considered to be clinically significant. However, the SI does not take into account the total number of reflux events and if a patient has many reflux events a high SI may be falsely obtained because of chance.

The SAP was hence developed as a statistical calculation that derives a P value and reduces the chance factor in association of symptoms with reflux episodes. The SAP calculation is based on constructing a 2×2 contingency table with symptoms and reflux. The Fisher exact test is then applied to calculate the probability that the observed association between reflux and symptoms occurred by chance or was significant. By understanding exactly which symptoms are most closely associated with the presence of a reflux episode, the surgeon can set expectations for the patient as to which symptoms are most likely to resolve with a procedure that inhibits reflux.

Over the last several years, the wireless pH monitoring system has become the new standard of care in pH monitoring (Bravo Capsule; Given Imaging, Yoqneam, Israel).[16] This study monitors acid reflux for 48 hours and is considered to be more accurate because the patient is more likely to go about their daily activities without a catheter in place.[17] The sensor can be placed endoscopically with sedation or transorally without sedation. The capsule is placed 6 cm above the gastroesophageal junction. The DeMeester score has been adapted to this study and scores and acid reflux time are reported for each day individually and in total for the 48 hours. This is one of the most important studies in objectively establishing the presence of GERD.

Nonacid Reflux Studies

If the traditional pH studies are all normal and the diagnosis of GERD is still being highly considered, then further testing to establish this diagnosis can be done. There is greater understanding now that in a certain group of patients the reflux may not be acidic. Traditionally, ambulatory pH testing has been designed with a cutoff pH of 4. It has been argued that this is an arbitrary cutoff and that some patients may have reflux disease even at a higher pH. This is where the role of multichannel intraluminal impedance (MII) in combination with conventional pH catheters (combined MII-pH) has come in, allowing a more comprehensive characterization of reflux episodes. Impedance technology allows assessment of bolus movement through the esophagus. When this is combined with pH monitoring, all episodes of reflux whether or not they are acid can be detected. The technology allows one to characterize the refluxate including physical properties (ie, liquid, gas, mixed), chemical properties (ie, acid or nonacid), height of the refluxate, and clearance of the refluxate. The study is similar to conventional catheter-based pH testing with a pH sensor located 5 cm above the gastroesophageal junction, combined with an impedance-measuring conductor at several levels in the esophagus. The main advantage of combined MII-pH over conventional pH monitoring is that it facilitates analysis of the relationship between symptoms and all types of reflux events, acid and nonacid. A negative combined MII-pH study is therefore more powerful in excluding reflux compared with regular pH monitoring. The most important reported datapoint is the symptom correlation seen with the presence of reflux (**Fig. 3**).

The impedance-pH study can also be helpful in patients who cannot stop medications but need better objective assessment of their reflux. These studies also allow for pH probes to be placed in the oropharynx and can be useful in evaluation of laryngopharyngeal reflux.

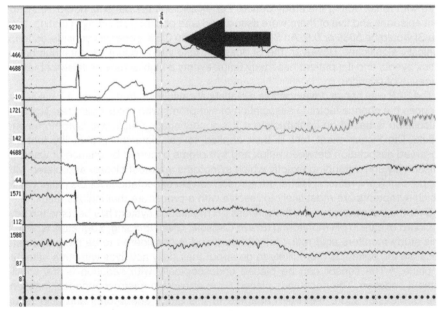

Fig. 3. Nonacid reflux episode detected by impedance. The *dashed line* is the pH of 4 threshold and the *arrow* points to proximal extent of reflux (20 cm).

Esophageal Function Testing (Used to Be Called Manometry)

The next study that every patient being considered for a procedure should have is an esophageal function study. Esophageal manometry is the gold standard esophageal function test (**Fig. 4**). Most modern machines can also perform high-resolution manometry. When combined with MII, it is referred to as esophageal function testing. This study allows evaluation of peristalsis and contraction amplitudes within the esophageal body, the pressure of LES, relaxation and length of the LES, and bolus transit through the esophagus. A normal LES pressure is between 10 and 45 mm Hg and relaxes with swallows. Peristalsis should be seen with greater than 70% of swallows and contraction amplitudes should be between 30 and 180 mm Hg. Abnormal LES can have pressure lower than 10 mm Hg, short total length (<2 cm), and less than 1 cm in the abdomen. Contraction amplitudes higher than 180 mm Hg may explain symptoms, such as chest pain and dysphagia. Contraction amplitudes lower than 30 mm Hg may suggest a weak esophagus and a partial fundoplication may be considered. It is imperative to rule out achalasia and other motility disorders before proceeding with a procedure for reflux disease (**Figs. 5** and **6**). This helps to guide further therapy based on the esophageal motility and the function of the LES. The new Chicago classification allows even better assessment of esophageal function. Esophageal motility disorders are discussed in detail elsewhere in this issue.

Lower Esophageal Sphincter Ultrasound

A high-frequency ultrasound probe has been used to study the LES. Mittal and colleagues[18] proposed the LES and esophageal muscle thickness and esophageal muscle cross-sectional area as parameters that are increased in patients with esophageal motility disorders.[19] The use of this evaluation is not widespread, being only used in specialized centers.

Gastric Emptying Study

A thorough assessment of gastric outlet obstruction should be done when assessing for reflux. This is because poor gastric emptying itself can be a cause of reflux with no dysfunction at the gastroesophageal junction and results from a backup in the "plumbing circuit." An initial screening can be done based on history alone looking

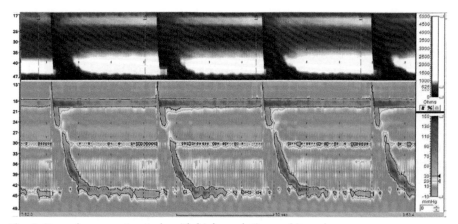

Fig. 4. Normal manometry study with high resolution and impedance.

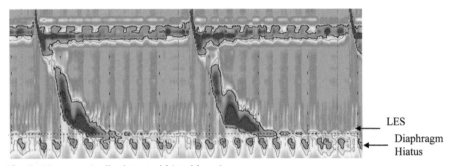

Fig. 5. Manometrically detected hiatal hernia.

for bloating, nausea, and vomiting. The upper endoscopy can help to see if there is any mechanical obstruction at the gastric outlet or if there is retained food in the stomach. The radiographic study can also be helpful in this regard. If these studies are not diagnostic, or if there is high suspicion of poor gastric function, then a gastric emptying study can be done. This study is done in nuclear medicine and should be taken into consideration in any patient undergoing surgery for GERD. Often gastric emptying may improve with the treatment of GERD. Very poor emptying on this study may prompt the surgeon to do a gastric emptying procedure or place a gastrostomy tube at the time of plication.

How Studies Help Choose the Proper Treatment

GERD is a common problem and affects a great portion of the population. The baseline treatments of lifestyle changes and acid-reducing medications can be used as diagnostic and therapeutic maneuvers. Patients for whom medications no longer work, those with side effects to medications, those with atypical symptoms, or those wishing to no longer take medications are candidates for an antireflux procedure. Also, patients with complications of reflux should be considered for a procedure. In this case further work-up for the disease should be done (**Fig. 7**). The first test that patients should have is an upper endoscopy. The exception is the patient with dysphagia. An esophagram first may alert the physician to conditions that may make the endoscopy

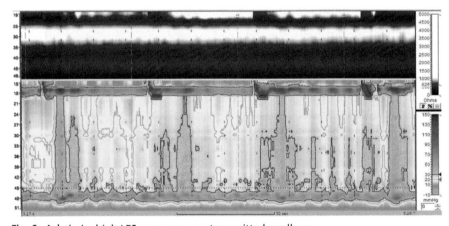

Fig. 6. Achalasia: high LES pressures, nontransmitted swallows.

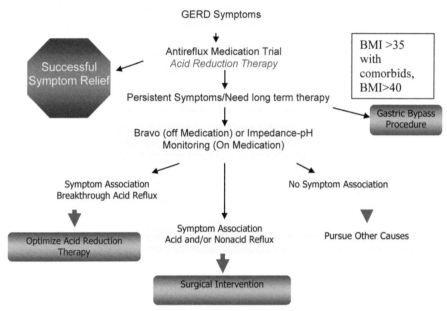

Fig. 7. Preoperative assessment for GERD. If the patient is morbidly obese, consider weight loss surgery. BMI, body mass index.

more complicated. If complications of GERD are seen then the authors suggest that interventional treatment should be considered. If patients were responsive to medications at one time but they no longer work, the patient may have progressive GERD and the patient can be considered for intervention. Before proceeding with any procedure the patient should undergo ambulatory pH testing, esophageal function testing, and esophagram. The other studies mentioned can be used as indicated. If the pH study is normal but the patient is suspected to have reflux, then consider a nonacid reflux study with impedance. If this study shows no symptom correlation and/or minimal reflux then a procedure should be aborted and other causes for the symptoms should be sought. Note that if at any point in the work-up the patient is noted to have a body mass index greater than 35 with comorbidities or more than 40, they are a candidate for weight loss surgery and all of the studies may not need to be done.

CLINICAL OUTCOMES IN THE LITERATURE

Preoperative studies are very important in predicting outcome following any procedure for GERD. This was pointed out early in the laparoscopic Nissen experience in 1999.[20] The authors noted that the key to a good outcome was proper diagnosis of GERD using the ambulatory pH study. The key outcome measures to note are the presence of reflux (whether it be acid or nonacid) and symptom correlation. Then the surgeon can have a discussion with the patient regarding expectations and outcomes. Additional predictors of outcome noted were typical symptoms and response to antireflux medications. Now that 15 years have passed since the publication of this paper, more and more patients are presenting for treatment that may have been responsive to medications at one time and now are seeking surgical intervention because the medications have stopped working. It is important to take a thorough history to elicit this information. The symptom for which a procedure can have the most impact is regurgitation. Procedures provide the mechanical approach to GERD that medications cannot provide. A more recent study looked at patients 10 years after fundoplication and noted similar conclusions.[21]

If a hiatal hernia is identified, it is likely to be contributing to the symptoms and should be repaired. All other procedures are designed to augment the LES. Dysfunctions of the LES found on evaluation, such as hypotensive LES or TLESR, can help to tailor which procedure should be used for augmentation of the LES. For hypotensive LES the patient has the option of Nissen fundoplication, endoscopic placation, or LINX. The LINX reflux management system is designed to augment LES pressure and gastric yield pressure. Transoral incisionless fundoplication is most helpful in the patient with a patulous flat LES seen on retroflexion with endoscopy. This procedure helps to reconstruct the angle of His. Radiofrequency ablation may be most helpful in those with TLESR as the cause of their reflux.

SUMMARY

GERD is a common problem. If prolonged therapy is needed, the patient should have at least an endoscopy to assess for complications of GERD. If a surgical treatment is being considered, a thorough preoperative evaluation should be done to confirm the presence of pathologic GERD. Studies that should be done before a procedure include ambulatory pH testing, esophageal function testing, endoscopy, and esophagram. Nonacid ambulatory studies can be done in those who seem to be suffering from nonacid reflux with careful note of symptom correlation. Gastric emptying studies should be done if gastroparesis or gastric outlet obstruction is suspected. Esophageal motility disorders should be assessed with manometry, especially to evaluate for achalasia, which can mimic reflux.

REFERENCES

1. Vakil N, van Zanten SV, Kahrilas P, et al. The Montreal definition and classification of gastroesophageal reflux disease: a global evidence-based consensus. Am J Gastroenterol 2006;101(8):1900–20 [quiz: 1943].
2. Clearinghouse TNNDDI. Digestive diseases statistics for the United States [Internet]. Available at: http://digestive.niddk.nih.gov/statistics/statistics.aspx. Accessed November 9, 2014.
3. Nebel OT, Fornes MF, Castell DO. Symptomatic gastroesophageal reflux: incidence and precipitating factors. Am J Dig Dis 1976;21(11):953–6.
4. Stein HJ, DeMeester TR. Outpatient physiologic testing and surgical management of foregut motility disorders. Curr Probl Surg 1992;29(7):413–555.
5. Schneider JH, Küper MA, Königsrainer A, et al. Transient lower esophageal sphincter relaxation and esophageal motor response. J Surg Res 2010;159(2): 714–9.
6. Taghavi SA, Ghasedi M, Saberi-Firoozi M, et al. Symptom association probability and symptom sensitivity index: preferable but still suboptimal predictors of response to high dose omeprazole. Gut 2005;54(8):1067–71.
7. Lord RV, Kaminski A, Oberg S, et al. Absence of gastroesophageal reflux disease in a majority of patients taking acid suppression medications after Nissen fundoplication. J Gastrointest Surg 2002;6(1):3–9 [discussion: 10].
8. Velanovich V. The development of the GERD-HRQL symptom severity instrument. Dis Esophagus 2007;20(2):130–4.
9. Wiklund I. Review of the quality of life and burden of illness in gastroesophageal reflux disease. Dig Dis 2004;22:108–14.

10. Katz P, Gerson L, Vela M. Guidelines for the diagnosis and management of gastroesophageal reflux disease. Am J Gastroenterol 2013;108:308–28.

11. Bello B, Zoccali M, Gullo R, et al. Gastroesophageal reflux disease and antireflux surgery: what is the proper preoperative work-up? J Gastrointest Surg 2013; 17(1):14–20 [discussion p. 20].

12. Ott DJ. Gastroesophageal reflux disease. Radiol Clin North Am 1994;32(6): 1147–66.

13. Johnson LF, Demeester TR. Twenty-four-hour pH monitoring of the distal esophagus. A quantitative measure of gastroesophageal reflux. Am J Gastroenterol 1974;62(4):325–32.

14. Wiener GJ, Richter JE, Copper JB, et al. The symptom index: a clinically important parameter of ambulatory 24-hour esophageal pH monitoring. Am J Gastroenterol 1988;83(4):358–61.

15. Weusten BL, Roelofs JM, Akkermans LM, et al. The symptom-association probability: an improved method for symptom analysis of 24-hour esophageal pH data. Gastroenterology 1994;107(6):1741–5.

16. Hirono I, Richter JE. Practice parameters committee of the American College of Gastroenterology. ACG practice guidelines: esophageal reflux testing. Am J Gastroenterol 2007;102(3):668–85.

17. Kahrilas PJ, Pandolfino JE. Review article: oesophageal pH monitoring-technologies, interpretation and correlation with clinical outcomes. Aliment Pharmacol Ther 2005;22(Suppl 3):2–9.

18. Mittal RK, Kassab G, Puckett JL, et al. Hypertrophy of the muscularis propria of the lower esophageal sphincter and the body of the esophagus in patients with primary motility disorders of the esophagus. Am J Gastroenterol 2003;98(8): 1705–12.

19. Mittal RK, Liu J, Puckett JL, et al. Sensory and motor function of the esophagus: lessons from ultrasound imaging. Gastroenterology 2005;128(2):487–97.

20. Campos GM, Peters JH, DeMeester TR, et al. Multivariate analysis of factors predicting outcome after laparoscopic Nissen fundoplication. J Gastrointest Surg 1999;3(3):292–300.

21. Morgenthal CB, Lin E, Shane MD, et al. Who will fail laparoscopic Nissen fundoplication? Preoperative prediction of longterm outcomes. Surg Endosc 2007;21: 1978–84.

Reoperative Antireflux Surgery

Brandon T. Grover, DO, Shanu N. Kothari, MD*

KEYWORDS

- Gastroesophageal reflux disease • Nissen fundoplication • Revisional surgery
- Roux-en-Y gastric bypass • Collis gastroplasty • Preoperative evaluation
- Outcomes

KEY POINTS

- The most common symptoms leading to reoperative antireflux surgery are recurrent heartburn, dysphagia, and regurgitation.
- The most common anatomic abnormalities found at the time of revisional surgery include slipped fundoplication, malpositioned wrap, intrathoracic wrap migration, and complete or partial wrap disruption.
- Success rates for revisional surgery are lower than primary antireflux surgery; despite this, greater than 80% of patients undergoing redo surgery are satisfied with their results.
- Reoperative antireflux surgery is technically challenging and should be performed by experienced foregut surgeons.

INTRODUCTION

Gastroesophageal reflux disease (GERD) is a common problem in the United States, affecting an estimated 40% of the adult population.[1] Since the widespread use of laparoscopic surgery, an increasing number of antireflux operations have been performed.[2] Surgical treatment of GERD has had mixed success. As many as 50% of patients resume antireflux medications after surgery,[3] often without objective evidence of true recurrent reflux disease.[4,5] Patient satisfaction up to 5 years after surgery is as high as 90%.[6–11] Between 3% and 10% of patients require reoperative antireflux surgery.[5,9,12–15]

No standard definition of what constitutes failure of antireflux surgery exists. Failure may be defined subjectively as return of symptoms, use of antacid

Dr B.T. Grover has nothing to disclose. Dr S.N. Kothari serves as a preceptor for Torax Medical, Inc.

Department of General and Vascular Surgery, Gundersen Health System, 1900 South Avenue, C05-001, La Crosse, WI 54601, USA

* Corresponding author.

E-mail address: snkothar@gundersenhealth.org

http://dx.doi.org/10.1016/j.suc.2015.02.014
surgical.theclinics.com
0039-6109/15/$ – see front matter © 2015 Elsevier Inc. All rights reserved.

medications, and patient dissatisfaction. Failure may also be defined objectively through esophagogastroduodenoscopy (EGD), pH studies, and radiographic imaging, which can identify recurrent hiatal hernias, wrap disruption, and/or recurrent reflux disease.

Revisional surgery is substantially more complex than initial antireflux surgery. A thorough preoperative evaluation is necessary to aid in operative planning and to ensure that the patient is an appropriate candidate for a particular revisional procedure. The most common indications for revisional surgery are recurrent symptoms of heartburn, recurrent hiatal hernia, and/or dysphagia. Other potential indications include misdiagnosis of initial symptoms and inadequate surgical technique.[16,17]

Several surgical approaches are available, including abdominal or thoracic access with either open or laparoscopic/thoracoscopic techniques. Options for revision surgery include redo fundoplication with or without a Collis gastroplasty, hiatal hernia repair if present, conversion to Roux-en-Y (RNY) anatomy, or esophagectomy. As surgeons have increased laparoscopic experience, minimally invasive redo antireflux surgery is becoming the gold standard, as is seen with primary antireflux surgery.

RISK FACTORS CONTRIBUTING TO SURGICAL FAILURE

Multiple reasons exist for failure of antireflux surgery. Both patient and technical factors can play a role in wrap failure or return of symptoms. Patient-specific risk factors include morbid obesity, atypical symptoms, lack of response to medications, chronic coughing, retching, preoperative poor esophageal peristalsis with excessive supine acid exposure, larger hiatal hernia, female gender, or age older than 50 years.[18–23]

Several technical errors at the time of initial operation can lead to failure. Common reasons include inadequate crural closure, misplaced wrap, failure to recognizing a short esophagus, and creation of a wrap that is too loose or too tight.[17,24,25]

CLINICAL PRESENTATION AND ETIOLOGY OF FAILURE

It is common for patients to have a variety of symptoms after Nissen fundoplication, such as bloating, increased flatus, inability to vomit or belch, and temporary mild dysphagia. These symptoms are usually self-limited and can be managed conservatively. The most common symptoms that lead to reoperative antireflux surgery are recurrent reflux, dysphagia, and regurgitation.[26]

Furnée and colleagues[16] performed a systematic review of the literature of failed antireflux surgery. They identified more than 4500 patients who underwent reoperative antireflux surgery. The most common indications for surgery were recurrent reflux and dysphagia. They reported wrap disruption, slipped fundoplication, and intrathoracic wrap migration as the most frequent anatomic abnormalities found at the time of reoperation (**Fig. 1**). Other less frequent abnormalities seen were hiatal disruptions, wraps that were too tight, and stricture. Several patients were thought to have had reflux surgery in error, with their actual diagnoses being achalasia, esophageal dysmotility or spasms, scleroderma, and esophageal cancer. Of the 81 studies included in their review, 5 summarized anatomic abnormalities based on the approach (open or laparoscopic) of the primary operation and the indications for reoperations (**Table 1**).[12,27–30] In patients with recurrent reflux as their presenting symptom, intrathoracic wrap migration and wrap disruption were most commonly seen. In patients with dysphagia as the presenting symptom, up to 40% of patients had no identified cause of failure at reoperation.

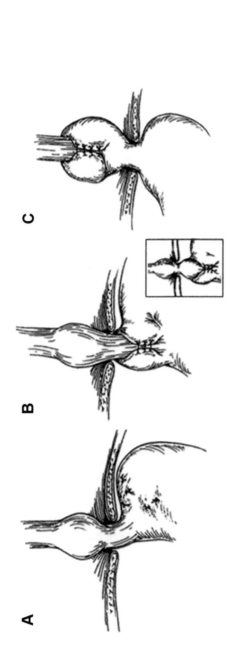

Fig. 1. Pattern of failure of primary repair. (*A*) Complete disruption, (*B*) slipped Nissen fundoplication, and (*C*) transhiatal herniation. (*From* Pennathur A, Awais O, Luketich JD. Minimally invasive redo antireflux surgery: lessons learned. Ann Thorac Surg 2010;89(6):S2175; with permission.)

Table 1
Anatomic abnormalities based on primary surgical approach and indication for reoperation

Anatomic Abnormality	Approach	
	Open, n = 120	Laparoscopic, n = 132
Wrap disruption	48 (40.0)	24 (18.2)
Telescoping	32 (26.6)	10 (7.6)
Hiatal disruption	23 (19.2)	42 (31.8)
Tight wrap	2 (1.7)	24 (18.2)
Miscellaneous	36 (30.0)	42 (31.8)

Anatomic Abnormality	Indication	
	Recurrent Reflux, n = 234	Dysphagia, n = 11
Intrathoracic wrap migration	104 (44.4)	18 (15.3)
Wrap disruption	109 (46.6)	12 (10.2)
No cause of failure	34 (14.5)	51 (43.2)
Miscellaneous	64 (27.4)	54 (45.8)

Data are presented as n (%). Totals do not equal 100% because some cases had multiple causes of failure.

Data from Furnée EJ, Draaisma WA, Broeders IA, et al. Surgical reintervention after failed antireflux surgery: a systematic review of the literature. J Gastrointest Surg 2009;13:1539–49.

EVALUATION

Because reoperative surgery is considerably more difficult than initial antireflux surgery, a thorough preoperative evaluation is essential. A comprehensive history and physical examination, with effort focused on identification of both initial and recurrent symptoms, is important. A review of the medical records, including pH and manometry studies, endoscopy reports, radiographic images, and operative reports, can offer insight into potential causes of recurrent symptoms. Details of the operative report must be carefully reviewed for the presence and size of hiatal hernia, management of hernia sac, extent of mediastinal dissection, identification and preservation of the vagus nerves, intra-abdominal esophageal length, division of short gastric vessels, crural closure (use of pledgets or mesh and type of mesh used), and type of fundoplication performed. This information can provide insight into the causes of failure and what to expect at reoperation. In addition, inquiring about symptom relief after the initial operation and any inciting events (ie, traumatic accident, episodes of retching, or significant weight gain) can be important in identifying potential cause of failure. As part of the physical examination, it is important to assess for morbid obesity because this condition is an independent risk factor for failed antireflux surgery.[18] Conversion to Roux-en-Y gastric bypass (RNYGB), as discussed later, should seriously be considered as the revision surgery of choice in this patient population.

An in-depth investigation with repeat EGD, upper gastrointestinal swallow study, and pH probe with impedance or Bravo probe should be obtained. If manometry was not performed before the initial operation, it should be considered to look for an esophageal motility disorder that could account for recurrent symptoms and affect future surgical care. A nuclear medicine gastric emptying study should be performed if there are symptoms of vomiting or severe gas bloat.

It is important to have objective evidence of reflux before undertaking revisional surgery in patients whose primary symptom is recurrent heartburn. Findings of esophagitis on endoscopy or an elevated DeMeester score on a pH study provide objective findings that support a diagnosis of recurrent reflux disease. Patients with dysphagia as the presenting symptom may not have an obvious cause, necessitating a thorough preoperative workup.

If a recurrent hiatal hernia is found in a symptomatic patient, it is not necessary to verify the presence of reflux disease; however, not all patients with recurrent hiatal hernia need reoperative surgery because many are asymptomatic or minimally symptomatic.

OPERATIVE APPROACHES

The conventional approach to reoperative antireflux surgery has been either open abdominal or open thoracic,[16,31] but with increasing experience and skill in laparoscopic surgery, minimally invasive techniques are being used more frequently. The complexity of the operation is far greater than the primary surgery, related to adhesion formation and altered anatomy. These operations should be performed by experienced laparoscopic foregut surgeons. Conversion to open surgery is occasionally required, but in experienced hands that rate can be as low as 1% to 2.5%.[25,26] The most common operation performed for failed antireflux surgery is redo fundoplication with hiatal hernia repair when needed.[25,26,32]

Description of Redo Laparoscopic Fundoplication

The patient is positioned in lithotomy and steep reverse Trendelenberg position. An open Hasson technique is used to gain access to the abdominal cavity, with care taken to avoid injury to intestines that may be adhered to the anterior abdominal wall from prior surgery. Following insufflation with CO_2, a 10-mm trocar is placed under direct visualization along the left mid-clavicular line just inferior to the costal margin. Two 5-mm trocars are also introduced, one in the left lateral abdomen and the other in the right upper abdomen, close enough to the falciform ligament to advance it from the right side of the abdomen to the left, if necessary, through the falciform. It is typical at this point to have significant adhesions of the liver to the stomach and prior wrap. The use of blunt and sharp dissection is used to carefully perform adhesiolysis. A thermal energy source can be used selectively and judiciously. Care should be taken to avoid inadvertent injury to the stomach or liver. It is helpful to dissect through the pars flaccida and use this posterior plane to advance the dissection toward the esophageal hiatus. Visualization of the caudate lobe of the liver can serve as a landmark for the dissection. Care is taken to not dissect behind this to prevent injury to the vena cava. As the liver and stomach are freed from adhesions, a liver retractor is placed through a separate incision to provide exposure for the remainder of the case. Once the crural pillars are identified, careful circumferential dissection of the distal esophagus and proximal stomach is performed. Once again, dense adhesions are typically encountered, and care must be taken to avoid injury to the visceral organs. Use of an endoscope or lighted bougie is extremely beneficial in helping to identify the esophagus during the mediastinal dissection. If there is recurrence of a hiatal hernia, complete hernia sac dissection and reduction is performed. This procedure can be technically challenging because of mediastinal adhesions. If a pneumothorax occurs, it is important to have good communication with the anesthesia team, owing to the potential for hemodynamic instability. It may be necessary to decrease pneumoperitoneum pressures. A chest tube is rarely needed, so long as there is no parenchymal lung injury. The anterior and posterior vagus nerves are identified and protected from injury. The goal is to restore normal anatomy, which includes ensuring that the gastroesophageal (GE) junction is intra-abdominal and that the prior fundoplication is taken down with the fundus returned to its normal position. Previously placed wrap sutures can often be visualized and can aid in identifying a plane to achieve wrap takedown. A useful technique is to use a linear stapler to divide the gastrogastric fundoplication. The fundus should be returned to its original anatomic position, which typically involves lysis of posterior adhesions where the wrap is adherent to the stomach and crus.

Once normal anatomy has been reestablished, assessing the intra-abdominal esophageal length is critical. There should be at least 2 to 3 cm of tension-free intra-abdominal esophagus. If this is not the case, continued mediastinal dissection of adhesions around the esophagus can often aid in mobilizing the GE junction further into the abdominal cavity. If this is not successful, a Collis gastroplasty should be performed; this can be accomplished with linear staples to fashion a wedge gastroplasty (**Fig. 2**) or with the use of an end-to-end stapler followed by the use of a linear stapler (**Fig. 3**). Crural repair is then undertaken and should follow the same surgical principles as used with primary hiatal closure. The authors use a permanent braided suture placed posteriorly, including the peritoneum that overlies the crural pillars. If closure requires more than 3 sutures or there is tension on the closure, the authors use an absorbable synthetic mesh (GORE Bio-A, W. L. Gore & Associates, Inc, Newark, DE, USA) to reinforce the repair. Care is taken to place the mesh such that it is not in direct contact with the esophagus. The fundus is again delivered posterior to the stomach, and a floppy 2.5-cm Nissen fundoplication is performed.

OUTCOMES

Long-term satisfaction rates after initial antireflux surgery are as high as 90%.[33] Satisfaction after primary revision antireflux surgery is lower but remains high at greater than 80% in multiple studies.[12,17,25,28,31] The GERD health-related quality of life (HRQL) questionnaire is the most commonly used tool to assess this. Several studies have reported on objective outcomes after laparoscopic reoperation, assessed by normal acid exposure on pH monitoring or lack of esophagitis on endoscopy, with a success rate greater than 80%.[25,27,31]

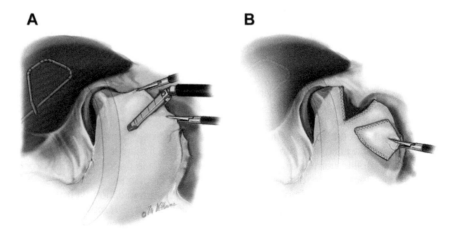

A   **B**

Fig. 2. (*A*) Collis lengthening procedure. Graspers are used to stabilize the stomach. (*B*) A reticulating Endo-GIA stapler (Covidien, Minneapolis, MN) is used to form a wedge of gastric cardia. (*Courtesy of* Marcia Williams, Santa FE, NM; with permission.)

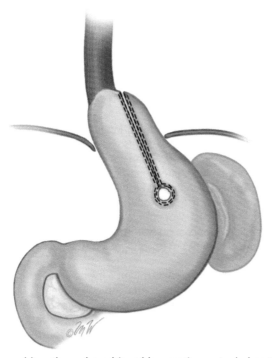

Fig. 3. Extraesophageal length can be achieved by creating a stapled gastric tube or Collis gastroplasty. This procedure can be done by using an end-to-end stapling technique. (*Courtesy of* Marcia Williams, Santa FE, NM; with permission.)

Intraoperative complication rates are higher with revisional surgery. In a systematic review of the literature, Furnée and colleagues[16] reported intraoperative and postoperative complication rates of 21.4% and 15.6%, respectively. The most common intraoperative complication was injury to the stomach or esophagus, which occurred in 13.1% of cases. Other specified intraoperative complications included pneumothorax (3.4%), hemorrhage (1.9%), and splenectomy (0.3%). The most frequent postoperative complications were infections and pulmonary and cardiac complications. Despite the high gastric or esophageal injury rates, a postoperative leak was reported in only 1.5% of patients. The researchers found a higher overall intraoperative complication rate in the laparoscopic group, 19.5% versus 5.4% in the open group. Alternatively, postoperative complication rates with open surgery were higher when compared with laparoscopic operation, 17.4% versus 15.3%, and 30-day mortality rates of 1.3% versus 0%, respectively. Conversion from laparoscopic to open surgery occurred in 8.7% of laparoscopic cases because of dense adhesions, intraoperative bleeding, and poor visualization.[16]

In a single-institution series of 275 redo operations by Awais and colleagues,[31] the most commonly identified cause of failure was recurrent hiatal hernia, found in 64% of patients. Other identified causes included short esophagus (43%), misplaced wrap (16%), wrap too loose or too tight (14%), and a disrupted wrap (4%). Laparoscopic surgery was attempted in 266 of these patients, with a rate of conversion to open surgery of 3%. With a median follow-up of 3.3 years, 11% of patients had failure of the redo operation, necessitating another surgical intervention. Although the investigators did not report on the frequency of intraoperative visceral injury, the postoperative leak rate was 3.3%. They reported no perioperative mortalities. From the GERD-HRQL questionnaire, 85% of patients were satisfied with their results. They concluded that minimally invasive redo antireflux procedures can be safely performed in an experienced center. Despite redo operations having poorer outcomes than initial surgery, they achieved a patient satisfaction rate of greater than 80%.

FAILURE OF REDO FUNDOPLICATION

Approximately 10% of patients undergoing laparoscopic reoperative antireflux surgery require another redo procedure.[31,34] Some patients have undergone as many as 4 revisional surgeries.[35,36] There is an increasing trend toward conversion to RNY anatomy with either a gastrojejunal (GJ) or esophagojejunal (EJ) anastomosis.[31,35–37] Other options include redo fundoplication with or without a Collis gastroplasty or esophagectomy. If a shortened esophagus is the cause of failure and was not treated during previous operative approaches, it may be appropriate to perform a second redo fundoplication with a Collis gastroplasty. In cases with significant esophageal dysfunction, an esophagectomy may be performed as a last resort.[24,26,31,37]

Performing a RNY reconstruction may become the operation of choice after failed primary or reoperative antireflux surgery. Little and colleagues[38] reported a satisfaction rate of only 42% in patients requiring 3 or more open operations. Rather than replication of the same procedure, conversion to RNY may be a better option. The RNY anatomy acts to separate most of the acid-producing parietal cells from the esophagus, thus preventing esophageal reflux disease. Creating a small gastric pouch, as is done in weight loss surgery, is important for successful treatment of reflux disease because retained parietal cells in a large gastric pouch can be a source of recurrent acid reflux. Obesity is a well-known independent risk factor for antireflux surgery failure, so conversion to RNYGB should seriously be considered as the operation of choice after failure of initial antireflux surgery[39–41] in the obese or morbidly obese population.

Another study by Awais and colleagues[37] reported on 25 patients with recurrent GERD after reflux surgery who underwent a "RNY near esophagojejunostomy", which they defined as a standard RNYGB, but with a smaller, 5- to 10-cm gastric pouch.[3] The goal of the small pouch is to have only gastric cardia, thus eliminating any acid production within the gastric pouch. In their series, 28% of patients had a body mass index less than 30 kg/m^2. About 44% of patients had more than 1 prior reflux operation. Patients reported significant improvements in heartburn, regurgitation, and dysphagia symptoms. Patient satisfaction rates after surgery were 80%, which far exceeds the 42% satisfaction rate after multiple redo fundoplications as reported by Little and colleagues.[38]

Makris and colleagues[36] reported on their single-institution experience with 72 patients who underwent conversion of failed fundoplication to RNY reconstruction; this included a combination of open and laparoscopic operations and reconstruction to a gastric pouch or the esophagus. Intraoperative complications were common, occurring in 43% of patients. Ten patients had intraoperative injury to the esophagus or GE junction. Despite the high complication rate, they reported zero 30-day mortality and a high patient satisfaction rate. With long-term follow-up, 89% of respondents indicated that they would refer a friend who was having similar symptoms.

Published perioperative major and minor complication rates with conversion to RNY reconstruction are high, ranging from 21% to 46%. Overall patient satisfaction rates from these same studies are similar to the initial antireflux surgery, 88% to 96% (**Table 2**).[35,36,39,42,43]

Table 2
Conversion of fundoplication to Roux-en-Y gastric bypass

Author, Publication Year	N	Preoperative BMI (kg/m^2)	Conversion to Open (n)	30-d Complication Rate (%)	30-d Mortality (n)	Patient Satisfaction (%)
Stefanidis et al,[35] 2012	25	24.4	2/24	40	0	96
Makris et al,[36] 2012	72	31.4	9/46	46	0	89
Houghton et al,[42] 2005	19	42.0	1/3	21	0	88
Kellogg et al,[43] 2007	11	44.0	0	45	0	NR
Zainabadi et al,[39] 2008	7	39.4	1/7	43	0	NR

Complication rate includes major and minor complications.
Abbreviations: BMI, body mass index; NR, not reported.
Data from Refs.[35,36,39,42,43]

RNYGB can be used in the nonobese patient, as excessive weight loss is typically not seen in patients of normal weight.[36,44] In this patient population, it has been the authors' practice to use this approach after 2 prior failed fundoplications. Esophagectomy is occasionally required in patients with multiple failed redo operations.[16,26,31] It is the authors' belief that earlier conversion to RNYGB can aid in preserving the esophagus.

SUMMARY

Antireflux surgery has a high success rate, with most patients being satisfied with their results. A small percentage of patients need reoperative treatment of new, persistent, or recurrent symptoms. Causes of failure include a variety of patient and technical factors. A complete patient evaluation and workup is necessary before proceeding with revisional surgery, including reviewing medical records, taking a detailed history, and obtaining appropriate studies and tests to verify recurrent disease. Attempts should be made to preserve the esophagus whenever possible. If a short esophagus is found, a Collis gastroplasty should be used to create adequate intra-abdominal esophageal length. If a hiatal hernia is present, the hernia sac must be completely dissected and reduced. If the patient has failed reoperative antireflux surgery or is considerably overweight, conversion to RNY anatomy should be performed. Success rates of reoperative surgery are inferior to those of primary surgery, and complications are considerably more common. Despite these challenges, surgeons with significant experience in foregut surgery can perform these complex operations, providing symptom relief and improved quality of life for a substantial majority of patients.

REFERENCES

1. Anand G, Katz PO. Gastroesophageal reflux disease and obesity. Gastroenterol Clin North Am 2010;39(1):39–46.
2. Finlayson SR, Birkmeyer JD, Laycock WS. Trends in surgery for gastroesophageal reflux disease: the effect of laparoscopic surgery on utilization. Surgery 2003;133(2):147–53.

3. Spechler SJ, Lee E, Ahnen D, et al. Long-term outcome of medical and surgical therapies for gastroesophageal reflux disease: follow-up of a randomized controlled trial. JAMA 2001;285(18):2331–8.
4. Lord RV, Kaminski A, Oberg S, et al. Absence of gastroesophageal reflux disease in a majority of patients taking acid suppression medications after Nissen fundoplication. J Gastrointest Surg 2002;6(1):3–9.
5. Thompson SK, Jamieson GG, Myers JC, et al. Recurrent heartburn after laparoscopic fundoplication is not always recurrent reflux. J Gastrointest Surg 2007; 11(5):642–7.
6. DeMeester TR, Bonavina L, Albertucci M. Nissen fundoplication for gastroesophageal reflux disease. Evaluation of primary repair in 100 consecutive patients. Ann Surg 1986;204(1):9–20.
7. Grande L, Toledo-Pimentel V, Manterola C, et al. Value of Nissen fundoplication in patients with gastro-oesophageal reflux judged by long-term symptom control. Br J Surg 1994;81(4):548–50.
8. Booth MI, Jones L, Stratford J, et al. Results of laparoscopic Nissen fundoplication at 2-8 years after surgery. Br J Surg 2002;89(4):476–81.
9. Anvari M, Allen C. Five-year comprehensive outcomes evaluation in 181 patients after laparoscopic Nissen fundoplication. J Am Coll Surg 2003;196(1):51–7.
10. Dallemagne B, Weerts J, Markiewicz S, et al. Clinical results of laparoscopic fundoplication at ten years after surgery. Surg Endosc 2006;20(1):159–65.
11. Granderath FA, Kamolz T, Schweiger UM, et al. Long-term results of laparoscopic antireflux surgery. Surg Endosc 2002;16(5):753–7.
12. Byrne JP, Smithers BM, Nathanson LK, et al. Symptomatic and functional outcome after laparoscopic reoperation for failed antireflux surgery. Br J Surg 2005;92(8):996–1001.
13. Luostarinen ME, Isolauri JO, Koskinen MO, et al. Refundoplication for recurrent gastroesophageal reflux. World J Surg 1993;17(5):587–93.
14. Dutta S, Bamehriz F, Boghossian T, et al. Outcome of laparoscopic redo fundoplication. Surg Endosc 2004;18(3):440–3.
15. Pessaux P, Arnaud JP, Delattre JF, et al. Laparoscopic antireflux surgery: five-year results and beyond in 1340 patients. Arch Surg 2005;140(10):946–51.
16. Furnee EJ, Draaisma WA, Broeders IA, et al. Surgical reintervention after failed antireflux surgery: a systematic review of the literature. J Gastrointest Surg 2009;13(8):1539–49.
17. Horgan S, Pohl D, Bogetti D, et al. Failed antireflux surgery: what have we learned from reoperations? Arch Surg 1999;134(8):809–15.
18. Morgenthal CB, Lin E, Shane MD, et al. Who will fail laparoscopic Nissen fundoplication? Preoperative prediction of long-term outcomes. Surg Endosc 2007; 21(11):1978–84.
19. Broeders JA, Roks DJ, Draaisma WA, et al. Predictors of objectively identified recurrent reflux after primary Nissen fundoplication. Br J Surg 2011;98(5):673–9.
20. Power C, Maguire D, McAnena O. Factors contributing to failure of laparoscopic Nissen fundoplication and the predictive value of preoperative assessment. Am J Surg 2004;187(4):457–63.
21. Soper NJ, Dunnegan D. Anatomic fundoplication failure after laparoscopic antireflux surgery. Ann Surg 1999;229(5):669–76.
22. O'Boyle CJ, Watson DI, DeBeaux AC, et al. Preoperative prediction of long-term outcome following laparoscopic fundoplication. ANZ J Surg 2002;72(7):471–5.
23. Jackson PG, Gleiber MA, Askari R, et al. Predictors of outcome in 100 consecutive laparoscopic antireflux procedures. Am J Surg 2001;181(3):231–5.

24. Morse C, Pennathur A, Luketich JD. Laparoscopic techniques in reoperation for failed antireflux repairs. In: Patterson GA, Pearson FG, Cooper JD, et al, editors. Pearson's thoracic and esophageal surgery, vol. 2, 3rd edition. Philadelphia: Churchill Livingstone; 2008. p. 367–75.

25. Khajanchee YS, O'Rourke R, Cassera MA, et al. Laparoscopic reintervention for failed antireflux surgery: subjective and objective outcomes in 176 consecutive patients. Arch Surg 2007;142(8):785–901.

26. Pennathur A, Awais O, Luketich JD. Minimally invasive redo antireflux surgery: lessons learned. Ann Thorac Surg 2010;89(6):S2174–9.

27. Furnée EJ, Draaisma WA, Broeders IA, et al. Surgical reintervention after antireflux surgery for gastroesophageal reflux disease: a prospective cohort study in 130 patients. Arch Surg 2008;143(3):267–74.

28. Coelho JC, Goncalves CG, Claus CM, et al. Late laparoscopic reoperation of failed antireflux procedures. Surg Laparosc Endosc Percutan Tech 2004; 14(3):113–7.

29. Safranek PM, Gifford CJ, Booth MI, et al. Results of laparoscopic reoperation for failed antireflux surgery: does the indication for redo surgery affect the outcome? Dis Esophagus 2007;20(4):341–5.

30. Leonardi HK, Crozier RE, Ellis FH Jr. Reoperation for complications of the Nissen fundoplication. J Thorac Cardiovasc Surg 1981;81(1):50–6.

31. Awais O, Luketich JD, Schuchert MJ, et al. Reoperative antireflux surgery for failed fundoplication: an analysis of outcomes in 275 patients. Ann Thorac Surg 2011;92(3):1083–9.

32. van Beek DB, Auyang ED, Soper NJ. A comprehensive review of laparoscopic redo fundoplication. Surg Endosc 2011;25(3):706–12.

33. Dallemagne B, Taziaux P, Weerts J, et al. Laparoscopic surgery of gastroesophageal reflux. Ann Chir 1995;49(1):30–6.

34. Deschamps C, Trastek VF, Allen MS, et al. Long-term results after reoperation for failed antireflux procedures. J Thorac Cardiovasc Surg 1997;113(3): 545–50.

35. Stefanidis D, Navarro F, Augenstein VA, et al. Laparoscopic fundoplication takedown with conversion to Roux-en-Y gastric bypass leads to excellent reflux control and quality of life after fundoplication failure. Surg Endosc 2012; 26(12):3521–7.

36. Makris KI, Panwar A, Willer BL, et al. The role of short-limb Roux-en-Y reconstruction for failed antireflux surgery: a single-center 5-year experience. Surg Endosc 2012;26(5):1279–86.

37. Awais O, Luketich JD, Tam J, et al. Roux-en-Y near esophagojejunostomy for intractable gastroesophageal reflux after antireflux surgery. Ann Thorac Surg 2008;85(6):1954–9.

38. Little AG, Ferguson MK, Skinner DB. Reoperation for failed antireflux operations. J Thorac Cardiovasc Surg 1986;91(4):511–7.

39. Zainabadi K, Courcoulas AP, Awais O, et al. Laparoscopic revision of Nissen fundoplication to Roux-en-Y gastric bypass in morbidly obese patients. Surg Endosc 2008;22(12):2737–40.

40. Frezza EE, Ikramuddin S, Gourash W, et al. Symptomatic improvement in gastroesophageal reflux disease (GERD) following laparoscopic Roux-en-Y gastric bypass. Surg Endosc 2002;16(7):1027–31.

41. Patterson EJ, Davis DG, Khajanchee Y, et al. Comparison of objective outcomes following laparoscopic Nissen fundoplication versus laparoscopic gastric bypass in the morbidly obese with heartburn. Surg Endosc 2003;17(10):1561–5.

42. Houghton SG, Nelson LG, Swain JM, et al. Is Roux-en-Y gastric bypass safe after previous antireflux surgery? Technical feasibility and postoperative symptom assessment. Surg Obes Relat Dis 2005;1(5):475–80.

43. Kellogg TA, Andrade R, Maddaus M, et al. Anatomic findings and outcomes after antireflux procedures in morbidly obese patients undergoing laparoscopic conversion to Roux-en-Y gastric bypass. Surg Obes Relat Dis 2007;3(1):52–7.

44. Makris KI, Lee T, Mittal SK. Roux-en-Y reconstruction for failed fundoplication. J Gastrointest Surg 2009;13(12):2226–32.

Short Esophagus

Nicholas R. Kunio, MD[a], James P. Dolan, MD[b],
John G. Hunter, MD[b],*

KEYWORDS

- Esophagus • Short esophagus • Gastroesophageal reflux disease • Hiatal hernia

KEY POINTS

- In the presence of long-standing and severe gastroesophageal reflux disease, patients can develop various complications, including a shortened esophagus.
- Standard preoperative testing in these patients should include endoscopy, esophagography, and manometry, whereas the objective diagnosis of a short esophagus must be made intraoperatively following adequate mediastinal mobilization.
- If left untreated, it is a contributing factor to the high recurrence rate following fundoplications or repair of large hiatal hernias.
- A laparoscopic Collis gastroplasty combined with an antireflux procedure offers safe and effective therapy.

INTRODUCTION

Hiatal hernias, paraesophageal hernias, and gastroesophageal reflux disease (GERD) are common problems.[1–4] Complications related to these disorders can occur in up to 40% of patients.[5] One of the most controversial complications is the acquired short esophagus. Although numerous studies have been published describing the short esophagus and its pathophysiology, diagnosis, and treatment,[6–10] various reputable investigators have challenged its existence.[11–14] Consequently, this dichotomy contributes to the confusion underlying this entity. This article considers the history, pathophysiology, diagnosis, and current treatment options for the shortened esophagus.

HISTORY

Some investigators have credited Dietlen and Knierim[15] with the first mention of a short esophagus in their description of a pregnant patient whose stomach was found to be intrathoracic on radiograph. However, others have attributed this description to

[a] Division of General and Vascular Surgery, Advocate Medical Group, 745 Fletcher Dr, Suite 302, Elgin, IL 60123, USA; [b] Division of Gastrointestinal and General Surgery, Digestive Health Center, Oregon Health & Science University, 3181 SW Sam Jackson Park Rd, L223A, Portland, OR 97239, USA
* Corresponding author.
E-mail address: hunterj@ohsu.edu

Surg Clin N Am 95 (2015) 641–652
http://dx.doi.org/10.1016/j.suc.2015.02.015
0039-6109/15/$ – see front matter © 2015 Elsevier Inc. All rights reserved.

Akerlund[16] or Findlay.[17,18] A shortened esophagus shown on esophagram was first reported by Fineman and Conner[19] in 1924,[18] whereas Woodburn Morison[20] provided the earliest endoscopic description in 1930.[18]

The grave operative challenges presented by a shortened esophagus was first shown in Plenk's description of a case of perforation and peritonitis in which the stomach could not be replaced into the abdomen, leading to a fatal situation.[18,21,22] This portrayal is consistent with the modern understanding of shortened esophagus in which esophageal length is insufficient to allow the esophagogastric junction to rest below the diaphragm, as first described by Barrett in 1950.[18,23,24] From this, the theory that chronic reflux disease was the underlying cause for acquired short esophagus was first proposed by Lortat-Jacob[25] a few years later.

INCIDENCE

Depending on the study, the incidence of shortened esophagus can vary widely. It has been reported to be as high as 60%[26] and as low as 0% in older open[11] and more recent laparoscopic series.[27] If the intraoperative requirement for extensive mediastinal dissection or the performance of a Collis gastroplasty is used to define the presence of shortened esophagus then the incidence in the open literature is between 8% and 10%.[28,29] Using the same definition, a wider range (7%–19%) has been documented in various laparoscopic series.[30–33] If the need for a Collis gastroplasty is used as the most restrictive definition, then retrospective review of the literature indicates that between 1% and 5% of patients undergoing GERD-related surgery meet criteria.[30,34–36]

PATHOPHYSIOLOGY

The most common entity associated with acquired short esophagus is chronic GERD, which results in a persistent inflammatory response.[7] In the setting of a dysfunctional lower esophageal sphincter the esophageal mucosa is exposed to either acidic or alkaline reflux and the normal esophageal squamous epithelium provides an inadequate barrier to the damaging effects of refluxed gastric juices. Animal models,[37,38] as well as in-vivo human[10] studies, have shown that refluxed gastric fluid leads to deeper penetration of hydrogen ions into the wall of the esophagus with localized cellular damage. The resulting inflammation causes tissue edema, migration of inflammatory cells into the damaged tissue, attempted healing, and ultimately tissue fibrosis. With repeated exposure over a period of time, the inflammatory process can extend transmurally. Transmural inflammation then leads to longitudinal contracture of the transmural scar and the clinical manifestation of esophageal shortening.[7]

PREOPERATIVE ASSESSMENT

Typical studies used in the preoperative evaluation of patients with GERD include dynamic esophagram, esophagogastroduodenoscopy, and esophageal manometry. Many prior attempts at identifying preoperative indicators of short esophagus have identified factors with low specificity.[31,39–41] Some investigators contend that evidence of a nonreducing type I hiatal hernia greater than 5 cm in length or a type III hiatal hernia on barium esophagram is predictive of short esophagus being present at surgery.[42] However, when a retrospective, blinded review of patients who had undergone Collis gastroplasty was performed, barium esophagram had a positive predictive value of only 50%.[7]

Other studies have attempted to improve on this finding. Awad and colleagues[31] performed a thorough evaluation of the predictive utility of all 3 diagnostic tests (esophagography, endoscopy, and manometry) individually and in conjunction with each other. When all were used together, the specificity for short esophagus was 100% but the sensitivity was only 28%. Esophagography and manometry used together had a 75% positive predictive value but, again, a low sensitivity of 28%. Manometric measurement alone had the best individual positive predictive value, but this was only 36%. Other investigators have also examined these 3 diagnostic modalities and reported that the presence of peptic stricture was the only significantly predictive factor for the need for Collis gastroplasty at surgery. Manometric esophageal length was associated with a short esophagus if the measurement was less than the fifth percentile, but was unable to yield a minimal cutoff in defining a short esophagus because of wide variability in measurements.[39]

Recently, Yano and colleagues[43] examined the utility of the esophageal length index (ELI), defined as the ratio of endoscopic esophageal length (in centimeters) to the patient's height (in meters) in order to help adjust for the variability in individual measurements caused by differences in height. They identified an ELI cutoff of 19.5 or less as having a positive predictive value of 81% (19% false-negative rate) and a negative predictive value of 83%. This index provides the most contemporary and useful tool in anticipating the need for an esophageal lengthening procedure during operation. Current preoperative diagnostic tests can only help surgeons anticipate the potential need for a Collis gastroplasty. They have not yet replaced intraoperative assessment and esophageal measurement as a requirement to make the final decision.

INTRAOPERATIVE ASSESSMENT

In order to define a shortened esophagus, the relationship of the esophagogastric junction to the hiatus must be assessed carefully. Most commonly, a shortened esophagus is associated with the presence of a large paraesophageal hernia. Consequently, after the stomach has been reduced, the hernia sac incised and pulled into the abdomen, and the short gastric vessels divided, mediastinal esophageal dissection is performed. Intra-abdominal esophageal length should be measured after the distal 3 to 4 cm of the mediastinal esophagus has been mobilized (type I dissection).[7] If insufficient length still exists after this, an extended (type II) dissection can be performed. Various investigators have described the limits of this dissection. Johnson and colleagues[34] described up to 8 cm of mediastinal length being mobilized, whereas O'Rourke and colleagues[32] stated that up to 10 cm of mediastinal dissection can be performed. Swanstrom and Hansen[44] used the level of the carina as their upper limit and DeMeester[45] the inferior pulmonary veins. Extended dissection may be necessary and beneficial in some cases. In their series of 106 patients, Bochkarev and colleagues[46] found that, with extended mediastinal dissection, adequate intra-abdominal esophageal length could be obtained, and this obviated a Collis gastroplasty.

Any traction on the esophagogastric junction should be relieved following the completion of the dissection. This relief should include removal of the nasogastric tube or bougie, because these can provide superior displacement and lead to inaccurate measurement of intra-abdominal esophageal length. Assuming the esophagogastric junction can be easily identified, the distance between it and the hiatus is measured.[7,34] The authors prefer to use the open jaws of a laparoscopic grasper for this measurement. When fully open, these measure 2.5 cm across. The graspers can then be placed alongside the dissected intra-abdominal esophagus to determine whether sufficient length for a fundoplication has been achieved (**Fig. 1**). If less than this distance is present after an extended mediastinal dissection, then a shortened esophagus is confirmed and a Collis-type gastroplasty is needed.

In situations in which the esophagogastric junction cannot easily be delineated, certain steps must be taken before intra-abdominal esophageal measurements are made. Conditions that can make visualization of the esophagogastric junction difficult include a large redundant hernia sac or a prominent junction fat pad that obscures the landmark. Dissection and removal of this excess tissue may be needed in order to properly identify the junction,[45,47] and this is commonly performed in our practice. When this proves insufficient for proper identification of the esophagogastric junction, endoscopic evaluation can be performed to aid with identification. By endoscopically identifying the junction and then transilluminating the esophageal wall the location can be seen laparoscopically and this can be successfully completed in almost all cases. Other investigators have also described how endoscopic measurement of the distance between the junction and the crural arch can also be used to determine whether sufficient length has been obtained.[7,40]

TREATMENT

The importance of identifying and correcting a short esophagus is underscored because the risk of fundoplication failure or crural disruption with wrap herniation is increased in cases in which a tension-free repair was not successfully performed.[48,49] This failure to treat a shortened esophagus is thought to be, in part, responsible for the 20% to 33% rate of repair failure in cases of giant paraesophageal hernias.[50–52]

The most commonly used method to obtain esophageal lengthening is the Collis gastroplasty and its current variation. Initially, this operation involved mobilization of the esophagus to the level of the aortic arch and was performed through a thoracoabdominal incision.[53] A dilator was inserted along the lesser curvature. Two clamps were then attached to the cardia parallel to the dilator and the stomach was divided, followed by oversewing the resection lines. The tubularized portion of the stomach then acted as a neoesophagus that, when combined with a standard antireflux procedure, allowed a tension-free repair.

With the advent of minimally invasive surgery as well as advances in surgical equipment, several novel adaptations of the Collis gastroplasty have evolved. Swanstrom and colleagues[30] first described their combination of a thoracoscopic and

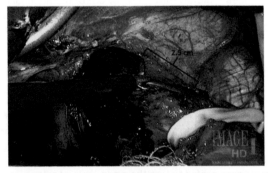

Fig. 1. Intra-abdominal esophageal length measurement using atraumatic grasper during a laparoscopic paraesophageal hernia repair. (*Courtesy of* Oregon Health & Science University, Portland, OR; with permission.)

laparoscopic gastroplasty with a Nissen fundoplication. In their approach an endoscopic linear stapler was introduced through the right chest, brought across the mediastinal pleura, and then brought trans-hiatally inserted into the abdomen. After a bougie had been inserted, the stapler was fired parallel to the lesser curvature against the left aspect of the bougie.[54] A similar technique, by means of a left-sided thoracoscopic stapler approach, was first described by Awad and colleagues[31] in 2000.[55] Taken together, the major disadvantage to these approaches was the need to enter 2 separate body cavities. In theory, this increased the risk of injury to intrathoracic structures.

The first totally laparoscopic approach to a modified Collis technique was described by Johnson and colleagues[34] in 1998. They used a laparoscopic version of the open approach initially described by Steichen.[56] With a 48-French bougie in place along the lesser curvature, a sealed transgastric window was created in the fundus using a circular stapling device. A linear stapler was then fired alongside the bougie dividing the fundus from the superior aspect of the fundal window to the angle of His, creating the neoesophagus. A floppy Nissen fundoplication was then created. After this description, an additional step, involving resection of the fundal apex, was described because of concerns for tissue ischemia.[57] This approach is technically challenging and involves a minilaparotomy in order to accommodate the circular stapler. In addition, Pierre and colleagues[58] reported a staple line leak in 3% of patients who underwent the procedure.

The fully laparoscopic approach to the Collis-type gastroplasty was made possible by the development of the articulating endoscopic linear stapler. Terry and colleagues[57] reported that this technique was first developed for a laparoscopic vertical banded gastroplasty by Champion,[59] and this remains our technique of choice. The wedge gastroplasty is performed using the same port placement as is used for standard laparoscopic fundoplication (**Fig. 2**). After completion of all dissection, a 48-French bougie is inserted alongside the lesser curvature. The assistant retracts the gastric fundus inferiorly while the surgeon maintains traction on the greater curvature just below the level of the angle of His. An articulating endoscopic linear stapler is then placed through the left subcostal port, maximally articulated and fired transversely

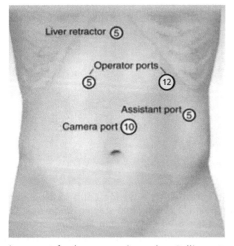

Fig. 2. Standard port placement for laparoscopic wedge Collis gastroplasty.

across the superior fundus to a point approximately 3 cm below the angle of His and abutting the bougie. While the assistant applies lateral traction on the wedge of fundus to be resected, a vertical firing of the linear stapler is then made parallel to the esophagus against the bougie, completing the wedge resection (**Fig. 3**). The resected portion is then removed from the stomach. A floppy fundoplication is then performed over a 56-French to 60-French bougie.

RESULTS OF OPERATIVE REPAIR

Before the advent of minimally invasive transabdominal surgery, the transthoracic Collis gastroplasty had been shown to have excellent long-term results. Symptomatic reflux control at 10 years following surgery was reported to be as high as 88%.[60,61] More recently, minimally invasive techniques have been used to perform a Collis gastroplasty from a transabdominal approach. Short-term results have been satisfactory. However, it is difficult to identify a single approach as producing superior outcomes given the paucity of long-term data.

As minimally invasive approaches to the Collis gastroplasty have evolved, an improvement in operative time has been seen. Mean operative time for the combined thoracoscopic/laparoscopic technique was 257 minutes.[54] It increased to 294 minutes with the challenging dual-stapler transabdominal approach.[34] At 184 minutes the transabdominal wedge gastroplasty showed the shortest mean operative time of all the minimally invasive techniques.[57]

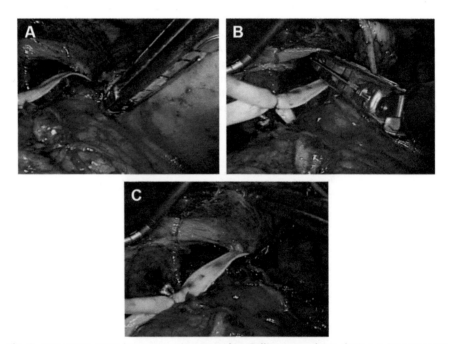

Fig. 3. Important steps in constructing a wedge Collis gastroplasty during a laparoscopic paraesophageal hernia repair. (*A*) Articulating stapler fired across fundus perpendicular to bougie. (*B*) Articulating stapler fired parallel and abutting bougie. (*C*) Completed wedge gastroplasty with creation of neoesophagus. (*Courtesy of* Oregon Health & Science University, Portland, OR; with permission.)

Perioperative morbidity following a Collis gastroplasty has been shown to occur in as few as 8% of cases,[62] but more commonly ranges between 19% and 36% (**Table 1**).[34,54,55,58,63–65] Complications commonly seen following a Collis gastroplasty included atelectasis, atrial fibrillation, ileus, pneumonia, and urinary tract infection,[34,55,62–64] whereas pneumothorax and pleural effusion were more often shown in series using a combined thoracoscopic/laparoscopic approach.[55,63] Of particular importance in Collis gastroplasty is the risk of postoperative leak. Houghton and colleagues[66] showed a similar incidence of perforation or leak when comparing patients having a Collis gastroplasty with those having a fundoplication alone, whereas Nason and colleagues[65] showed a significantly increased risk of leak (2.7% vs 0.6%) when comparing patients after Collis and standard fundoplication. Both studies showed similar overall morbidity between groups. All studies to date have shown a very low incidence of perioperative mortality, similar to that seen with standard fundoplication (see **Table 1**).

Clinical outcomes have shown consistent improvement across studies following performance of a Collis gastroplasty. The incidence of persistent or recurrent reflux symptoms following a Collis gastroplasty since the advent of minimally invasive techniques ranges between 7% and 24%. Postoperative dysphagia rates have been shown to be between 10% and 28% (see **Table 1**). Comparing standard fundoplication with Collis gastroplasty, Houghton and colleagues[66] showed a significantly increased incidence of requiring postoperative dilatation in patients after Collis gastroplasty (6% vs 2%). Overall the Collis gastroplasty has shown good patient satisfaction, ranging from 77%[63] to 93%,[58] and this is comparable with that seen in patients undergoing fundoplication alone.

As shown in **Table 1**, the incidence of postoperative hernia recurrence or wrap failure following a Collis gastroplasty and antireflux procedure can be low (0% to 18%). These reported rates are in contrast with prior studies examining the risk of hernia recurrence following laparoscopic paraesophageal hernia repair. The patients included in these studies did not undergo esophageal lengthening procedures and recurrence rates seen in those having a minimally invasive approach ranged from 32% to 42%.[67–69] It has been suggested that these high rates of recurrence can be attributed to the failure to identify a short esophagus and perform a lengthening procedure.[50–52,58] This theory is reinforced by the significant reduction in recurrence rates seen to date in series examining patients undergoing a Collis gastroplasty and antireflux procedure.

Two main concerns have been raised with regard to the Collis gastroplasty. The first is that the neoesophagus lacks motility and in theory may contribute to postoperative dysphagia. Although postoperative dysphagia rates range between 3% and 13%,[31,34,54,58,62–64] dysphagia was generally improved in comparisons between postoperative and preoperative incidence. The second concern centers on the presence of acid-secreting gastric mucosa within the neoesophagus, which can potentially contribute to ongoing esophagitis. During 24-hour pH testing, Jobe and colleagues[54] found that 7 out of 14 patients in their series of combined thoracoscopic/laparoscopic gastroplasty had abnormal findings, with a mean DeMeester score of 100. More recently, Mor and colleagues[70] compared the acid clearance time between normal patients, those following Nissen fundoplication, and those following Nissen-Collis gastroplasty. Esophageal acid clearance time was significantly greater in the Nissen-Collis group. Pathologic esophageal acid exposure was seen in 10% of patients after Nissen fundoplication and 22% of patients after Nissen-Collis gastroplasty; however, this difference was not statistically significant.

Table 1
Postoperative functional results after Collis gastroplasty

Study	Type	Approach	n	n, Follow-up	Follow-up	Antireflux Procedure	Mortality, n (%)	Morbidity, n (%)	Outcomes		
									Reflux Symptoms, n (%)	Dysphagia, n (%)	Recurrence, n (%)
Pearson et al,[26] 1987	Open	Thoracic	215	NA	1–15 y	Toupet	NA	NA	6 (3)	24 (11)	6 (3)
Stirling & Orringer,[60] 1989	Open	Thoracic	353	261	44 mo	Nissen	4 (1.1)	28 (8)	65 (25)	44 (17)	26 (10)
Swanstrom et al,[30] 1996 & Jobe et al,[54] 1998	Laparoscopic	Thoracic/Abdominal	15	14	14 mo	Nissen or Toupet	0	3 (20)	2 (14)	2 (14)	0
Johnson et al,[34] 1998	Laparoscopic	Abdominal	9	9	12 mo	Nissen	0	2 (22)	1 (11)	1 (11)	NA
Awad et al,[31] 2001 & Awad et al,[55] 2000	Laparoscopic	Thoracic/Abdominal	11	11	6–35 mo	Nissen or Toupet	0	4 (36)	1 (9)	0	2 (18)
Pierre et al,[58] 2002	Laparoscopic	Abdominal	112	NA	1–78 mo	Nissen	1 (0.8)	31 (28)	NA	NA	3 (3)
Garg et al,[63] 2009	Open/Laparoscopic	Thoracic/Abdominal	85	50	9–111 mo	Nissen or Toupet	1 (1)	26 (31)	12 (24)	14 (28)	NA
Houghton et al,[64] 2007	Open/Laparoscopic	Abdominal	63	62	1–64 mo	Nissen or Toupet	0	12 (19)	12 (20)	6 (10)	1 (2)
Nason et al,[65] 2011	Laparoscopic	Abdominal	454	368	33 mo	Nissen, Toupet, Dor	7 (1.5)	89 (20)	NA	NA	53 (16)
Zehetner et al,[62] 2014	Laparoscopic	Abdominal	85	NA	12 mo	Nissen or Toupet	0	7 (8)	6 (7)	14 (16)	2 (2.4)

Abbreviation: NA, not available.
Data from Refs.[26,30,31,34,55,58,60,62–65]

SUMMARY

In the presence of long-standing and severe GERD, patients can develop various complications, including a shortened esophagus. Standard preoperative testing in these patients should include endoscopy, esophagography, and manometry, whereas the objective diagnosis of a short esophagus must be made intraoperatively following adequate mediastinal mobilization. Some debate still persists as to the validity of this entity but there are now significant data available to support its existence. If left untreated, it is a contributing factor to the high recurrence rate following fundoplications or repair of large hiatal hernias. A laparoscopic Collis gastroplasty combined with an antireflux procedure offers safe and effective therapy.

REFERENCES

1. Draaisma WA, Gooszen HG, Tournoij E, et al. Controversies in paraesophageal hernia repair. Surg Endosc 2005;19:1300–8.
2. Altorki NK, Yankelevitz D, Skinner DB. Massive hiatal hernias: the anatomic basis of repair. J Thorac Cardiovasc Surg 1998;115:828–35.
3. Andujar JJ, Papasavas PK, Birdas T, et al. Laparoscopic repair of large paraesophageal hernia is associated with a low incidence of recurrence and reoperation. Surg Endosc 2004;18:444–7.
4. Spechler SJ. Epidemiology and natural history of gastro-oesophageal reflux disease. Digestion 1992;51(Suppl 1):24–9.
5. Stein HJ, Barlow AP, DeMeester TR, et al. Complications of gastroesophageal reflux disease. Role of the lower esophageal sphincter, esophageal acid and acid/alkaline exposure, and duodenogastric reflux. Ann Surg 1992;216:35–43.
6. Durand L, De Antón R, Caracoche M, et al. Short esophagus: selection of patients for surgery and long-term results. Surg Endosc 2012;26:704–13.
7. Horvath K, Swanström L, Jobe B. The short esophagus: pathophysiology, incidence, presentation, and treatment in the era of laparoscopic antireflux surgery. Ann Surg 2000;232:630–40.
8. Paterson WG, Kolyn DM. Esophageal shortening induced by short-term intraluminal acid perfusion in opossum: a cause for hiatus hernia? Gastroenterology 1994;107:1736–40.
9. Paterson WG. Role of mast cell-derived mediators in acid induced shortening of the esophagus. Am J Physiol Gastrointest Liver Physiol 1998;274:385–8.
10. Gozzetti G, Pilotti V, Spangaro M, et al. Pathophysiology and natural history of acquired short esophagus. Surgery 1987;102:507–14.
11. Hill LD, Gelfand M, Bauermeister D. Simplified management of reflux esophagitis with stricture. Ann Surg 1970;172:638–51.
12. Korn O, Csendes A, Burdiles P, et al. Length of the esophagus in patients with gastroesophageal reflux disease and Barrett's esophagus compared to controls. Surgery 2003;133:358–63.
13. Madan AK, Frantzides CT, Patsavas KL. The myth of the short esophagus. Surg Endosc 2004;18:31–4.
14. Larrain A, Csendes A, Strauszer T. The short esophagus: a surgical myth? Acta Gastroenterol Latinoam 1971;3:125–33.
15. Dietlen H, Knierim G. Hernia diaphragmatica dextra. Berl klin Wchnschr 1910;1:1174–7.
16. Akerlund AI. Hernia diaphragmatica Hiatus oesophagei vom anatomischen und roentgenologischen Gesichtspunkt. Acta Radiol 1926;6:3–22.

17. Findlay L, Kelly B. Congenital shortening of the oesophagus and the thoracic stomach resulting therefrom. J Laryng & Otol 1931;46:797–816.
18. Herbella FM, Patti MG, Del Grande JC. When did the esophagus start shrinking? The history of the short esophagus. Dis Esophagus 2009;22:550–8.
19. Fineman S, Conner HM. Right diaphragmatic hernia of the short esophagus type. Am J Med Sci 1924;3:672.
20. Woodburn Morison JM. Diaphragmatic hernia. Proc R Soc Med 1930;23(11): 1615–34.
21. Plenk A. Zur Kazuistik der Zwechfellhernien. Wien klin Wchnschr 1922;35: 339–41.
22. Barrett NR. Chronic peptic ulcer of the esophagus and 'oesophagitis'. Br J Surg 1950;38:175–82.
23. Large AM. The problem of short oesophagus with oesophagitis. Br J Surg 1962; 49:527–32.
24. Spechler SJ, Goyal RK. The columnar-lined esophagus, intestinal metaplasia, and Norman Barrett. Gastroenterology 1996;110:614–21.
25. Lortat-Jacob JL. L'endo-brachyesophage [Barrett's esophagus]. Ann Chir 1957; 11:1247 [in French].
26. Pearson FG, Cooper JD, Patterson GA, et al. Gastroplasty and fundoplication for complex reflux problems. Long-term results. Ann Surg 1987;206:473–81.
27. Coster DD, Bower W, Wilson VT, et al. Laparoscopic partial fundoplication vs. laparoscopic Nissen-Rossetti fundoplication: short-term results of 231 cases. Surg Endosc 1997;11:625–31.
28. Polk HC. Fundoplication for reflux esophagitis: misadventures with the operation of choice. Ann Surg 1976;183:645–52.
29. Kauer WK, Peters JH, DeMeester TR, et al. A tailored approach to antireflux surgery. J Thorac Cardiovasc Surg 1995;110:141–7.
30. Swanstrom LL, Marcus DR, Galloway GQ. Laparoscopic Collis gastroplasty is the treatment of choice for the shortened esophagus. Am J Surg 1996;171:477–81.
31. Awad ZT, Mittal SK, Roth TA, et al. Esophageal shortening during the era of laparoscopic surgery. World J Surg 2001;25:558–61.
32. O'Rourke RW, Khajanchee YS, Urbach DR, et al. Extended transmediastinal dissection: an alternative to gastroplasty for short esophagus. Arch Surg 2003; 138:735–40.
33. Mattioli S, Lugaresi M, Costantini M, et al. The short esophagus: intraoperative assessment of esophageal length. J Thorac Cardiovasc Surg 2008;136:834–41.
34. Johnson AB, Oddsdottir M, Hunter JG. Laparoscopic Collis gastroplasty and Nissen fundoplication: a new technique for the management of esophageal foreshortening. Surg Endosc 1998;12:1055–60.
35. Terry M, Smith CD, Branum GD, et al. Outcomes of laparoscopic fundoplication for gastroesophageal reflux disease and paraesophageal hernia. Surg Endosc 2001;15:691–9.
36. Richardson JD, Richardson RL. Collis-Nissen gastroplasty for shortened esophagus: longterm evaluation. Ann Surg 1998;227:735–40 [discussion: 740–2].
37. Lillemoe KD, Johnson LF, Harmon JW. Role of the components of the gastroduodenal contents in experimental acid esophagitis. Surgery 1982;92: 276–84.
38. Lillemoe KD, Johnson LF, Harmon JW. Taurodeoxycholate modulates the effects of pepsin and trypsin in experimental esophagitis. Surgery 1985;97:662–7.
39. Gastal OL, Hagen JA, Peters JH, et al. Short esophagus: analysis of predictors and clinical implications. Arch Surg 1999;134:633–6 [discussion: 637–8].

40. Mittal SK, Awad ZT, Tasset M, et al. The preoperative predictability of the short esophagus in patients with stricture or paraesophageal hernia. Surg Endosc 2000;14:464–8.

41. Yau P, Watson DI, Jamieson GG, et al. The influence of esophageal length on outcomes after laparoscopic fundoplication. J Am Coll Surg 2000;191:360–5.

42. Bremner RM, Bremner CG, Peters JH. Fundamentals of antireflux surgery. In: Peters JH, DeMeester TR, editors. Minimally invasive surgery of the foregut. 1st edition. St Louis (MO): Quality Medical Publishing; 1994. p. 119–243.

43. Yano F, Stadlhuber RJ, Tsuboi K, et al. Preoperative predictability of the short esophagus: endoscopic criteria. Surg Endosc 2009;23:1308–12.

44. Swanstrom LL, Hansen P. Laparoscopic total esophagectomy. Arch Surg 1997; 132:943–9.

45. DeMeester SR. Laparoscopic paraesophageal hernia repair: critical steps and adjunct techniques to minimize recurrence. Surg Laparosc Endosc Percutan Tech 2013;23:429–35.

46. Bochkarev V, Lee Y, Vitamvas M, et al. Short esophagus: how much length can we get? Surg Endosc 2008;22:2123–7.

47. Maziak DE, Todd TR, Pearson FG. Massive hiatus hernia: evaluation and surgical management. J Thorac Cardiovasc Surg 1998;115:53–60 [discussion: 61–2].

48. Peters JH, DeMeester TR. The lessons of failed antireflux repairs. In: Peters JH, DeMeester TR, editors. Minimally invasive therapy of the foregut. 1st edition. St Louis (MO): Quality Medical Publishing; 1994. p. 190–200.

49. Juhasz A, Sundaram A, Hoshino M, et al. Outcomes of surgical management of symptomatic large recurrent hiatus hernia. Surg Endosc 2012;26:1501–8.

50. Ellis FH Jr, Gibb SP, Heatley GJ. Reoperation after failed antireflux surgery. Review of 101 cases. Eur J Cardiothorac Surg 1996;10:225–31 [discussion: 231–2].

51. Siewert JR, Isolauri J, Feussner H. Reoperation following failed fundoplication. World J Surg 1989;13:791–6 [discussion: 796–7].

52. DePaula AL, Hashiba K, Bafutto M, et al. Laparoscopic reoperations after failed and complicated antireflux operations. Surg Endosc 1995;9:681–6.

53. Collis JL. An operation for hiatus hernia with short esophagus. Thorax 1957;12: 181–8.

54. Jobe BA, Horvath KD, Swanstrom LL. Postoperative function following laparoscopic Collis gastroplasty for shortened esophagus. Arch Surg 1998;133:867–74.

55. Awad ZT, Filipi CJ, Mittal SK, et al. Left side thoracoscopically assisted gastroplasty: a new technique for managing the shortened esophagus. Surg Endosc 2000;14:508–12.

56. Steichen FM. Abdominal approach to the Collis gastroplasty and Nissen fundoplication. Surg Gynecol Obstet 1986;162:372–4.

57. Terry ML, Vernon A, Hunter JG. Stapled-wedge Collis gastroplasty for the shortened esophagus. Am J Surg 2004;188:195–9.

58. Pierre AF, Luketich JD, Fernando HC, et al. Results of laparoscopic repair of giant paraesophageal hernias: 200 consecutive patients. Ann Thorac Surg 2002;74: 1909–15 [discussion: 1915–6].

59. Champion JK. Laparoscopic vertical banded gastroplasty with wedge resection of gastric fundus. Obes Surg 2003;13:465 [author reply: 465].

60. Stirling MC, Orringer MB. Continued assessment of the combined Collis-Nissen operation. Ann Thorac Surg 1989;47:224–30.

61. Orringer MB, Sloan H. Combined Collis-Nissen reconstruction of the esophagogastric junction. Ann Thorac Surg 1978;25:16–21.

62. Zehetner J, DeMeester S, Ayazi S, et al. Laparoscopic wedge fundectomy for Collis gastroplasty creation in patients with a foreshortened esophagus. Ann Surg 2014;00:1–4.

63. Garg N, Yano F, Filipi C, et al. Long-term symptomatic outcomes after Collis gastroplasty with fundoplication. Dis Esophagus 2009;22:532–8.

64. Houghton S, Deschamps C, Cassivi S, et al. The influence of transabdominal gastroplasty: early outcomes of hiatal hernia repair. J Gastrointest Surg 2007;11: 101–6.

65. Nason K, Luketich J, Awais O, et al. Quality of life after Collis gastroplasty for short esophagus in patients with paraesophageal hernia. Ann Thorac Surg 2011;92:1854–61.

66. Houghton S, Deschamps C, Cassivi S, et al. Combined transabdominal gastroplasty and fundoplication for shortened esophagus: impact on reflux-related and overall quality of life. Ann Thorac Surg 2008;85:1947–53.

67. Hashemi M, Peters JH, DeMeester TR, et al. Laparoscopic repair of large type III hiatal hernia: objective followup reveals high recurrence rate. J Am Coll Surg 2000;190:553–60 [discussion: 560–1].

68. Khaitan L, Houston H, Sharp K, et al. Laparoscopic paraesophageal hernia repair has an acceptable recurrence rate. Am Surg 2002;68:546–51 [discussion: 551–2].

69. Jobe BA, Aye RW, Deveney CW, et al. Laparoscopic management of giant type III hiatal hernia and short esophagus. Objective follow-up at three years. J Gastrointest Surg 2002;6:181–8 [discussion: 188].

70. Mor A, Lutfi R, Torquati A. Esophageal acid-clearance physiology is altered after Nissen-Collis gastroplasty. Surg Endosc 2013;27:1334–8.

Endoscopic Treatment of Gastroesophageal Reflux Disease

 CrossMark

Kristin Hummel, DO, William Richards, MD*

KEYWORDS

- Gastroesophageal reflux disease • Endoluminal devices • Stretta • EsophyX

KEY POINTS

- Gastroesophageal reflux disease (GERD) is a disease that affects over 20% of the US population on at least a weekly basis.
- Laparoscopic Nissen fundoplication has been the gold standard for treatment of refractory GERD, but endoluminal therapies are gaining popularity and showing significant symptom control, at least in short-term data.
- There are 2 predominant devices currently in production for endoluminal treatment of GERD: Stretta, using radiofrequency ablation, and EsophyX, a transoral incisionless fundoplication; studies show improved symptom control and decreased proton pump inhibitors use but lack consistent long-term data demonstrating a decrease in esophageal acid exposure.
- Future studies are needed to demonstrate long-term efficacy of radiofrequency ablation (Stretta) and transoral incisionless fundoplication (EsophyX).

INTRODUCTION

Gastroesophageal reflux disease (GERD) is the most common disorder of the esophagus, affecting over 20% of the North American and Western European populations. More recent studies indicate the prevalence of GERD, defined as at least weekly heartburn and/or regurgitation, to be as high as 18% to 27% in the United States alone.[1] Current treatment of GERD costs close to $10 billion annually, with antireflux medication accounting for over one-half of the total cost.[2]

GERD is a chronic medical condition stemming from one or more factors:

1. Incompetent lower esophageal sphincter (LES) secondary to a hypotensive LES, increased intra-abdominal pressure that overwhelms a near normal LES, or inappropriate transient LES relaxations (TLESRs)

Disclosures: The authors have no financial disclosures or conflicts of interest.
Department of Surgery, University of South Alabama College of Medicine, Mastin Building, 2451 Fillingim Street, Mobile, AL 36617, USA
* Corresponding author.
E-mail address: brichards@health.southalabama.edu

2. Decreased contractile response of the diaphragmatic sphincter
3. Hiatal hernia
4. Poor esophageal clearance of acid as is seen in scleroderma

These physiologic disturbances cause a burning sensation in the chest or throat and/or regurgitation as the most common symptoms but may also be associated with extra-esophageal symptoms including chest pain, cough, hoarseness, and aspiration pneumonia. Prolonged acid exposure or bile reflux also increases the susceptibility of strictures, erosion, ulceration, Barrett esophagus, and even esophageal cancer.

Medical treatment consists of proton pump inhibitors (PPIs), which largely replaced the role of H2-blockers discovered in the 1970s. PPIs are effective in reducing gastric secretion of acid, yielding symptom relief in the majority of patients compliant with a daily or twice daily regimen. Many PPIs are now available over the counter and have affordable generic counterparts. In 2012, Nexium alone earned nearly $6 billion in sales, making it a top seller among all US medications.[3] Adjuncts to medical therapy include lifestyle changes such as smoking cessation and limiting meal sizes and alcohol intake. Overall, PPIs have adequate long-term safety, although the prolonged use has been linked to osteoporosis and susceptibility to *Clostridium difficile* colitis and, committing patients to a lifetime of PPI therapy can be expensive over time, and even cost-prohibitive in some patients. Also, despite lifestyle changes and optimized medical treatment, up to 20% of GERD patients have refractory or recurrent symptoms.[4]

Surgery for GERD is indicated when medical treatment fails or is no longer feasible (because of adverse effects, patient intolerance, or cost), when complications of GERD such as strictures, aspiration pneumonia, refractory asthma, esophageal bleeding occur, or at the patient's request when objective evidence of pathologic GERD has been diagnosed. The gold standard for surgical treatment of GERD is the laparoscopic Nissen fundoplication with hiatal hernia repair if indicated. The fundoplication increases lower esophageal sphincter pressure, decreases compliance of the gastroesophageal junction (GEJ), decreases frequency of TLESRs, increases the length of the intra-abdominal segment of the LES, reduces the sliding hiatal hernia, and restores the angle of His.[5] Although laparoscopic Nissen fundoplication (LNF) has excellent outcomes, with average cure rates in line with Kellokumpu's data of 87.7% at 5 years and 72.9% at 10 years,[6] it does carry inherent surgical and anesthetic risks. Postoperative dysphagia is the most commonly reported complication (although often transient, this may affect over 70% of patients in some studies),[6] followed by bloating, inability to belch, increased flatus, and need for repeat antireflux surgery. In a large cohort analysis based on 7531 patients between 2005 and 2009 from the National Surgical Quality Improvement Program (NSQIP) database, overall surgical mortality was less than a fraction of a percent, and in patients younger than 70 years of age, it was less than 0.05%.[7]

While the laparoscopic Nissen fundoplication was introduced into clinical practice in 1991 and remains the most frequently utilized operation for GERD,[8] the risks associated with surgery and adverse effects of dysphagia, bloating, and increased flatus are deterrents for many patients, thereby urging the surgical community to further pursue laparoscopic and endoscopic alternatives. Endoluminal techniques fall into 3 major categories: implantation or injection of foreign materials, radiofrequency ablation, and endoscopic tissue apposition techniques. Most endoluminal procedures are reserved for patients with documented symptomatic GERD, positive esophageal pH studies, and hiatal hernias less than 2 to 3 cm. Patients with evidence of pulmonary disease, Barrett esophagus, large hiatal hernias, obesity or morbid obesity, severe medical comorbidities, or esophageal dysmotility disorders are often excluded.

IMPLANTATIONS AND INJECTIONS

The theory of implantation and injection devices is to instill a bulking agent to augment the natural mechanical barrier to reflux. In 1984, O'Conner and colleagues,[9,10] reported an experimental model to control reflux using a bulk-forming agent of either bovine dermal collagen or Teflon (DuPont, Wilmington, Delaware) (PTFE resin) in the distal esophagus of dogs with surgically induced GERD. This required multiple, sometimes large-volume injections with fleeting results. Over the years, further attempts were made, but none remain on the market secondary to serious adverse events and/or lack of sustainable clinical efficacy.[11–13] These 4 products included

  Enteryx (Boston Scientific Corporation, Marlborough, MA): biopolymer of ethylene vinyl alcohol
  Gatekeeper (Medtronic Europe, Tolochenaz, Switzerland, Incorporated): hydrogel prosthesis
  Plexiglas microspheres (Artes Medical, San Diego, CA, Incorporated): polymethyl methacrylate
  Polytef (Mentor O&O, Santa Barbara, CA): polytetrafluoroethelyne

Radiofrequency Ablation

The Stretta system (Mederi Therapeutics, Norwalk, Connecticut, previously Curon Medical) was approved in April 2000 as an endoscopic procedure for treatment of GERD patients. The device uses a flexible catheter with a balloon–basket assembly fitted with needle–titanium electrodes to deliver the radiofrequency energy by way of a 4-channel generator into the esophageal wall and LES complex while irrigating the overlying mucosa to prevent thermal injury as shown in **Fig. 1**. The ablation is repeated by rotating the device and varying its linear position between 2 cm above and 2 cm below the Z-line (video: https://www.youtube.com/watch?v=Ibsn7VhBJXE&feature=youtu.be). The mechanisms of action are complex and not fully understood, but involve tissue

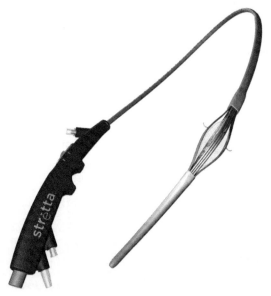

Fig. 1. The Stretta device used for radiofrequency energy treatment of GERD. (*Courtesy of* Mederi Therapeutics Inc., Norwalk, CT; with permission. © 2015 Mederi Therapeutics Inc.)

remodeling and contraction at the LES, causing reduced compliance and tightening of the sphincter (see **Fig. 1; Fig. 2**).

Decreased frequency of TLESRs has also been demonstrated, likely a sequela of alterations to vagal efferent fibers, inhibiting the motor component of reflux episodes.[14–16] The Stretta procedure has been proven safe, with few adverse events being reported early, and after 2005, major adverse reactions were reported in less than 0.1% of patients.[14,17]

Review of Recent Literature

Perry and colleagues[18] performed a systematic review and meta-analysis of radiofrequency energy from 20 studies (2 randomized controls and 18 cohort studies) including 1441 patients between 2001 and 2010. Investigators found an overall decrease in heartburn symptoms in 525 patients over 24.1 months, decreased GERD health-related quality-of-life (GERD-HRQL) scores in 433 patients in 9 studies over average follow-up of 19.8 months, and improved DeMeester scores from 44.37 pre-Stretta to 28.53 post-Stretta in 267 patients evaluated over an average of 13.1 months. Average LES pressure in 263 patients over 7 studies increased from 16.54 to 20.24, with a mean follow-up of 8.7 months. Overall conclusions were that Stretta improves GERD symptoms, improves but does not normalize esophageal acid exposure, and does not significantly increase LES pressure.

In another article by Dughera and colleagues,[19] investigators reported 8-year follow-up of 26 patients (from 56 with 4-year follow-up and 86 patients originally studied). Primary outcomes were GERD-related symptoms and GERD-HQRL. Secondary outcomes were medication use, LES pressure at esophageal manometry, and esophageal acid exposure at pH-metry. There was a significant decrease in heartburn scores (6-point Likert scale), with mean decrease of 2.8 points at 4 years and 1.8 points at 8 years. GERD-HQRL scores also decreased by a mean of 14 points at 4 years and 11 points at 8 years. The median LES pressure did not show significant changes at either 4 or 8 years. Mean esophageal acid exposure time initially improved at 4 years but returned to baseline at 8 years. None of the patients at 4 or 8 years had esophagitis on esophagoscopy. After 4 and 8 years, 21 and 20 of 26 patients, respectively, were completely off PPIs, with the remainder using occasional oral antacids or PPIs. The only complication reported was a case of severe gastroparesis requiring long-term hospitalization (3 weeks); this patient reached full recovery at 8 weeks post-Stretta. Overall conclusions were that Stretta is safe, with some long-term improvement in GERD-HQRL.

SAGES (Society of American Gastrointestinal and Endoscopic Surgeons) Recommendations

"Stretta is considered appropriate therapy for patients being treated for GERD who are 18 years of age or older, who have had symptoms of heartburn, regurgitation, or

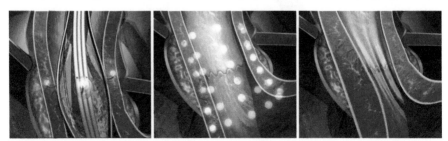

Fig. 2. Artist depiction of the mechanism of action of Stretta. (*Courtesy of* Mederi Therapeutics Inc., Norwalk, CT; with permission. © 2015 Mederi Therapeutics Inc.)

both for 6 months or more, who have been partially or completely responsive to anti-secretory pharmacologic, and who have declined laparoscopic fundoplication. Quality of evidence ++++, Recommendation strong."[20]

ENDOSCOPIC TISSUE APPOSITION TECHNIQUES

Several endoscopic suturing and apposition devices have come to market. The goal of these procedures is to mechanically bolster the lower esophageal sphincter or improve the antireflux barrier by creating plication of tissue at or just below the GEJ.

Endoscopic Submucosal Suturing System

The EndoCinch (Bard Endoscopic Technologies, Murray Hill, NJ) suture system is attached to the end of a standard flexible endoscope and has a cavity into which a tissue fold can be suctioned. A T-tag secures the submucosal tissue, and the physician lowers the suturing system to the GEJ, where a series of adjacent sutures are placed below the LES. The 2 sutures are then opposed, resulting in stomach plication. The plicated tissues tighten the GEJ and LES, forming a valve to create a barrier against GERD. Additional plication may be performed below the sphincter.[21] Although it had a good safety profile, long-term efficacy was lacking, and EndoCinch is no longer manufactured.

Endoscopic Full-Thickness Plication System

The NDO Plicator (NDO Surgical, Inc., Mansfield, MA) was designed to create a transmural, full-thickness, serosa-to-serosa plication below the GEJ at the angle of His. The plication is created under direct retroflexed visualization provided by a pediatric gastroscope that is inserted through a dedicated channel of the instrument. A pretied, suture-based pledget is delivered to create the plication, which is typically placed between the anterior gastric wall and the fundus, thereby avoiding major branches of the gastric arteries and vagus nerves.[22] The procedure was relatively safe but is no longer available for commercial use.[21]

Endoluminal Fundoplication

The EsophyX device (Endogastric Solutions, Redmond, WA) enables the creation of a 270°, 2 to 3 cm esophagogastric fundoplication by using proprietary tissue-manipulating elements and a minimum of 12 full-thickness polypropylene H-fasteners in conjunction with a flexible video endoscope providing visualization throughout the procedure. The procedure is fully described Bell and Cadière,[23] and illustrations of the procedure are shown in **Figs. 3–5**.

The procedure, transoral incisionless fundoplication (TIF), attempts to mimic the effects of the laparoscopic fundoplication by elongating the intra-abdominal esophagus, reducing a small (<2–3 cm) hiatal hernia if present by positioning the distal esophagus and stomach below the diaphragm, approximating and tightening the fundus around the distal esophagus, recreating the dynamics of the angle of His, and restoring the distal high pressure zone. Manufacturers claim benefits of TIF over traditional LNF:

TIF provides a more physiologic repair than a 360° wrap, allowing for decreased dysphagia or gas bloat after the procedure.
No dissection is performed.
It has a better safety profile than LNF.
It can be revised if required.
Comparable outcomes to LNF have been reported.[24]

A   B

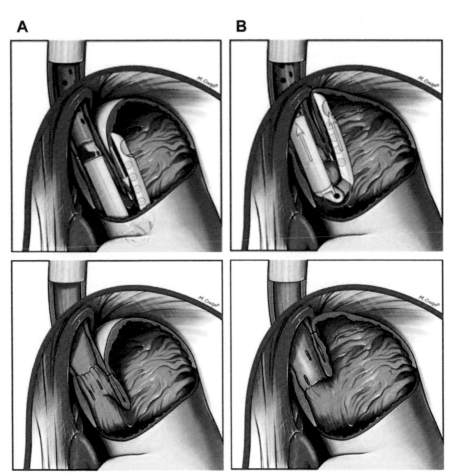

Fig. 3. Artist depiction of the EsophyX device creating the transoral incisionless fundoplication. (*A*) TIF 1 procedure with gastrogastric plications placed at the level of the Z-line. (*B*) TIF 2 technique creates an esophagogastric fundoplication proximal to the Z-line. (*From* Bell RC, Cadiere GB. Transoral rotational esophagogastric fundoplication: technical, anatomical, and safety considerations. Surg Endosc 2011;25(7):2390.)

Review of Recent Literature

In 2011, Bell and Freeman[25] retrospectively evaluated clinical and pH-metric outcomes after TIF for the treatment of GERD in 37 consecutive patients. Sixty-eight percent of patients had GERD-associated cough, asthma, or aspiration, and 32% of patients had heartburn or regurgitation. All patients remained on PPIs for 2 weeks after the procedure, then stopped administration of all antacid therapy. There were 2 complications (1 mediastinal abscess and 1 patient with postoperative bleeding). Outcomes at 6 months showed improvement in atypical symptoms in 64% of patients and typical symptoms in 70% to 80% of patients, measured by greater than or equal to 50% reduction in either GERD-HRQL or reflux symptom index (RSI), compared with baseline on PPIs. Eighty-two percent of patients were off PPIs at the 6-month interval. Of the 37 patients enrolled, 24 were evaluated endoscopically and with pH probe at 6 months. The mean esophageal acid exposure decreased from 10.4 to 5.2 and normalized in 61% of patients. Four patients had increased esophageal acid

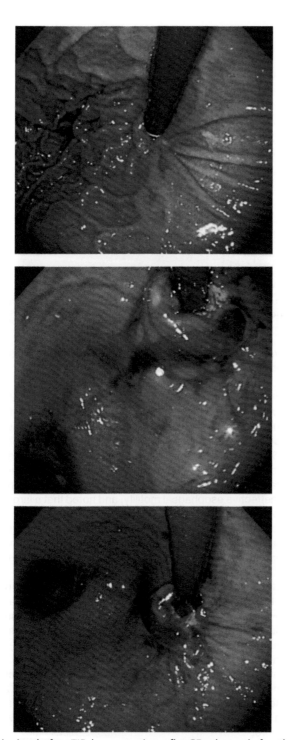

Fig. 4. Endoscopic view before TIF demonstrating a flat GE valve and after the TIF procedure demonstrating the 270° fundoplication.

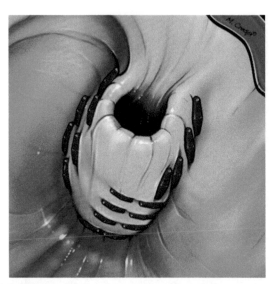

Fig. 5. Artist depiction of the plications inserted into the gastric mucosa creating the transoral incisionless fundoplication. (*Courtesy of* EndoGastric Solutions, Inc., San Mateo, CA. © 2015 EndoGastric Solutions, Inc.)

exposure. The average reflux episodes per 24-hour period decreased from 82.4 to 20.8 and normalized in 89% of patients. DeMeester scores reduced from 37.1 to 16.9 and normalized in 56% of patients.

Testoni and colleagues[26] reported on 42 patients followed at 6, 12, and 24 months after TIF. Thirty-five completed the 6 month follow-up, and 26 patients completed the 24-month follow up. At 6 months, 60% of patients were off PPIs completely, and 17% of patients were on one-half of their previous dose. At 24 months, only 42% remained off PPIs, and 27% were on one-half dose. There was no significant difference in DeMeester scores, and there were 2 complications (both pneumothoraces). Authors also found correlation between increased risk of recurrent symptoms in those with hiatal hernia and ineffective esophageal motility, and noted that a larger number of fasteners placed is predictive of positive outcomes.

In a prospective multi-institutional cohort study enrolling 100 patients from January 2010 until February 2011, Bell and colleagues[27] evaluated outcomes at 6 months. Seventy three percent of patients with typical GERD normalized their GERD-HRQL score, and 71% completely discontinued PPI usage. In atypical GERD patients, 65% experienced elimination of daily bothersome symptoms and 69% normalized their RSI scores. Eighty-two percent of atypical GERD symptom patients were able to discontinue PPIs at 6 months. Of the 35 patients with elevated percent total time of esophageal acid exposure, 28 underwent postoperative testing. A significant reduction in the mean number of refluxes, fraction of time pH less than 4 (%), and DeMeester score was demonstrated. A decreased duration of the longest reflux (55–24 minutes) was not significant. On endoscopy, 6 months after procedure, Hill grade classification of the GEJ was improved compared with baseline in 80% of patients, and hiatal hernia was either completely reduced (29 of 43 patients, 67%) or partially reduced (7 of 43 patients, 16%) in 84% (36 of 43 patients) of patients diagnosed with Hiatal hernia before the procedure.

More recently, Rinsma and colleagues[28] reported on the effects of TIF on TLESRs from the Netherlands. From 2008 to 2012, TIF was performed on 60 patients. Only

15 agreed to participate in the investigation of the effects of TIF on reflux mechanisms, focused on TLESRs and esophagogastric junction (EGJ) distensibility. Stationary esophageal manometry and impedance pH monitoring (90 min postprandial) were performed. TIF resulted in reduction of both the number of TLESRs (mean 16.8 to 9.2) and the number of TLESRs associated with liquid-containing reflux after the procedure (mean 11.1 to 5.6). Basal LES pressure in the fasted state was also increased after TIF, from mean of 13.9 to 20.5 mm Hg. As in previous studies, TIF did not significantly reduce mean esophageal acid exposure time, but analysis of 24-h impedance pH tracings showed a reduction in the number of liquid-containing reflux episodes after TIF without affecting the number of gas reflux episodes. Authors also observed a reduction in the proximal extent of reflux episodes during postprandial and ambulatory settings, leading to a significant improvement of acid exposure in the upright position but not the supine position.

In a systematic review by Welding and colleagues,[29] researchers evaluated 4 retrospective and 11 prospective studies on endoscopic fundoplication for GERD. They found that GERD-HRQL scores reduced on average from 21.9 on PPI therapy to 5.9 after TIF. RSI scores fell (in 4 retrospective studies) from 24.5 to 5.4 after TIF with a mean follow-up of 7.6 months. Cessation of PPI therapy in 14 studies yielded an overall rate of 67% at a mean follow-up of 8.3 months. pH data collected from 7 studies showed a statistically significant decrease in acid exposure, but no data demonstrated normal esophageal acid exposures. Overall complications in 559 total patients were hemorrhage (6, 1.1%), mediastinal abscess (1, 0.2%), esophageal perforation (4, 0.7%), dysphagia (3, 0.5%), and bloating (7, 1.3%). Forty patients (7.2%) failed treatment with TIF and later required Nissen fundoplication. Five patients required a redo TIF procedure, and the overall failure rate requiring reintervention was 8.1% at 9.5 months.

Trad and colleagues[30] reported on the TEMPO trial (TIF EsophyX vs Medical PPI Open label trial), a randomized clinical trial involving 63 patients at 7 US community hospitals. Forty patients were randomized to the TIF arm (performed by general surgeons in 4 centers and gastroenterologists at 3 centers), and 23 were randomized to the PPI arm (maximum standard dose) using a 2 to 1 ratio. Three patients were lost to follow-up at 6 months, leaving 39 in the TIF arm and 21 in the PPI arm. Primary outcomes were measured by GERD-HRQL, RSI, and RDQ (reflux disease questionnaire) instruments. Troublesome regurgitation was eliminated in 97% of patients in the TIF group versus 50% of patients in the PPI group. GERD-HQRL scores decreased from 19 to 2 on average in the TIF group and from 17 to 11 in the PPI group. Secondary outcomes were measured by normalization of esophageal acid exposure, PPI usage, and healing of esophagitis. At 6 months, 90% of patients were off PPIs. Fifty-four percent of TIF patients had normalized esophageal acid exposure, compared with 52% of patients on maximum-dose PPIs. There was also complete healing of esophagitis in 90% of TIF patients compared with 38% in the PPI group. TIF had significant improvement in 48-hour pH parameters but did not reach levels of pH normalization reported after laparoscopic fundoplication. The authors concluded that TIF was more effective than PPIs in elimination of troublesome regurgitation and that TIF was equivalent to PPIs in normalizing distal esophageal acid exposures (EAEs).

Sufficient long-term data are lacking, but Muls and colleagues[31] reported results from a multicenter prospective study enrolling 86 patients, with 66 available for 3-year follow-up. Twelve of those patients underwent repeat operation (2 laparoscopic fundoplication, 10 TIF) for treatment failure. Compared with median and mean scores at baseline off PPIs, they demonstrated clinically significant improvement in GERD-HRQL scores in 80% of patients at 3 years. Patient satisfaction was maintained at

Table 1
Summary of studies

Author	Study Type	Symptom Improvement	Esophageal Studies	PPI Use	Complications
Bell and Cadière,[23] 2011	Retrospective 37 patients 6 mo follow-up	Improved atypical symptoms in 64% and typical symptoms: 70%–80% (improved = >50% reduction in RSI or GERD-HRQL score)	Mean EAE (% time pH<4) decreased from 10.4 to 5.2 and normalized in 61% patients Average reflux episodes/24-h decline from 82.4 to 20.8 & normalized in 89% of patients DeMeester scores reduced from 37.1 to 16.9 & normalized in 56% of patients	82% off PPI @ 6 mo	Mediastinal abscess (1) Postoperative bleeding (1)
Testoni et al,[26] 2012	Prospective cohort 42 patients 35 at 6 mo 26 at 24 mo 6 & 24 mo follow-up	Improved mean GERD-HRQL scores from 22 pre-TIF on PPIs to 15 at 6 mo 18 at 24 mo off PPI therapy	Improved Hill grade at 6, 12 and 24 mo compared with before TIF	At 6 mo: 60% off PPIs 17% on half-dose PPI At 24 mo: 42% off PPIs 26.9% on half-dose PPI 30.8% on same dose as pre-procedure	Pneumothorax (2) 4 patients unresponsive to TIF underwent LNF
Bell et al,[27] 2012	Multi-institutional cohort 100 patients 6 mo follow-up	73% normalized GERD-HRQL scores 69% normalized RSI scores	Of 35 patients with elevated EAE, 28 underwent postoperative testing and demonstrated a significant reduction in mean number of refluxes, fraction of time pH<4, and DeMeester scores Hiatal hernia completely reduced in 29/43 patients and partially reduced in 7/43 patients	At 6 mo: 71% total off PPI (82% of atypical GERD patients off PPI)	No serious adverse reactions Nausea, pain, and anxiety in 12% of patients requiring prolonged stay Urinary retention in 1 patient

| Rinsma et al,[28] 2013 | Prospective cohort 60 patients (15 underwent post-TIF endoscopic evaluation) 6 mo follow-up | 80% normalized GERD-HRQL scores mean GERD-HQRL score reduced from 27.5 to 13.2 | Reduction in: Number of TLESRs from (mean 16.8 to 9.2) Number of TLESRs associated with liquid containing reflux (mean 11.1 to 5.6) Increased basal LES in fasting state (mean 13.9–20.5 mm Hg) No significant decrease in mean EAE | At 6 mo 67% off PPI 1/15 patients used antacids daily for mild symptoms 27% (4/15) continued daily PPI 3/15 were at lower doses | None reported |
| Wendling et al,[29] 2013 | Systematic review 563 patients Mean follow-up 9.5 mo | Overall decrease in mean GERD-HRQL compared with baseline on PPIs (decreased 21.9 to 5.9) Overall decrease in RSI score from 24.5 to 5.4 after TIF at average follow-up of 7.6 mo | Significant improvement in DeMeester scores in 3 of 4 studies None demonstrated normal post-procedure esophageal acid exposures or mean esophageal acid exposure time | Overall rate of PPI discontinuation was 67% at mean follow-up of 8.3 mo | Overall major complication rate 3.2% Hemorrhage in 6 patients Mediastinal abscess in 1 patient Esophageal perforation in 4 patients Overall patient failure 7.2% |

(continued on next page)

Table 1
(continued)

Author	Study Type	Symptom Improvement	Esophageal Studies	PPI Use	Complications
Trad et al,[30] 2015	RCT 63 patients 6 mo follow-up	Regurgitation eliminated in 97% TIF patients vs 50% PPI patients GERD-HRQL scores decreased from a mean of 19 to 2 in TIF patients vs 17 to 11 in PPI group	54% TIF patients had normalized EAEs 52% PPI patients had normalized EAEs Complete healing in esophagitis in 90% TIF patients vs 52% of patients on max PPI	90% TIF patients off PPI at 6 mo	No serious adverse events reported
Muls et al,[31] 2013	Multicenter prospective study 86 patients 66 @ 3-y follow-up	Improved GERD-HRQL scores in 80% of patients at 3 y. Patient satisfaction 70% at 3 y post-TIF vs 36% on PPI therapy alone	Esophagitis reduced from 78% to 38% at 3 y with complete resolution in 62% of patients Of 11 patients who underwent pH testing at 3 y, 9 demonstrated normalized pH (% time pH<4); the other 2 underwent a revisional procedure	86% off daily PPI at 1 y 74% off daily PPI at 3 y	12 patients underwent repeat operation (2 LNF, 10 repeat TIF) for treatment failure

Data from Refs.[23,26–31]

70% after 3 years compared with 36% on PPI therapy at baseline. Discontinuation of daily PPI use was maintained in 74% of patients at 3 years compared with 86% at 1 year. Overall esophagitis was reduced from 78% to 38% at 3 years, with complete resolution in 62% of those patients.

Data from recently reviewed articles are summarized in **Table 1**.

SAGES Recommendations

"Long term data is not yet available for EsophyX. In short-term follow-up, from 6 months to 2-years, EsophyX may be effective in patients with a hiatal hernia <2 cm with typical and atypical GERD. Further studies are required to define optimal techniques and most appropriate patient selection criteria, and to further evaluate device and technique safety. Quality of evidence (++), Grade recommendation: weak."[20]

DISCUSSION

The evolution of GERD treatment over the last 40 years has seen many therapeutic options come and go. From H2 blockers and PPIs, to the current surgical and endoscopic procedures, physicians have a variety of tools to attain symptom control of a life-changing disease. Despite recent advances, however, there is not a treatment with sustained efficacy and minimal risk. Endoscopic approaches including implants and injectables used as bulking agents have come and gone, while simple suturing or plicating techniques along with radiofrequency ablation have lacked sustainable efficacy. The EsophyX, which attempts to mimic LNF, has shown the most promise, reducing or eliminating need for antacid therapy, improving symptom control, and decreasing the number of TLESRs. Despite symptom improvement, trials have failed to show significant reduction of esophageal acid exposure, leaving laparoscopic Nissen fundoplication as the gold standard for management of refractory GERD. Other limitations of endoscopic therapies are the restrictive criteria, which exclude patients with hiatal hernias greater than 2 or 3 cm, significant pulmonary disease, Barrett esophagus, and moderate-to-severe esophageal dysmotility disorders. While data on endoscopic therapies slowly accumulates, proceduralists are improving their techniques, and devices are undergoing revisions to attempt the recreation of physiologic lower esophageal barrier in the management of GERD. While in this interim, TIF and Stretta both appear to be safe and have at least short term evidence to support use in patients refractory to medical therapy unwilling or unable to undergo LNF.[32,33]

REFERENCES

1. El-Serag HB, Sweet S, Winchester CC, et al. Update on the epidemiology of gastro-esophageal reflux disease: a systematic review. Gut 2014;63(6):871–80.
2. Richards WO, Houston HL, Torquati A, et al. Paradigm shift in the management of gastroesophgeal reflux disease. Ann Surg 2003;237:638–47.
3. Drugs to treat heartburn and acid reflux; the proton pump inhibitors comparing effectiveness, safety and pumps. 2013. Available at: http://consumerreports.org/health/resources/pdf/best-buy-drugs/PPIsUpdate-FINAL.pdf. Accessed August 2, 2014.
4. Gerson LB, Boparai V, Ullah N, et al. Oesophageal and gastric pH profiles in patients with gastro-oesophageal reflux disease and Barrett's oesophagus treated with proton pump inhibitors. Aliment Pharmacol Ther 2004;20:637–43.
5. Ryou M, Thompson CC. Endoscopic therapy for GERD: does it have a future? Curr Gastroenterol Rep 2008;10:215–21.

6. Kellokumpu I, Voutilainen M, Haglund C, et al. Outcomes following laparoscopic Nissen Fundoplication: assessing short-term and long-term outcomes. World J Gastroenterol 2013;19(24):3810–8.

7. Niebisch S, Fleming F, Galey K, et al. Perioperative risk of laparoscopic fundoplication: safer than previously reported - analysis of the American College of Surgeons National Surgical quality improvement program 2005 to 2009. J Am Coll Surg 2012;215(1):61–8.

8. Broeders JA, Rijnhart-de Jong HG, Draaisma WA, et al. Ten-year outcome of laparoscopic and conventional Nissen Fundoplication: randomized clinical trial. Ann Surg 2009;250:698–706.

9. O'Connor KW, Madison ST, Smith DJ, et al. An experimental endoscopic technique for reversing gastroesophageal reflux in dogs by injecting inert material in the distal esophagus. Gastrointest Endosc 1984;30:275–80.

10. O'Connor KW, Lehman GA. Endoscopic placement of collagen at the lower esophageal sphincter to inhibit gastroesophageal reflux: a pilot study of 10 medically intractable patients. Gastrointest Endosc 1988;34:106–12.

11. Lehman GA. Injectable and bulk-forming agents for enhancing the lower esophageal sphincter. Am J Med 2003;115(Suppl 3A):188S–91S.

12. Wong RF, Davis TV, Peterson KA. Complications involving the mediastinum after injection of Enteryx for GERD. Gastrointest Endosc 2005;62:752–6.

13. Fokens P, Bruno MJ, Gabbrielli A, et al. Endoscopic augmentation for the lower esophageal sphincter for the treatment of gastroesophageal reflux disease: multicenter study of the Gatekeeper reflux repair system. Endoscopy 2004;36: 682–9.

14. Galmich JP, Bruley des Varannes S. Endoluminal therapies for gastroesophageal reflux disease. Lancet 2003;361:1119–21.

15. DiBaise JK, Brand RE, Quigley EM. Endoluminal delivery of radiofrequency energy to the gastroesophageal junction in uncomplicated GERD: efficacy and potential mechanism of action. Am J Gastroenterol 2002;97:833–42.

16. Yeh RW, Triadafilopoulos G. Endoscopic antireflux therapy: the Stretta procedure. Thorac Surg Clin 2005;15:395–403.

17. Franciosa M, Triadafilopoulos G, Mashimo H. Stretta radiofrequency treatment for GERD: a safe and effective modality. Gastroenterol Res Pract 2013;2013:783815. Available at: http://www.hindawi.com/journals/grp/2013/783815/.

18. Perry K, Banerjee A, Melvin WS, et al. Radiofrequency energy delivered to lower esophageal sphincter reduces esophageal acid exposure and improves GERD symptoms: a systematic review and meta-analysis. Surg Laparosc Endosc Percutan Tech 2012;22(4):283–8.

19. Dughera L, Rotondano G, De Cento M, et al. Durability of Stretta radiofrequency treatment for GERD: results of an 8-year follow-up. Gastroenterol Res Pract 2014; 2014:531907.

20. Auyang E, Carter P, Rauth T, et al, the SAGES Guidelines committee. Endoluminal treatments for gastroesophageal reflux disease. SAGES. Available at: http://www. sagescms.org. Accessed August 9, 2014.

21. Vassiliou MC, von Renteln D, Rothstein RI. Recent advances in endoscopic reflux techniques. Gastrointest Endosc Clin N Am 2010;20:89–101.

22. Chuttani R. Endoscopic full-thickness plication: the device, technique, preclinical and early clinical experience. Gastrointest Endosc Clin N Am 2003;13: 109–16.

23. Bell RC, Cadière GB. Transoral rotational esophagogastric fundoplication: technical, anatomical and safety considerations. Surg Endosc 2011;25:2387–99.

24. Available at: www.endogastricsolutions.com/technology/esophyx-device/www.endogastricsolutions.com/tif-procedure/tif-vs-antireflux-surgery/. Accessed August 2, 2014.

25. Bell R, Freeman KD. Clinical and pH-metric outcomes of transoral esophagogastric fundoplication for the treatment of GERD. Surg Endosc 2011;25:1975–84.

26. Testoni PA, Vailati C, Testoni S, et al. Transoral incisionless fundoplication (TIF 2.0) with EsophyX for gastroesophageal reflux disease: long-term results and findings affecting outcome. Surg Endosc 2012;26:1425–35.

27. Bell R, Mavrelis PG, Barnes WE, et al. A prospective multicenter registry of patients with chronic gastroesophageal reflux disease receiving transoral incisionless fundoplication. J Am Coll Surg 2012;215(6):794–809.

28. Rinsma NF, Smeets FG, Bruls DW, et al. Effect of transoral incisionless fundoplication on reflux mechanisms. Surg Endosc 2013;28:941–9.

29. Wendling MR, Melvin S, Perry KA. Impact of transoral incisionless fundoplication (TIF) on subjective and objective indices: a systematic review of the published literature. Surg Endosc 2013;27:3754–61.

30. Trad K, Barnes WE, Simoni G, et al. Transoral incisionless fundoplication effective in eliminating GERD symptoms in partial responders to proton pump inhibitor therapy at 6 months: the TEMPO randomized clinical trial. Surg Innov 2015; 22(1):26–40.

31. Muls V, Eckardt AJ, Marchese M, et al. Three-year results of a multicenter prospective study of transoral incisionless fundoplication. Surg Innov 2013;20:321. Available at: http://sri.sagepub.com/content/20/4/321.

32. Torquati A, Richards WO. Endoluminal GERD treatments: critical appraisal of current literature with evidence-based medicine instruments. Surg Endosc 2007;21: 697–706.

33. Auyang ED, Carter P, Rauth T, et al. SAGES clinical spotlight review: endoluminal treatments for gastroesophageal reflux disease. Surg Endosc 2013;27:2658–72.

Esophageal Strictures and Diverticula

C. Daniel Smith, MD

KEYWORDS

- Esophageal stricture • Esophageal diverticula • Esophageal surgery
- GERD complications • Esophageal stricture management
- Esophageal diverticulectomy

KEY POINTS

- Esophageal disease, and in particular, dysfunction of the lower esophageal sphincter (LES) manifesting as gastroesophageal flux disease, is the most common of all gastrointestinal conditions impacting patients daily.
- Conditions leading impairment of esophageal outflow can be categorized into 2 broad categories, esophageal stricture or narrowing, and disorders of esophageal motility and LES function.
- Management focuses on the diverticulum itself, and relieving the underlying sphincter dysfunction.
- Many conditions can cause esophageal luminal narrowing or stricture; the most common are peptic, malignant, and congenital. Other causes include autoimmune, iatrogenic, medication induced, radiation induced, infectious, caustic, and idiopathic.

INTRODUCTION

The topics of this article can best be understood in the context of impairment of esophageal outflow and its consequences. Conditions that lead to impairment of esophageal outflow can best be categorized into 2 broad categories: esophageal stricture or narrowing and disorders of esophageal motility and lower esophageal sphincter (LES) function. The consequence of esophageal stricture most often involves the immediate mechanical impact of the esophageal narrowing, and treatment focuses on relieving the stricture and control of the underlying process, which lead to the stricture. Esophageal diverticula are most commonly the result of pressurization of the esophagus above a dysfunctional sphincter that fails to open appropriately (lower esophageal and cricopharyngeal), leading to the development of a false diverticulum just proximal to the sphincter. Management focuses on the diverticulum itself, and relieving the underlying sphincter dysfunction. One type of diverticulum not related

Piedmont Clinic, 2795 Peachtree Road, Unit 1808, Atlanta, GA 30305, USA
E-mail address: cdanielsmith@icloud.com

Surg Clin N Am 95 (2015) 669–681
http://dx.doi.org/10.1016/j.suc.2015.02.017
0039-6109/15/$ – see front matter © 2015 Elsevier Inc. All rights reserved.

to esophageal motor dysfunction, a midesophageal diverticulum is also discussed in this article. In contrast with the false diverticula of the esophagus, a midesophageal diverticulum is a true diverticulum and the result of mediastinal inflammatory processes and the resulting focal traction on the esophageal wall, and is therefore not related to esophageal outflow obstruction.

Many conditions can cause esophageal luminal narrowing or stricture. The most common causes are peptic, malignant, and congenital; other causes include autoimmune, iatrogenic, medication induced, radiation induced, infectious, caustic, and idiopathic.

ESOPHAGEAL STRICTURE

The term 'esophageal stricture' is reserved typically for intrinsic diseases of the esophagus causing luminal narrowing through inflammation, fibrosis, or neoplasia. Strictures are grouped typically into benign and malignant categories, with treatment varying depending on the underlying cause. Other causes of esophageal narrowing sometimes considered under the category of esophageal stricture include extrinsic compromise of the esophageal lumen by direct invasion, lymph node enlargement, or direct compression. This article focuses on the intrinsic causes of esophageal narrowing/stricture.

Presentation

Regardless of the nature of a stricture, the clinical presentation typically involves any or all of the following: dysphagia, food impaction, odynophagia, chest pain, and weight loss. Of these, progressive dysphagia to solids is the most common presenting symptom, with benign strictures following a more slow and insidious progression (eg, months to years), whereas dysphagia of a malignant stricture tends to progress more rapidly (eg, in weeks to months).

The clinical history may help to determine the cause of the dysphagia, although 25% of patient presenting with peptic strictures have no prior heartburn or other symptoms of gastroesophageal reflux disease (GERD). A known history of use of medications known to cause peptic ulcers or irritation, or caustic ingestion, are other examples of clinical history that might suggest the underlying cause.

Diagnosis

Esophagogastroduodenoscopy and contrast swallow are the mainstays of the initial workup and diagnosis for esophageal strictures. Although a contrast swallow is obtained most easily, esophagogastroduodenoscopy can provide more overall information and establish not only the diagnosis of a stricture or esophageal narrowing, but also allow visualization of the esophageal mucosa, including biopsy to establish definitively the underlying cause of the stricture. This becomes especially important in determining whether a stricture is benign or malignant. Contrast swallow may be particularly useful in defining the overall esophageal anatomy and identifying other associated pathology, such as an esophageal diverticulum. Esophageal pH testing, esophageal motility may be needed to confirm a diagnosis of GERD or an underlying esophageal motor abnormality (see Esophageal Diverticula section). Finally, when a stricture is determined to be malignant, or extrinsic pathology is thought to be the cause of esophageal narrowing, CT of the chest and abdomen is indicated to establish the cause of extrinsic narrowing and/or to stage a biopsy-proven malignant stricture. Endoscopic ultrasonography has emerged as a useful diagnostic tool to characterize the nature of a stricture and assess the stage and severity of a malignant or infiltrating process. This has become the mainstay of staging malignant disease of the esophagus.

Benign Esophageal Stricture

Benign strictures are by far the most common, and peptic strictures account for 70% to 80% of all causes of esophageal stricture. Peptic strictures are the result of gastroesophageal reflux–induced esophagitis and scarring.[1–4] With this, peptic strictures usually occur in the distal esophagus within 4 cm of the squamocolumnar junction. The associated mucosal inflammation and submucosal fibrosis give an appearance of inflammation and smooth narrowing without mass effect (**Fig. 1**).

Another common cause of benign stricture is a Schotski's ring, a ringlike constriction of the distal esophagus, often described as a "bandlike" ring of constriction. The etiology of a Schotski's ring remains elusive. Theories include that (1) the ring is a pleat of redundant mucosa that forms when the esophagus for unknown reasons shortens transiently or permanently, (2) the ring is congenital, (3) the ring is a short peptic stricture related to GERD, and (4) the ring is the result of pill-induced esophagitis.

The treatment of benign stricture is dilation (see details elsewhere in this article) and management of any underlying inflammatory process.[1–4] The treatment of the underlying cause cannot be overemphasized.[5] Patients on maximum medical therapy for GERD have lower redilation rates and better resolution of dysphagia than those who are not on maximal medical GERD therapy. Twice daily dosing of a proton pump inhibitor is more effective than H2 blockers alone and for patients with breakthrough evening GERD symptoms, adding a single evening dose of an H2 blocker is indicated. This regimen is continued for at least 1 month, at which time a repeat esophagogastroduodenoscopy is undertaken to reassess. It may be necessary to repeat the dilation at that time and continue maximum medical therapy until the stricture and inflammatory process has completely resolved. At that time, medication can be tapered to a level for symptom control and an endoscopy planned for 12 months later.[6] For more severe strictures, this plan may be compressed to repeat endoscopy and

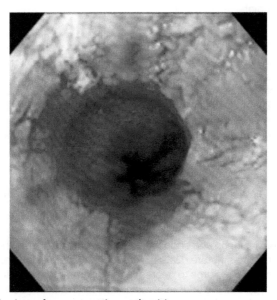

Fig. 1. Endoscopic view of severe peptic esophagitis.

dilation within 1 to 2 weeks of an initial dilation, and more frequent reassessments. Adjuncts such as steroid injections in and around the stricture have been used, especially for more chronic fibrotic strictures. Stenting (see elsewhere in this article) has little role in benign strictures unless the underlying issue with the stricture is anastomotic breakdown and leak from a recent esophageal procedure (which is beyond the scope of this article).

Surgery is indicated for peptic stricture that recurs despite maximal medical therapy, in which case an antireflux procedure is indicated, or for nondilatable fibrotic strictures, which typically requires resection and reconstruction to resolve.[7] One should be cautioned about using a segmental resection of the distal esophagus and esophagogastrostomy to manage a benign stricture because the majority of these patients will have severe GERD after such a procedure, leaving the patient with ongoing issues with peptic injury to the esophagus.[8] If a resection is needed, it is best to use an esophagojejunostomy to avoid severe GERD.

Malignant Esophageal Stricture

The most common cause of malignant esophageal stricture is adenocarcinoma associated with Barrett's esophagus. This is a change from decades ago when most malignant disease of the esophagus was squamous cancer associated with alcohol and tobacco use. The management of malignant stricture centers on tissue diagnosis, staging, and definitive therapy versus palliation. In contrast with benign strictures, dilation plays only a temporizing role, typically to facilitate placement of a stent or prepare for definitive therapy (resection). Stenting (see elsewhere in this article) is much more common in malignant stricture, either as permanent management for advanced disease or temporary management to allow completion of neoadjuvant therapy before undergoing resection.

Management

Dilation
Esophageal dilation[9] for stricture involves selection of technique of dilation, use of adjuncts and endpoint.

Techniques
Mercury-filled bougies (Maloney or Hurst dilators) are reasonable for uncomplicated strictures with an initial diameter of greater than 10 mm. These dilators are inexpensive and fluoroscopy is not needed. This is the technique used for self, at-home dilations.

Wire-guided polyvinyl bougies (Savary-Gilliard dilators) are stiff dilators appropriate for strictures 5 to 20 mm in diameter and are best suited for long, tight strictures. Fluoroscopy is typically needed to assess guidewire placement and to visualize safe passage of the dilator. Use usually requires sedation and is more traumatic on the larynx than other techniques of dilation.[10]

Through-the-scope balloon dilators allow visualized placement and dilation. Although more expensive, balloon dilation seems to result in safe management of more complicated and tighter strictures with fewer sessions and a lower recurrence rate.[11]

Adjuncts
Intralesional steroid injection and endoscopic stricturoplasty are the 2 most commonly talked about adjuncts to stricture dilation. Although few data exist to support a mechanism of action, the first ventures to decrease the inflammatory reaction to the trauma of dilation and thereby limit the degree of restenosis after dilation. Several studies have achieved larger final luminal diameter and lower stricture recurrence with the use of

intralesional steroid.[12] It seems reasonable to use this in a benign stricture where dysphagia persists despite dilations and maximal medical management of GERD.

Four-quadrant stricturoplasty followed by dilation has been described for more fibrotic strictures with limited success.[13] Concern with stricturoplasty relates to perforation making the fibrotic strictures most appealing for this adjunct.

Endpoint of Dilation

How much dilation can be achieved in a single session of dilation, and what luminal diameter should be the goal remain controversial. Most would agree that gaining 1 to 2 mm of luminal diameter through 3 consecutive passes of dilators of increasing size during 1 session is a good general rule. Use of balloon dilators may allow even more increase in luminal diameter during a session. Obviously, perforation remains the concern, and balloon dilation provides real-time, direct visualization of the mechanical effects of the dilation and may allow more aggressive, safe dilation. Most patient experience complete relief of dysphagia when a luminal diameter of 40 to 54F is achieved.

Stenting

Stenting for esophageal structure is used most commonly for malignant strictures, either to provide permanent palliation for advanced disease or temporary palliation while a patient is treated with neoadjuvant therapy in preparation for curative resection.[14,15] Permanent stents are usually self-expanding metal or plastic stents, and temporary stents have the stent itself covered so as to limit tissue ingrowth, allowing the stent to be removed more easily. The details of stent design and placement are beyond the scope of this article.

Surgery

Finally, surgery has a primary role for a malignant stricture where staging reveals a potentially curable cancer. In this case, esophagectomy with either high thoracic or cervical esophageal anastomosis to tubularized stomach or colon interposition is preferred. Distal esophageal segmental resection with esophagogastrectomy should be avoided owing to the severe GERD that often results with the LES gone and an intrathoracic anastomosis to stomach. If it is desirable to preserve as much esophagus as possible, it is better to use jejunum for reestablishing intestinal continuity.

The role of surgery in benign stricture is largely limited to antireflux procedures to manage the GERD that is etiologic in most benign strictures. For a nondilatable benign stricture, segmental resection is reasonable so long as an esophagojejunostomy is performed rather than an esophagogastrostomy (see elsewhere in this article).

ESOPHAGEAL DIVERTICULA

An esophageal diverticulum is an epithelial-lined mucosal pouch that protrudes from the esophageal lumen.[16] Esophageal diverticula are classified according to their location (pharyngoesophageal, midesophageal, or epiphrenic), the layers of the esophagus that accompany them (true diverticulum, which contain all layers, or false diverticulum, containing only mucosa and submucosa), or mechanism of formation (pulsion or traction; **Table 1**). Most esophageal diverticula are pulsion diverticula and are the consequence of a dysfunctional esophageal sphincter that fails to open appropriately, resulting in pressurization of the esophageal lumen forcing the mucosa and submucosa to herniate through the esophageal musculature (false diverticulum). Pharyngoesophageal and epiphrenic diverticula are pulsion diverticula. Less

Table 1
Classification of esophageal diverticula

Diverticulum	Location	Mechanism	Type
Pharyngoesophageal	UES	Pulsion	False
Midesophageal	Tracheal bifurcation	Traction	True
Epiphrenic	Distal esophagus	Pulsion	False

Abbreviation: UES, upper esophageal sphincter.

commonly, a periesophageal inflammatory process adheres to the esophagus and subsequently pulls the esophageal wall focally, resulting in all layers of the esophagus comprising the diverticulum (true diverticulum). Midesophageal diverticula are usually traction diverticula resulting from inflammatory changes in mediastinal lymph nodes.

Pharyngoesophageal Diverticulum (Zenker's)

In 1878, Zenker described 27 cases of pharyngoesophageal diverticulum, and thus his name is associated with this condition. This is the most common of the esophageal diverticula. Pharyngoesophageal diverticula consistently arise within the inferior pharyngeal constrictor, between the oblique fibers of the thyropharyngeus muscle and through or above the more horizontal fibers of the cricopharyngeus muscle (the upper esophageal sphincter; **Fig. 2**). Killian's triangle is the area of weakness through which most pharyngoesophageal diverticula protrude. These diverticula seem to be acquired owing to some degree of incoordination in the swallowing mechanism with

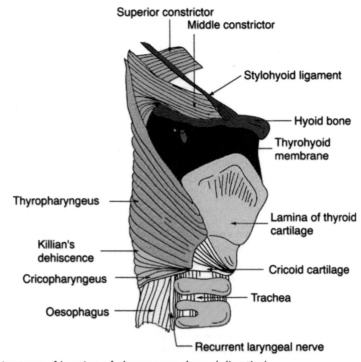

Fig. 2. Anatomy of location of pharyngoesophageal diverticula.

an abnormally high intrapharyngeal pressure leading to protrusion of esophageal mucosa and submucosa through the esophageal wall with subsequent diverticulum formation.

Diagnosis

The presenting symptoms of pharyngoesophageal diverticulum are usually characteristic, and consist of cervical esophageal dysphagia, regurgitation of bland undigested food, frequent aspiration, noisy deglutition (gurgling), halitosis, and voice changes. Dysphagia is present in 98% of patients, and pulmonary aspiration occurs in up to one-third of patients.

The diagnosis of pharyngoesophageal diverticulum is made easily with a barium esophagram (**Fig. 3**). Endoscopy, 24-hour pH monitoring, and esophageal manometry are not indicated unless some features of the symptoms or the esophagram raise suspicion of other conditions (malignancy or GERD). Although these diverticula can reach impressive sizes, it is the degree of upper esophageal sphincter dysfunction that determines the severity of symptoms, not the absolute size of the diverticulum. In most symptomatic cases, treatment is indicated regardless of the size of the diverticulum.

Treatment

As is the case with all pulsion diverticula, proper treatment must be directed at relieving the underlying neuromotor abnormality responsible for the increased intraluminal pressure and then managing the diverticulum.[17] Most techniques described have used division of the cricopharyngeus muscle followed by resection, imbrication, obliteration, or fenestration of the diverticulum (**Table 2**). Most approaches to management agree that relief of the relative obstruction distal to the pouch through cricopharyngeal myotomy is the most important aspect of treatment. Early surgical

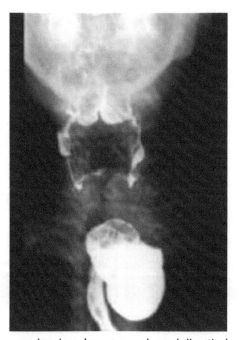

Fig. 3. Barium esophagram showing pharyngoesophageal diverticulum.

Table 2
Treatment options for pharyngoesophageal diverticula

Treatment	Description
Endoscopic diverticulotomy	Endoscopic division of cricopharyngeus and common wall between diverticulum and esophagus (electrocautery, stapler, laser, etc)
Operative myotomy and diverticulectomy	Cricopharyngeal myotomy and excision of diverticulum
Operative myotomy and diverticulopexy	Cricopharyngeal myotomy and mobilization of sac with suture fixation of the sac above the neck of the diverticulum
Operative myotomy alone	Cricopharyngeal myotomy only

strategies using diverticulectomy only, without myotomy, had high failure rates because of esophageal leaks from the suture line, or recurrence. More recently, endoscopic management has emerged as the preferred method of managing these diverticula (ref). Dividing the septum between the esophagus and diverticulum and the cricopharyngeus muscle using either an energy device (eg, cautery, laser; **Fig. 4**) or a stapling device (**Fig. 5**) allows a minimally invasive approach that both addresses the cricopharyngeus muscle and the trapping of content in the diverticulum. The typical advanced age of many who suffer with this condition also makes the endoscopic approach appealing. Success is achieved in more than 90% of patients undergoing endoscopic management with a low morbidity and mortality. Twenty percent of patients may require 2 treatments to achieve these results.[18–21]

Midesophageal Diverticulum

Midesophageal diverticula are rare and most commonly associated with mediastinal granulomatous disease (histoplasmosis or tuberculosis). They are thought to arise because of adhesions between inflamed mediastinal lymph nodes and the esophagus. By contraction, the adhesions exert "traction" on the esophagus with eventual localized diverticulum development. These are true diverticula with all layers of the esophagus present in the diverticulum.

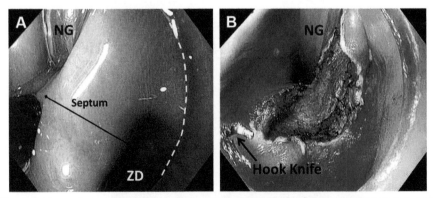

Fig. 4. Endoscopic management of pharyngoesophageal diverticulum. Yellow dashes indicate lateral edge of diverticulum. (*A*) Endoscopic view before diverticulotomy. NG, nasogastric tube in esophagus; ZD, lumen of Zenker's diverticulum. (*B*) Completed diverticulotomy.

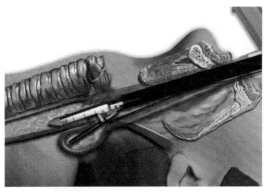

Fig. 5. Stapled endoscopic management of pharyngoesophageal diverticulum.

Diagnosis/treatment

A midesophageal diverticulum is typically asymptomatic and diagnosed incidentally on a barium esophagram undertaken for other reasons. When such an asymptomatic diverticulum is found, no treatment is necessary. In patients with symptoms, esophageal manometry is indicated to ensure that the LES function is normal and that there is not a pulsion diverticulum. Symptomatic diverticula require treatment. Larger diverticula usually require an accompanying resection or diverticulopexy. In the absence of a motor abnormality, diverticulectomy alone may be adequate. Many surgeons will add an esophagogastric myotomy (Heller myotomy) for any esophageal diverticulectomy to minimize the risk of staple line leak that may accompany any early postoperative esophageal lumen pressurization. Data in the literature are mixed related to the requirement of esophagogastric myotomy for true traction diverticula.[22,23] It is this author's preference to add an esophagogastric myotomy (Heller myotomy) myotomy to all cases where esophageal diverticulectomy is indicated (of course, not including pharyngoesophageal diverticula).

Epiphrenic (Pulsion) Diverticulum

An epiphrenic diverticulum typically occurs within the distal 10 cm of the esophagus and is a pulsion type. It is most commonly associated with esophageal motor abnormalities (achalasia, hypertensive LES, diffuse esophageal spasm, nonspecific motor disorders), but may be the result of other causes of increased esophageal pressure (eg, after fundoplication with esophageal outflow obstruction). I have managed several epiphrenic diverticula in patients who have undergone endoluminal fundoplication, in particular transoral incisionless fundoplication, where the esophageal wall has been weakened by the transmural fixation and outflow obstruction has allowed pressurization of the esophagus above and at the fundoplication with subsequent diverticulum formation.

Diagnosis/treatment

Most epiphrenic diverticula are symptomatic because of the underlying esophageal motor disorder. Diagnosis of the diverticulum is made during barium esophagram (**Fig. 6**). Manometry, esophagoscopy, and 24-hour pH testing may be necessary to diagnose associated conditions and direct specific treatments. Most epiphrenic diverticula require esophageal myotomy extending from the neck of the diverticulum

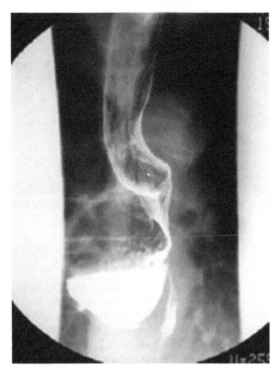

Fig. 6. Barium esophagram showing a large epiphrenic diverticulum.

onto the gastric cardia for a distance of 1.5 to 3.0 cm (see Myotomy for Achalasia). Diverticulectomy, fundoplication, or repair of hiatal hernia may also be necessary, depending on the size of the diverticulum or associated conditions.

Technique of midesophageal and epiphrenic diverticulectomy

In the past, an open thoracic approach has been the preferred approach to these diverticula. Today, a laparoscopic or combined laparoscopic/thoracoscopic approach allows a minimally invasive approach to these diverticula, significantly decreasing the morbidity and mortality of management of these diverticula (ref). If the neck of the diverticulum is above the esophageal hiatus and/or the diverticulum itself is very large and extends up into the chest, the operation commences with a thoracoscopic approach. Prone thoracoscopy[24] significantly facilitates mobilization of the diverticulum (**Figs. 7** and **8**) and stapled transection of the neck (**Figs. 9** and **10**). Once the diverticulum is resected, the patient is flipped into the supine position for laparoscopic esophagogastric myotomy and partial fundoplication. If the neck of the diverticulum is at the level of the esophageal hiatus and the diverticulum does not extend far into the chest, an entirely laparoscopic approach may be adequate. As we have gained experience with prone thoracoscopy, we now approach most epiphrenic diverticula with the combined thoracoscopic/laparoscopic approach.

Several series have documented the feasibility of this approach.[25,26] We have experience in the management of more than 40 cases using laparoscopic/thoracoscopic approach. As stated, we prefer to add an esophagogastric myotomy to all cases to minimize the risk of staple line leak postoperatively.[27]

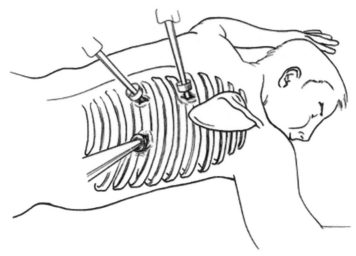

Fig. 7. Illustration of prone thoracoscopy used to approach mid- and large epiphrenic diverticula.

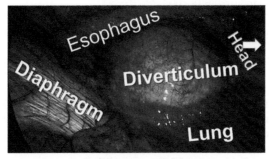

Fig. 8. Prone thoracoscopic view of epiphrenic diverticulum.

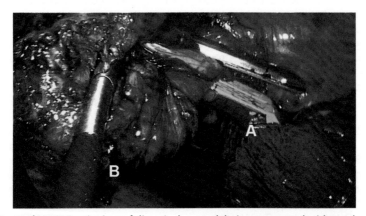

Fig. 9. Prone thoracoscopic view of diverticulum neck being transected with stapler. (A) Stapler across diverticulum neck. (B) Grasper holding diverticulum.

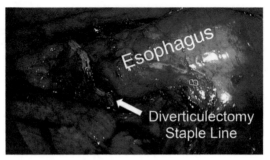

Fig. 10. Completed diverticulectomy.

REFERENCES

1. Pregun I, Hritz I, Tulassay Z, et al. Peptic esophageal stricture: medical treatment. Dig Dis 2009;27:31–7.
2. Pace F, Antinori S, Repici A. What is new in esophageal injury (infection, drug-induced, caustic, stricture, perforation)? Curr Opin Gastroenterol 2009;25:372–9.
3. Guda NM, Vakil N. Proton pump inhibitors and the time trends for esophageal dilation. Am J Gastroenterol 2004;99:797–800.
4. Marks RD, Richter JE, Rizzo J, et al. Omeprazole versus H2-receptor antagonists in treating patients with peptic stricture and esophagitis. Gastroenterology 1994; 106:907–15.
5. Dakkak M, Hoare RC, Maslin SC, et al. Oesophagitis is as important as oesophageal stricture diameter in determining dysphagia. Gut 1993;34:152–5.
6. Patterson DJ, Graham DY, Smith JL, et al. Natural history of benign esophageal stricture treated by dilatation. Gastroenterology 1983;85:346–50.
7. Smith CD. Antireflux surgery. Surg Clin North Am 2008;88:943–58.
8. Smith CD. Surgical therapy for gastroesophageal reflux disease: indications, evaluation, and procedures. Gastrointest Endosc Clin N Am 2009;19:35–48, v–vi.
9. de Wijkerslooth LR, Vleggaar FP, Siersema PD. Endoscopic management of difficult or recurrent esophageal strictures. Am J Gastroenterol 2011;106:2080–91 [quiz: 2092].
10. Fan Y, Song HY, Kim JH, et al. Fluoroscopically guided balloon dilation of benign esophageal strictures: incidence of esophageal rupture and its management in 589 patients. AJR Am J Roentgenol 2011;197:1481–6.
11. Saeed ZA, Winchester CB, Ferro PS, et al. Prospective randomized comparison of polyvinyl bougies and through-the-scope balloons for dilation of peptic strictures of the esophagus. Gastrointest Endosc 1995;41:189–95.
12. Ramage JI Jr, Rumalla A, Baron TH, et al. A prospective, randomized, double-blind, placebo-controlled trial of endoscopic steroid injection therapy for recalcitrant esophageal peptic strictures. Am J Gastroenterol 2005;100:2419–25.
13. Raijman I, Siddique I, Rachcal LT. Endoscopic stricturoplasty in the management of recurrent benign esophageal strictures. Gastrointest Endosc 1999; 49:AB172.
14. Sharma P, Kozarek R. Practice Parameters Committee of American College of G. Role of esophageal stents in benign and malignant diseases. Am J Gastroenterol 2010;105:258–73 [quiz: 274].
15. Hindy P, Hong J, Lam-Tsai Y, et al. A comprehensive review of esophageal stents. Gastroenterol Hepatol (N Y) 2012;8:526–34.

16. Smith CD. Esophagus. In: Norton JA, Chang AE, Lowry SF, et al, editors. Essential practice of surgery basic science and clinical evidence. New York: Springer - Verlag; 2003. p. 167–84.
17. Zaninotto G, Narne S, Costantini M, et al. Tailored approach to Zenker's diverticula. Surg Endosc 2003;17:129–33.
18. Tang SJ. Flexible endoscopic Zenker's diverticulotomy: approach that involves thinking outside the box (with videos). Surg Endosc 2014;28:1355–9.
19. Parker NP, Misono S. Carbon dioxide laser versus stapler-assisted endoscopic Zenker's diverticulotomy: a systematic review and meta-analysis. Otolaryngol Head Neck Surg 2014;150:750–3.
20. Law R, Baron TH. Transoral flexible endoscopic therapy of Zenker's diverticulum. Dig Surg 2013;30:393.
21. Huberty V, El Bacha S, Blero D, et al. Endoscopic treatment for Zenker's diverticulum: long-term results (with video). Gastrointest Endosc 2013;77:701–7.
22. Isaacs KE, Graham SA, Berney CR. Laparoscopic transhiatal approach for resection of midesophageal diverticula. Ann Thorac Surg 2012;94:e17–9.
23. Galata CL, Bruns CJ, Pratschke S, et al. Thoracoscopic resection of a giant midesophageal diverticulum. Ann Thorac Surg 2012;94:293–5.
24. Goldberg RF, Bowers SP, Parker M, et al. Technical and perioperative outcomes of minimally invasive esophagectomy in the prone position. Surg Endosc 2013; 27:553–7.
25. Herbella FA, Patti MG. Modern pathophysiology and treatment of esophageal diverticula. Langenbecks Arch Surg 2012;397:29–35.
26. Soares RV, Montenovo M, Pellegrini CA, et al. Laparoscopy as the initial approach for epiphrenic diverticula. Surg Endosc 2011;25:3740–6.
27. Melman L, Quinlan J, Robertson B, et al. Esophageal manometric characteristics and outcomes for laparoscopic esophageal diverticulectomy, myotomy, and partial fundoplication for epiphrenic diverticula. Surg Endosc 2009;23:1337–41.

Index

Note: Page numbers of article titles are in **boldface** type.

Surg Clin N Am 95 (2015) 683–693
http://dx.doi.org/10.1016/S0039-6109(15)00057-2
0039-6109/15/$ – see front matter © 2015 Elsevier Inc. All rights reserved.

surgical.theclinics.com

Moving?

Make sure your subscription moves with you!

To notify us of your new address, find your **Clinics Account Number** (located on your mailing label above your name), and contact customer service at:

Email: journalscustomerservice-usa@elsevier.com

800-654-2452 (subscribers in the U.S. & Canada)
314-447-8871 (subscribers outside of the U.S. & Canada)

Fax number: 314-447-8029

Elsevier Health Sciences Division
Subscription Customer Service
3251 Riverport Lane
Maryland Heights, MO 63043

*To ensure uninterrupted delivery of your subscription, please notify us at least 4 weeks in advance of move.

Printed and bound by CPI Group (UK) Ltd, Croydon, CR0 4YY

14/10/2024

01773722-0001